T0257230

Patient's Progress

To the Memory of Our Fathers

Patient's Progress

*Doctors and Doctoring
in Eighteenth-century England*

DOROTHY PORTER
and
ROY PORTER

Polity Press

First published 1989 by Polity Press in association with Basil Blackwell.

Editorial Office:
Polity Press, Dales Brewery, Gwydir Street,
Cambridge CB1 2LJ, UK

Basil Blackwell Ltd
108 Cowley Road, Oxford OX4 1JF, UK

British Library Cataloguing in Publication Data

Porter, Dorothy
    Patient's progress: doctors and doctoring
    in eighteenth-century England
    1. England.   Medicine, 1650–1850.
    Social aspects
    I. Title II. Porter, Roy, *1946–*
    362.1'0942

ISBN: 978-0-7456-0251-6

Typeset in 10 on 12 pt Garamond
by Photo·graphics, Honiton, Devon

Contents

Preface

It may be worth clarifying at the outset what kind of a work this is. It is not a history of medicine, nor even a social history of medicine, in the couple of centuries before Victorian professionalization and the birth of scientific medicine. It is, rather, an exploration of the relations between sick people and their doctors in the pre-modern era. We aim to show that the patients were the making of the doctors, and the doctors the making of the patients. It is this quasi-contractual symbiosis that we have attempted to analyse.

We have not given systematic, structural accounts of the epidemiology of the times, the social distribution of sickness, or of the various layers of the medical profession which developed to meet the challenge of the sick. We have tried something altogether more subjective and impressionistic: exploring consciousness, the mind of the times. What did the sick think about their doctors? How did doctors regard their patients? And we have attempted this analysis of an emergent culture largely through presentation and evaluation of first-hand attitudes and experiences, as recorded in letters, diaries, autobiographies and table-talk.

It will be clear from the text, but it may be worth emphasizing here, that this approach means that we concentrate almost wholly on those strata of society which left ample documentary remains of their opinions: that is, the urban middle classes and the 'Quality'. A great deal of additional research using different techniques would be required to recover the experiences of the bulk of the population in respect of their treatment by doctors and healers. It has, furthermore, been our practice in this book to lump together evidence from widely spaced decades. This has been a deliberate decision, for we believe that, in most salient respects, attitudes and practices did not fundamentally transform themselves in the generations under discussion: there was continuity over 'la longue durée'.

Acknowledgements

We have written this book in the happy environment of the Wellcome Institute for the History of Medicine, and are glad to acknowledge the immense help we have received from the library staff, and from the gallant xeroxer, Andy Foley. Anne Darlington and Petra Westphal have perfected the art of high-velocity word-perfect typing: our thanks go to them. Mary Fissell, Marie Roberts, Sylvana Tomaselli, Jane Walsh and Andrew Wear have been most generous with comments on earlier drafts of this book; all errors are of course our own.

For researching the illustrations we are extremely grateful to William Schupbach of the Wellcome Institute. At Polity Press, Tony Giddens and the series editor, Andrew Scull, have supported us with their great enthusiasm for the project, and Claire Andrews has saved us from many errors while seeing it into production. As ever, Jean Runciman has proved the perfect copy-editor and indexer: our thanks to her.

We are grateful to the Wellcome Institute for the History of Medicine for permission to reproduce the photographs that appear in this book. Plate 1 – Coloured etching by Isaac Cruikshank, 1804. Plate 2 – Engraving by P.F. Tardieu (1711–1771) after J.B. Oudry (1686–1755) after Lafontaine. Plate 3 –Exhib.: Amsterdam, 6th internat. congress of the history of medicine, 1927, drawings no. 69 (as by W. Hendriks (1744–1831) and coll. the Print Room, Rijksmuseum, Amsterdam). Plate 4 – German lithograph, c. 1830. Plate 5 – Painting in the Wellcome Institute (n. CC5083), attributed to John Kay (1742–1826). The physician may be William Cullen. Plate 6 – Goldsmith, the physician, leaves in a huff because the patient prefers to follow the advice of the apothecary. Painting in the Wellcome Institute Library by T.P. Hall (Victorian). Plate 7 – Coloured stipple engraving by J. Cary after H. Taylor, 1786.

We are grateful to the publishers concerned for permission to reproduce material from the following: Bagley, J. J. (ed.), *The Great Diurnal of Nicholas Blundell*, transcr. and annot. by F. Tyrer, 3 vols (Record Society of Lancashire and Cheshire, 110 (1968); 112 (1970);

114 (1972)); Beresford, J. (ed.), _The Diary of a Country Parson: the Rev. James Woodforde, 1758–1802_, 5 vols (reprinted Oxford, Oxford University Press, 1978–8); Bessborough, Earl of, and Aspinall, A. (eds), _Lady Bessborough and her Family Circle_ (London, Murray, 1940); Brockbank, W., and Kenworthy, F. (eds), _The Diary of Richard Kay (1716–51) of Baldingstone, near Bury_ (Manchester; Chetham Society, 1968); Cave, K. (ed.), _The Diary of Joseph Farington_, vols VII–XVI (New Haven, Yale University Press, 1982–4); Chapman, R. W. (ed.), _The Letters of Samuel Johnson_, 3 vols (Oxford, Clarendon Press, 1984); Corner, B. C. and Booth, C. (eds), _Chain of Friendship: Selected Letters of Dr John Fothergill_ (Cambridge, Mass., Harvard University Press, 1971); Cozens-Hardy, B. (ed.), _The Diary of Sylas Neville 1767–1788_ (London, Oxford University Press, 1950); Greig, J. Y. T. (ed.), _The Letters of David Hume_, 2 vols (Oxford, Clarendon Press, 1969); Griggs, E. L. (ed.), _Collected Letters of Samuel Taylore Coleridge_, 6 vols (Oxford, Clarendon Press, 1956–68); Hemlow, J. (ed.), _The Journals and Letters of Fanny Burney (Madame D'Arblay)_, 12 vols (Oxford, Clarendon Press, 1972–84); Johnson, R. B. (ed.), _Letters from the Right Honorable Lady Mary Wortley Montagu, 1709–1762_ (London, Dent, 1906); LeFanu, W. (ed.), _Betsy Sheridan's Journal_ (London, Eyre & Spottiswoode, 1960); Little, D. and Kahrl, G. (eds), _The Letters of David Garrick_, 3 vols (London, Oxford University Press, 1963); Marchand, L. A. (ed.), _Byron's Letters and Journals_, 12 vols (London, John Murray, 1973–81); North, R., _General Preface and Life of Dr John North_, ed. by P. Millard (Toronto, University of Toronto Press, 1984); Norton, J. E. (ed.), _The Letters of Edward Gibbon_, 3 vols (London, Cassell, 1956); Sorlien, R. P. (ed.), _The Diary of John Manningham_ (New Hampshire, University Press of New England, 1976); Vaisey, D. (ed.), _The Diary of Thomas Turner_ (Oxford, Oxford University Press, 1984); Verney, Lady F. P., and Verney Lady M. M. (eds), _Memoirs of The Verney Family_, 4 vols (London, Tabard, 1970); Verney, Lady M. M. (ed.), _Verney Letters of the Eighteenth Century from the MSS at Clayton House_, 2 vols (London, Ernest Benn, 1930).

PART I

Context

1

Facing Sickness

INTRODUCTION

What did people in England a couple of centuries ago do when they fell sick?[1]

It happened often enough. For the world we have lost was a society of sickness. Disease descended, sudden and deadly, picking individual victims or gathering a bumper harvest from households and the community at large.[2] Threats to health took many forms. A series of letters exchanged between a medical student at St Thomas's Hospital and his country doctor father in the Sussex village of Hurstpierpoint gives evidence of a great diversity of medical conditions handled by the father during the years 1801 and 1802, including:[3]

Tap old mother Clark [for dropsy]
Typhus
Inflammation of the pleura, treated by bleeding
A strong convulsive fit. She had two previously
'Yellow fever' [presumably jaundice]
Leeches applied to Grace's [Grace Weekes] eyes on two occasions
Inflammatory rheumatism
Scarlatina
Aphtha alba [diphtheria]
A sore throat
Dysentery accompanied by a high fever
Haemorrhage from the intestines, unaccompanied by diarrhoea
Crope [Croup]
Ptysis. Pulmon. [Pulmonary tuberculosis.] Three patients died of it
Post partum white leg leading to death
Nervous disorder
Louisa Newnham ill: 'I see her three times a day'

Toothache
Tumefaction of the thigh
Fever, two died
Hydrocephalic fever
Diabetes

Some serious, some trivial, not a few fatal – a typical mixed bag. Plenty of surgical problems also found their way into the correspondence. The village doctor told his son of the following cases:[4]

Fall off a horse and killed on the spot
Shattered hand from exploding gun
Burns from clothes set on fire
Gunshot wound to abdomen
Compound [fracture] tibia and fibula in a boy of 13
Bad compound [fracture], at Henfield
Sprained wrist from chaise overturning
Sprained foot in a lady staying at Danny
Fractured rib or two. Bled for treatment
Sprained ankle which confined Richard Weekes to the house for a few days. It
    happened when he fell off his horse and was in the same ankle he broke
    fifteen years previously
Dislocated humerus
Compound fracture of leg and arm when run over by a roller
Drowning in a petit (water closet) [!]
Death from concussion after chaise overturned

These were, doubtless, simply the more interesting, serious – or bizarre! – cases, worthy of report, the merest tip of the iceberg in respect to the practice as a whole; but they do offer a random sample of the dangers to health in whose shadow pre-moderns lived, and of which, all too commonly, they died.

Sickness and medicine often filled the home: 'Rydal Mount is at present a *Hospital*', complained Mary Wordsworth in 1835.[5] Illness forms a constant threnody in the letters, journals and diaries of earlier centuries.[6] Take a few days in December 1724, as recorded by the Lancashire gentleman, Nicholas Blundell:[7]

6   Fanny took a Vomit after Supper
7   I took a Purge and Kept my Roome
8   I was something Aguish so we went to the Doctor to let him see how I
    was. . . .
9   Mrs Diconson of Wrightington sent a How-do-you to Fanny
    Fanny took a Doce of Phisick.

People could expect to be assailed, from early in life, by a battery of disorders, many of which might possibly prove fatal. At least before inoculation was commonly adopted from the mid-eighteenth century, a high proportion of the population caught smallpox. It was so prevalent that prudent parents took active steps to ensure their children had it early, in a mild form, to get it over and done with. Yet in severe local outbreaks, anything up to 10 per cent of cases could prove fatal; even in cases of recovery, it often left its victim permanently disfigured – loss of looks was damaging to a girl's attractiveness. (It was scant compensation that smallpox left others blind.)

Unlike many of life's afflictions, disease was no respecter of rank. Smallpox carried away Queen Mary, wife of William III, no less than wiping out scores of thousands of village Hampdens. (Inoculation in turn killed Augustus, one of George III's sons.)[8] Numerous other fevers – contemporaries called them by various names ('continuing', 'hectic', 'intermittent', 'relapsing', etc.) and we can tentatively identify them as typhoid, typhus, measles, scarlatina, diphtheria, and so forth – took a toll which was not, perhaps, individually as high as that for smallpox, but which, nevertheless, frequently created 'crisis mortality' in particular villages or market towns. Though the plague ceased its visitations after 1666, 'new diseases' such as rickets, whooping-cough and tuberculosis assumed ever more menacing proportions, especially amongst the urban poor; and cholera was to become, from 1831 onwards, the new plague of the Victorian era.[9]

Studies of parish records and bills of mortality by historical demographers and epidemiologists have given some quantitative dimension to the ubiquity of sickness in earlier society. A substantial proportion – probably over one-fifth – of new-born babies did not even survive infancy. Disease depressed life expectations to an average of under forty years, comparable to that in many Third World societies today. And records of individual experiences bear out this dismal picture.

The diary of Richard Kay, a doctor from Bury in Lancashire, ends suddenly on 19 July 1750, presumably because of illness. Three months later his father died; a sister died at the beginning of the next year, as did another sister in the following October, together with the diarist himself, at the age of thirty-five. The Kay family seems to have succumbed to 'spotted fever', probably typhus.[10] Some infections were doubly fearsome because they could not even be given a familiar name. In 1657 an unknown fever broke out in the southern counties. Spreading steadily, it reached Claydon in Buckinghamshire, seat of the prominent gentry family, the Verneys. Many fled, but Sir Ralph Verney returned to his manor to help out with 'this new disease, or a longe tertian or a Quaterne, be which it will'. He apologized to Lady Warwick:

> Madame, I had not a servant to send to satisfie my selfe of the condition of your health, for all these parts have been sorely visited, and particularly this very Towne, in soe high a manner, that since I writ last to your

Ladishipp, heere hath been 40 or 50 sick at a time, whereof the Parson, and 8, or 9 more are already dead, and at this hower many are dangerously sick, and still sicken dayly. I thanke God my selfe & sonne are well, but (excepting one) there is not a man servant in my house that hath not been very ill, and are yet soe weake, that I am forced to hier others to assist & tend them.[11]

Serious indeed. Yet the apparently trivial could prove equally fatal. 'The Quene of Portugall dyed', Lady Gardiner reported in 1699, 'with only making A holl in her yeare for to wear pendants, & by whot accydent they due not give an Account, more then that humors fell so fast on the plac as it could not be stayed bot senc gangrened notwithstanding all the helps shee had.'[12]

Everyone knew that, despite all endeavours, once an infant had a severe bout of diarrhoea, or a teenager developed smallpox, there was nothing to be done which, with any assurance, would tip the balance between life and death. For that reason, the pre-moderns needed all possible resources – religious, philosophical, moral and personal – for coping with affliction and death. Theirs was hence also a culture bound to take all steps to prevent sickness in the first place. Through word of mouth and via books, a great quantity of advice was disseminated about health promotion and disease prevention. People were urged to look to their diets and their life-styles, to take exercise and to spot, avoid and rectify environmental hazards. Popular, if not elite, culture continued to fend off sickness by recourse to magic: spells, charms, incantations and ritual practices.[13] The fact that people fell sick after all that highlighted the need for eternal vigilance, and confirmed the vice-like grip sickness exerted on that society, the shadow it cast over vulnerable lives. Suffering was Everyman's lot.[14] The sick were enjoined to 'mix Stoicism with Christianity', as the Cambridge philosopher, Henry More, put it in the mid-seventeenth century;[15] resignation to the mysterious ways of Providence taught endurance of what could not be changed.

This, however, is not to imply that people were fatalistic or apathetic (in either the popular or the philosophical sense). As we shall see, in cases of sickness, there was no want of therapeutic heroism, of the desperate deployment of desperate remedies. In a few well-documented cases (for example, the last days of Charles ii and of Queen Caroline) the medical bombardment would surely have been saluted by General Haig.[16] Moreover, it would be false to suppose that the paths of sickness inevitably led to the grave. For every disease that killed, dozens merely caused pain, disrupted lives or disabled sufferers, temporarily or permanently, from work, physical mobility, pleasure or peace of mind.

Ignorance, poverty, malnutrition, overwork, accidents, poor personal hygiene and umpteen other factors produced scores of conditions which today rarely arise, or, if they do, are easily corrected or cured.[17] Bad teeth were omnipresent (England was becoming a sugar-consuming society) and led to secondary, internal infections.[18] Intestinal worms, piles, skin ulcers and running sores were all common. Multiple difficult childbirths left women with gynaecological disorders, including vaginal tears and anal fissures. Skin disease was extremely frequent. Ulcerations, running sores, subcutaneous parasites and scrofulous swellings readily became infected, causing further complications, including blood-poisoning and tetanus. Those working outside in all weathers – most of the workforce – were crippled with bronchial complaints, rheumatism and lameness. Nobody, not even 'the Quality', was safe from environmental hazards that made life painful. 'I am all over bug-bites, in such a condition as you never saw', complained the Marchioness of Kildare in 1761; 'the Doctor and Mrs Moss advise me to . . . have my bed taken to pieces and examined.'[19] Even the King kept his bug-destroyer royal. Thus, alongside the killer diseases, people were also plagued with innumerable endemic medical conditions which often crippled, typically discomforted and sometimes proved chronic. Those disorders you lived with rather than died of demanded a stoicism of their own, but they also spurred active strategies in reaction.

For if pre-modern England was a 'sickness society', it was also, equally, a 'medicine society'. Things might have been different. A culture might be so captivated by its faith in Divine Providence as to believe all sickness to be heaven-sent, whereupon interference with the mysterious ways of God would be impious. Islamic attitudes towards plague, and, in the nineteenth century, the opposition of religious sects such as the Peculiar People to smallpox vaccination, smack of such higher fatalism.[20] Or a society might simply lack the resources and resourcefulness to combat visitations of sickness with counter-measures. Yet pre-modern England's dominant value system was just the reverse of this. Practical activity was prized to counter sickness. When his friend, Henry Thrale, was seriously ill with apoplexy, Samuel Johnson asked point-blank, 'Does [the physician] direct any regimen, or does Mr Thrale regulate himself?' One or the other was necessary: capitulating was inadmissible.[21]

AN OPPORTUNITY SOCIETY

The society emerging in England after the Civil War and political turmoils of the late Stuart age took its cue from its capitalist economy, with thriving agricultural, commercial, and manufacturing sectors. Apologists and opinion-makers promoted an ethos that commended the

busy, energetic, and practical.[22] Worldly success was highly prized,
failure despised and punished by destitution, shame and, ultimately, the
debtors' jail or the penalties of the Poor Law.[23] The Protestant work
ethic and the possessive individualism codified by Locke and early
political economists thrust the onus for surviving and thriving in the
competitive and often cut-throat market-place squarely upon the
individual. Baconian maxims such as *quisquis faber fortunae suae* (every
man the maker of his own fortune) carried weight long before Samuel
Smiles systematized them into *Self Help*. Helping yourself was an
opportunity – almost an incitement – yet it was also a duty and a
warning.[24]

Sturdy individualism was thus valued. Families, kinship networks and
friends all provided succour in times of trouble, but recent research has
emphasized the *limits* of traditional family support systems in early
modern England.[25] Families were nuclear rather than extended. Every
marriage created a new household, and the old were commonly expected
to live separately from their offspring. From the young journeyman on
the tramp, to the widow or widower, self-sufficiency was enjoined,
heeding the harsh law of reality that the weak went to the wall. English
Protestantism no more romanticized poverty and mortification as holy
states than it encouraged indiscriminate and boundless charity. People
were expected to look after themselves and their own.[26]

True, the parish system served as an ultimate safety-net for the
'virtuous poor', the unfortunate, those unavoidably without work or
incapable of earning their own living, and the house of correction would
handle sturdy rogues. Recent studies have confirmed that the Old Poor
Law – that in operation before the universal implementation of the
workhouse system in 1834 – was commonly humane and even generous.
Parishes laid out money not just on food but on the varied necessities
of life: clothes, shelter, fuel, and medical treatment. Quite large sums
– not infrequently, £20 on a single patient – were sometimes spent by
overseers on doctors' fees to treat their paupers. Enlightened self-
interest, after all, dictated it: a guinea spent on medicines promptly
might put a parishioner back at work, saving the £50 otherwise later
required for the relief of his family.[27] Yet the stigma of the Poor Law
was omnipresent; even before 'less eligibility', the pauper's life was
hardly eligible. And for those industrious and virtuous poor who kept
their chins above the breadline, society provided little back-up in the
way of services, charity and aid.

For, before the modern 'welfare state', before hospital facilities became
generally available and statutory public health agencies developed in the
mid-nineteenth century, the maintenance of health and the battle against
disease remained essentially individual responsibilities.

On the negative side, people enjoyed an almost unlimited freedom (by today's standards) to destroy their own health and that of their fellows. There were no laws restricting the sale of poisons, no licensing laws – at least before the decimating 'gin craze' of the 1730s and 1740s. Workshops and industrial premises could pollute the environment and create multiple health hazards without penalty. Despite agitation by would-be reformers, environmental and occupational diseases attracted little legislation till the second half of the nineteenth century.[28]

On the positive side, all were left at liberty to follow whatever form of health care and medical system they chose or could afford. People were free to achieve as they pleased that goal increasingly articulated in the *siècle des lumières*, the pursuit of happiness within the utilitarian programme of maximizing pleasures and avoiding pains.[29]

The harsh fate Nature doled out through disease, distress and disaster was thus matched by the hard-bitten tone of English society. But misery's edge was blunted by other characteristics of England's emergent capitalist order, fast becoming the envy of the world. For one thing, the economy was enjoying sustained and accelerating growth, especially from the 1740s, culminating in rapid industrialization. The physical penalties suffered by large sectors of the work-force through the occupational evils of a manufacturing economy still ultra-dependent upon muscle-power must never be underestimated.[30] All the same, from the late seventeenth century, economic growth was producing a society in which – in noticeable contrast to most Continental rivals – a large and growing number of the work-force were living above the breadline and had expectations of improvement. In contrast to the French, English people no longer starved to death *en masse*; there is little evidence that the waves of epidemics in Georgian England were triggered by times of severe dearth.[31]

From artisans upwards, more people had money in their pockets to spend. As consumers, they increasingly tasted the pleasures of buying items hitherto available only to the rich – inventories show even humble small-town stores stocking a veritable cornucopia of goods, many imported.[32] Demand for services likewise spread. Many functions traditionally undertaken within the household – by the master, his wife or, amongst the better-off, by retinues of servants – came to be performed, or purchased from outside. In middle-class households, commodities like soap and starch, traditionally made at home, were increasingly bought ready-made; activities such as making clothes and furnishings, styling hair or educating children were increasingly put out to experts and professionals. Within the framework of individual enterprise, 'the helping professions' achieved a presence. This is fundamental to our theme; for, within the service economy, though wealth could not buy health, it could command a widening range of medical services, including proprietary medicines and the skills of doctors.[33]

In ways closely connected with this extension of market-based consumerism, England became a society notable for high levels of literacy, and, especially from the 1690s, for the wide, cheap and legally unfettered circulation of information. Alongside printed books, pamphlets enjoyed their golden age, while newspapers, magazines, almanacs, and primers diffused information and ideas to the millions. Knowledge became a trade, and the much-despised Grub Street multiplied publications instructing people in useful knowledge, practical skills, sciences and self-help.

Health proved no exception. Shelvesfull of books appeared in the 'Every Man his Own Doctor' genre.[34] Addressing the proliferation of such instruction manuals (cookbooks, for example), scholars have pondered whether they were indeed read and followed, or merely purchased for show. But there is, as we shall see, plenty of evidence that household health books were widely put to use by sufferers, who also drew upon theories and practices acquired by word of mouth, and from personal, first-hand experience. Foreign visitors were then impressed, as historians are today, by Georgian England as the land of the resilient and inventive, attuned to practical business, and at the cutting-edge of intellectual and cultural innovation.[35]

Such energetic diffusion and advancement of knowledge might, of course, be variously interpreted. The permeation of print can be construed as aiding attempts by the guardians of official culture to silence, purify or reform popular beliefs and practices. Yet there is more to the diffusion of knowledge than stifling and suppression.[36] For literacy and education are enabling as well as controlling media. The net effect of the spread of literacy and of the increasing availability of ideas in print was an authentic ferment of thinking, fresh convictions about the 'priesthood' of all readers, the democratic intellect, and thus a reinforcement of individualism.

Stimulated (both positively and negatively) by a thriving market economy and by a practical freedom from censorship, permitting freedom of information, English society transformed Enlightenment ideals into their most practical embodiment. Economic growth, social change and the march of mind in turn played their parts in shaping responses to the threats to health, livelihood and even life itself posed by rampant disease. It is precisely these responses that we propose to examine in this book.

RESPONSES TO SICKNESS

The measures people took on falling ill were diverse and often drew upon a variety of systems. For, as suggested already, responses to sickness lay along a broad spectrum. At one end, there was the sturdiest of individualisms, which presumed everyman's responsibility for his own body, health and sickness; *treatments* lay in one's own hands, since one's *life* was. Such individualism could be the child of choice or necessity. At the other end, there was growing recourse to expert advice and professional services. These were in themselves multifarious; for, as we shall explore in the next chapter, many different types of operators were able to obtain credit, or at least a hearing, for their claims to medical knowledge or know-how, and – unlike in France – neither the state nor the law significantly circumscribed the freedom to dispense medical services.

It would be misleading to convey the impression that an ideological gulf separated those practising self-healing and domestic medicine from those drawing upon professional services. Very few made the unswerving recourse to auto-medication a matter of pride and principle.[37] Obviously, many could never afford the services of a regular doctor, and even the middling sort – shopkeepers, curates, smallholders and craftsmen – had to ration their use of professionals. Yet we must not forget that there were hosts of empirics and itinerants providing cheap, if unqualified and unreliable, medical services to the lower classes, to those who could afford medicines costing no more than a glass of ale: Samuel Johnson's lodger and friend, Robert Levet, is a good example. Neither should it be forgotten that the very poor, and the servant classes, often received treatment gratis from rather superior doctors, provided via charity, the dispensary or hospital, or paid for by their masters or through the Poor Law.

People drew upon multifarious medical services as the need arose. Some help was self-generated; other assistance came from friends, family and acquaintances, and was dispensed free of charge. Services were provided by recognized, regular medical men who had had a university education or an apprenticeship, but also by all manner of other healers who would charge or be recompensed for their efforts – nurses, itinerants, midwives, mountebanks, so-called 'empirics' and 'wise women' (the dividing line between the latter and 'witches' was a fine one). Choosing one rather than the other would depend upon a host of factors, such as availability, cost, distance, the perceived seriousness of the condition, past experience and so forth. Very commonly, it was a matter not of either/or but of both; and when sickness persisted, diverse forms of medical aid would be tried, either simultaneously or in a despairing succession as various expedients failed.

The sick had to balance many desiderata. Survival and recovery were paramount, and would obviously sanction putting one's life into other people's hands and the recourse to desperate remedies. Yet sufferers commonly strove to retain maximum personal control over their own bodies and the medicaments they swallowed. Doctors of all stripes were often treated with deep distrust, the sick fearing they would prove no less perilous than the disease itself. 'Met Mr Forbes the surgeon going to kill a few patients', recorded Parson William Holland in 1800; yet Holland himself drew routinely, albeit grumblingly, upon Forbes's 'homicidal' services.[38]

This book will not examine in any detail the attitudes sick people displayed towards health in general, their bodies or disease, or towards suffering and its rationales, though we take it for granted that sufferers entertained strong and reasoned views on these issues: we have attempted to do that elsewhere.[39] Rather, we aim to examine attitudes and actions with respect to the *treatment* of illness. We shall look at the basic dilemma: should one treat at all? And if so, should one self-treat or seek external aid? We shall also examine the particular issue: what specific form of treatment was sought? How did people define and recognize a good doctor? Above all, we shall explore the momentous, but by no means inevitable, step of becoming a *patient*,[40] the moment when a sick person puts himself under a doctor.

In other words, central to this book will be examination of the structure and dynamics of doctor/patient relations, or, as it seems more sensible to speak of them, patient/doctor relations, since they were typically *initiated* by the sick person or patient-to-be.

In the loom of our language, the patient is, definitionally, etymologically passive. But in the real world, that clearly was not so. Nowadays, medical authority, medical institutions and medical science and technology (all deploying the 'medical model', which regards the body as a mechanism, the sum of its parts) combine to render the patient paradigmatically passive, with the doctor on top – the position preferred by the medical profession for treatment. Nevertheless, medical sociology has shown that even nowadays, patient/doctor relations constitute a contested dialectic process, in which the formal arrow of authority, coming from the doctor, constantly refracts and ricochets, thanks to the redoubtable capacity of patients to play the system. In the last resort, sickness itself guarantees the patient a certain residual power in the encounter.[41]

This applied, all the more so, in the pre-modern medical world. Many factors gave pull to the affluent patient. He would do the summoning.

He would pay the bill, and so expect to have that say, that sway, which the power of the purse conferred. He might well be of higher social status than the practitioner.

The pre-modern practitioner had no miracle cures in his bag to command the unqualified submission and lasting gratitude of his patients. Everyone saw that the doctor's common experience was one of failure, or at best partial success; patients often died or did not respond to treatment. Moreover, within traditional medicine, the physician was fundamentally beholden to his patient for divulging all those clues – the medical history – indispensable for an astute diagnosis. He was also highly dependent upon the patient's co-operation in executing the prescribed course of treatment (few captive hospital patients in those days!), particularly as this might require considerable patient initiative, such as exercise, travel or a change of diet.[42]

In this book we examine lay people's attitudes towards doctors and to the therapeutic encounters initiated with them. We shall explore how patient/doctor relations were moulded around and modelled upon other familiar and well-established social relations – for example, those obtaining within the family hierarchy, or echoing other kinds of ties of service, patronage and employment.

We shall then, in some detail, scrutinize what actually happened in such encounters. We shall do this largely from the sick person's, rather than the doctor's, viewpoint. We have chosen this perspective for several reasons. In part it is because, as traditionally written, the history of medicine has been strangely silent about the patient's role in the clinical encounter. The bedside acumen of great doctors from Galen to Moran has been justly celebrated;[43] but such a style of history tends to reduce the patient to something akin to the corpse in a detective story. It is time to acknowledge how far the procedures and outcomes of pre-modern medicine depended upon a dialogue, a co-operative relationship established between the sick person and his medical attendant.

Second, we believe it important to stress that the pivotal figure in the clinical encounter truly is the patient. The story of sickness begins with a person falling ill, leads to decisions that draw in the doctor, and rises to a resolution in recovery, relapse or, on occasion, in death. The doctor stars in one episode of a larger epic which opens and ends with the sick person.

Third, there is a wider range of ampler sources available written by patients than by doctors. They are simply more abundant. Moreover, the sources typically drawn upon in this book – the autobiographies, diaries, journals, letters etc., of the sick – are more revealing about the ramifications and resonances of individual encounters than the remains left by doctors, which rarely go beyond notes of diagnosis and treatment, and are mainly in standardized form, following the conventions governing medical perception and practice. Presumably because being sick is such an existentially precarious state, patients seize upon the virtues and vices of the doctor – out of gratitude, rage or a desire to forewarn others. By contrast, doctors' case-books – mainly quite laconic – occasionally tell us much about the patient's history, but next to nothing about the practitioners' attitudes towards him and the clinical encounter as a whole.[44] Nevertheless, we have tried not to ignore the doctor's view: indeed, chapter 8 below is devoted to it. In some cases we are doubly fortunate, possessing two-way patient/doctor correspondence that enables us to gauge from both sides the clinical dynamics.[45]

We conceive this book as a contribution to the micro-social history of pre-modern medicine.[46] It presupposes many developments in society at large and in medicine in particular, studied by other historians. These can neither be researched nor even more than baldly restated here: the operations of a flourishing market society; the aspirations of enterprising professionals eager to benefit from prosperity and the potentialities of active consumerism; the transmission of medical knowledge and skills through publishing outlets;[47] the free market in medical practice in early modern England;[48] beliefs, taboos and practices governing control of the body, involving notions of privacy, ownership, honour and gender;[49] etiquette regulating gentlemanly and ladylike behaviour and the ethics of medicine;[50] the role of knowledge and expertise, money and exchange, in an Enlightenment society; and so forth. Against these lightly sketched-in backgrounds, we investigate the attitudes and actions of people who fell sick, and the social relations to which sickness led.

Of course, we examine only a sprinkling of people, hailing from a restricted segment of society, primarily those wealthy, leisured and literate – indeed, self-conscious and self-confident – enough to leave behind substantial written remains. Likewise, most of our records of doctors' doings are those of relatively conspicuous physicians. No harm is done by this selectivity, so long as no pretence is made that their experience is representative of society as a whole.

We draw upon evidence ranging from the mid-seventeenth to the mid-nineteenth century. Believing that, for the most part, attitudes and practices did not change fundamentally during that period, we have not scrupled to juxtapose scattered evidence, quite widely separated in time, in the course of this *longue durée*. Historians have argued that patient/doctor relationships possibly changed considerably in the second half of the nineteenth century, as the medical profession consolidated itself, as a fringe culture proliferated and as diagnostic technology and surgical interventions grew more sophisticated.[51]

This is a work of micro-history, the politics of face-to-face relations in a familiar society; it is about small things, how a person treated himself, how family groups pooled medical knowledge and, above all, how sick people entered into webs of relations with their doctors. All too often, historians have simply accepted the doctor as the agent of primary care. People, however, took *care* before they took *physic*. What we habitually call primary care is in fact secondary care, once the sufferer has become a patient, has entered the medical arena. And even under medical control, patients have by no means been so passive as the various 'medicalization' theories advanced by Michel Foucault, Ivan Illich and others might lead us to believe. From their distinct points of view, Thomas Szasz's pleas for the autonomy of the afflicted, and Erving Goffman's studies of the Brechtian survival strategies of the inmates of total institutions, offer salutary counter-balances, views of lay initiative, resilience and capacity to play the system.[52]

These names raise big issues – matters of life and death – and they are at the very heart of the medical enterprise. After all, no patients, no doctors. Or, as Frank Wedgwood observed in the Victorian era, in a dark phrase to which we shall return, 'no doubt the final cause of patients *is* the doctor'.[53]

2

Healing in Society

We habitually think in terms of polar opposites: patient and doctor, or more broadly, layman and professional. By starting from these dichotomies, we can easily go on to suppose that, medically speaking, pre-modern England was a two-culture society, structured around a pair of alternatives. When you fell sick, either you treated yourself or you got a doctor to treat you. And from here it is tempting to assume that the decision must have been, at bottom, economic (could you afford the physician?), tempered by a touch of the pragmatic (was there a doctor in the village or vicinity, close enough to make consulting him practical?).[1]

Thus construed, the treatment of sickness would nestle neatly into the general model of cultural bifurcation widely and plausibly applied by historians to many other sectors of material culture and ideology during the long eighteenth century. Such an interpretation argues that 'polite' or 'patrician' culture on the one hand, and 'popular' culture on the other, were becoming increasingly polarized from each other, moving into 'separate spheres'. This divorce was set in motion by elite desires for cultural dominance and hegemony; and it was accomplished through the divisive power of money. For although 'polite culture' was nominally open to all within the free market, the cost of participating in 'Georgian delights' (having your portrait painted, enjoying the 'season', joining a circulating library, or whatever) in reality debarred the majority from becoming effective consumers.[2] Georgian England was becoming, it is argued, a society whose cultural boundaries were being drawn more sharply by purchasing power.

Of course, as noted earlier, many in England indeed had money to spend; even mere tradesmen could participate in polite pursuits, such as going to the theatre, precisely because they could pay the admission.

But those lacking the wherewithal were excluded, and would continue with their old plebeian rites (their wassailings, their Valentine kisses and Mayday revels, their wakes and plough-Monday, their blood sports, their Morris dancing on the green).[3] We might assume, along these lines, that a similar divide applied in medicine. Those who could afford to, consulted a professional doctor when they fell sick; those who could not, treated themselves. But reality proves far more complicated.

For one thing, the decision in case of sickness whether to self-dose or to call the doctor typically hinged upon factors other than mere ability to pay: personal preferences and the perceived seriousness of the complaint, for instance. For another, it would be a major mistake to assume (as old-fashioned medical historians did) that in early modern England medical practitioners were few and far between, and that only the well-off could afford them (most of the populace being left to fend for themselves, or to resort to the ministrations of witches, layers-out, wise women and other such amateurs.)[4]

Of course, this conventional picture contains a grain of truth: certain top medical practitioners cultivated practices amongst fashionable members of society, who could afford a guinea or more per consultation. Yet even they would also treat less affluent patients, charging a sliding scale of fees according to ability to pay. Top physicians such as John Coakley Lettsom held charity surgeries for the poor. And it is wrong to assume – as has happened all too often – that medical practitioners were thin on the ground before the nineteenth century, and confined chiefly to London and a scatter of fashionable centres, corporate and cathedral cities.

This misconception arises from assuming that the ideal type of the tripartite professional hierarchy, commonly set out in medical propaganda from Tudor times onwards, corresponded with reality. This schema presupposed a professional pyramid lorded over by a closed clique of physicians, liberally educated at Oxford and Cambridge, cultivating a gentlemanly ethos and dignified by fellowships at the Royal College of Physicians in London. Such privileged physicians would look down upon their distant cousins, the surgeons, who had trained for their primarily manual craft through mere apprenticeship.[5] The traditionally inferior status of surgery is indicated by the fact that until 1745, the Company of Surgeons had been formally yoked with the barbers' trade. Lower still, and under the supervision of the College of Physicians, were the apothecaries, whose job was to dispense physicians' prescriptions: theirs was a trade reeking of the counter. It was not until the turn of the eighteenth century that apothecaries established the legal right to prescribe medicines in their own right. Traditional histories emphasized how this hierarchical structure was regulated through three corporate bodies, regulating admission and the right to practise: the College of Physicians, the Corporation of Surgeons and the Society of Apothecaries.

MEDICINE IN THE MARKET-PLACE

Yet this neat and tidy picture of a hierarchically organized, corporate profession – upheld by some as an ethical career ideal, denounced by others as a sinister closed shop – hardly corresponds to reality, especially beyond the boundaries of the metropolis. Certainly the three separate branches did preserve distinct profiles in London, and there was endemic intraprofessional rivalry. Through the seventeenth century, the College of Physicians strove with some success to oversee the apothecaries and to drive interlopers – those lacking its licence – out of practice. In the eighteenth century, the College pettily excluded from its fellowship those without Oxbridge degrees, including the increasing numbers of highly trained, skilled and successful Scottish graduates, such as John Fothergill and William Hunter.[6]

But the attempt to create a medical monopoly had largely broken down, even in London, by the eighteenth century. Following the Rose Case judgment in the House of Lords (1704), apothecaries basked in their newly-won right to prescribe (provided they maintained the legal fiction of charging only for their medicines, not for advice). Moreover, a plague of irregular practitioners – nostrum-mongers and mesmerists, for instance – practised without hindrance from the College, despite the formal licensing requirements. In a climate of public opinion increasingly wedded to *laissez faire*, the corporations presumably chose to turn a blind eye to unlicensed practice, rather than pursue highly unpopular and utterly futile attempts to enforce their legal monopolies.[7]

Outside London, practitioners never had existed in sufficient concentrations to make the tripartite hierarchical structure relevant or workable. In traditional corporate cities such as Norwich, guilds for surgeons and apothecaries had long existed, designed to regulate outsiders and enforce apprenticeship; these continued in existence, though their long-term effectiveness is unclear. But the norm in the typical small market town or industrial village was increasingly for medical practitioners to set up shop or put down roots wherever they felt demand for their services existed, or could be excited, having an eye chiefly to market opportunity, regardless of formal jurisdictions. In some places their numbers went up by leaps and bounds, as classically in Bath, where, according to Richard Steele, 'The Physicians here are very numerous' – he added, with a sting in the tail, 'they had almost killed me with their humanity'.[8]

Indeed, all watering places and spa towns, enjoying their apogee in the Georgian age, attracted doctors. 'Physicians swarm here like pickpockets at a fair', Ned Ward noted of early eighteenth-century Tunbridge Wells, 'and quality neither eat, drink, or exonerate [*sic*] without the advice of a doctor.'[9]

For the great mass of Georgian doctors, corporate affiliation was relatively irrelevant to achieving individual advancement. They were barely bound (despite the traditional picture) by membership of a closed corporation. Neither were they operating within the modern peer-regulating norms definitive of a qualified profession, as understood by medical sociologists. Their success or failure depended, rather, principally upon their credit not with their peers but with their patients. In his influential *Medical Ethics*, written at the close of the eighteenth century, the Mancunian physician, Thomas Percival, certainly took for granted the desirability of a professional *esprit de corps*. But he did so in the light of his experience of its opposite: competition, even undercutting, which would ultimately, in his view, preclude medicine being what it should be by rights, a 'lucrative' profession. Percival notably did not look to corporate policing as the royal road forward; the desired *esprit* would have to be upheld by informal consensus.[10]

Recent research has indicated that far more were engaged in medicine as a remunerative occupation than was formerly believed. Robert Burton had complained early in the seventeenth century of the swarms of irregular practitioners: 'for there be many Mountebanks, Quacksalvers, Empiricks, in every street almost, and in every village, that take upon them this name, make this noble and profitable Art to be evil spoken of, and contemned, by reason of these base and illiterate Artificers.'[11] But there were also far more regulars than membership totals for the various corporations might lead one to expect. Local research, for example, has revealed no fewer than a hundred practitioners active in Norwich between 1550 and 1600. It has been suggested that in seventeenth-century East Anglia there was at least one medical practitioner (of some kind) for every 400 members of the population.[12]

By 1779 the first nationwide commercial *Medical Register* was published – itself a sign of the times, suggesting that consumers would find such information helpful when choosing a practitioner. It listed a grand total of some 3000 regular practitioners (physicians, surgeons and apothecaries) in England, a tally that is demonstrably a considerable understatement.[13] Of these, only a minuscule fraction were Oxbridge-educated gentleman physicians, though this cadre exercised sway over fashionable medicine out of all proportion to their numbers and skills.[14] But the vast majority were everyday surgeons and apothecaries, sprung from the provincial middle classes, the sons of farmers or tradesmen, or sometimes the cadets of good family or clergy. Most had trained by up to seven years' apprenticeship, learning their trade the hard way at the elbow of a proverbially demanding task-master; the premium for that would be a modest £100 or so.[15]

Medicine was attracting plenty of trainees throughout the eighteenth century, so much so that the wail went up early in the nineteenth century that the profession was becoming overstocked.[16] Everything points to an expanding demand for medical services. In the early eighteenth century, Claver Morris, a graduate physician in the cathedral city of Wells, Somerset, was netting some £200 a year – a modest income, because he was apparently attending just a few cases a day. About half a century afterwards, in the same region, William Pulsford, a humble surgeon-apothecary, or medical jack-of-all-trades, who was, in effect, a general practitioner *avant la lettre*, was leading an extremely busy life, treating clients from all ranks and occupations and earning at least twice as much. Pulsford's greater success is an index of the fact, amongst other things, that his services were simply in greater demand.[17] Certainly doctors' diaries suggest they became very busy men. The Midlands physician, Erasmus Darwin, claimed to cover some 10,000 miles on calls per annum. It was nothing for the Kay family practice of Bury in Lancashire, to see a score or more patients a day. On 13 August 1746, Richard Kay listed his day's work:

> Besides the Patients Father has attended upon at Home, I shall give a short Account of those I have visited to Day in about 12 or 14 Miles ride; A young Woman under a bad Fever 5 Days . . . I bled her this Morning, applied a Blister Plaister to her Back, and left her proper Medicines. A young Woman mentioned July 2d seized very bad in her Belly who has had a dangerous Fever, and been very much threatened, from the Violence of her Pain at first, . . . [but who now] is much better, and we hope will be very well again. A young Man beginning a Fever who I bled, and ordered to sweat. A Girle with a Strumous Disorder under her Chin. An Antient Woman with a Bad Pain in her Hip. A young Wife near the Time of her Delivery and under some Discouragement lest she shou'd not do well. A Brother and Sister both consumptive. A Woman with a sore Leg. A young Women with a very sore stinking Leg. A Man under a Strumous Disorder in his Arm. These Particulars have been the Occurrences of the Day, and to mention which every Day wou'd be abundantly too tedious and prolix.[18]

Regular practitioners became a more visible presence. Geoffrey Holmes has argued that rising demand for doctors not only increased their numbers but also raised their quality. For in buoyant times, the ambitious surgeon, apothecary or surgeon-apothecary had incentives to improve on the traditional training by apprenticeship in the quest for advancement. Many served as army or navy surgeons, thereby gaining invaluable front-line expertise in operative techniques. Some acquired a medical education at one of the Scottish universities, which were cheap, open – unlike Oxford and Cambridge – to Dissenters and of tiptop quality (droves of Scottish-born graduates of Scottish universities came to England). Others walked the wards at one of London's expanding hospitals, fast emerging as leading teaching centres. Richard Kay was deeply impressed by the operative skills he witnessed while a medical student in the capital.[19]

Overall the rewards were rising, and there is no doubt that the occupation of medicine was thriving by the close of the eighteenth century. Top London physicians such as Matthew Baillie were earning some £10,000 a year, as was the 'mere' surgeon, Astley Cooper (knighted in 1821): such was the income of a minor peer. It was nothing unusual for a provincial physician to be pocketing in excess of £1,000. Even a few apothecaries were in the four-figure income bracket – for example, William Broderip of Bristol, who at one stage of his career apparently grossed over £2,000 a year, keeping a carriage and a country retreat. On the death of the fourth Duke of Queensbury in 1810, his heirs were sent an apothecary's bill for £16,000, for constant attendance over many years. A court reduced the sum to a paltry £7,500 plus costs.[20]

In this bubbling world of opportunity, practitioners alerted themselves to opportunities for advancement. Sensing the advantages of engaging in a riding practice in the manner of a true country practitioner, the traditional apothecary abandoned his vulgar shop-counter and turned bedside-visiting into the most visible aspect of his craft. Thereby the nation became stocked with general practitioners (forerunners of the Victorian family doctor), a breed anomalous to the traditional tripartite hierarchy. At the close of the eighteenth century, Thomas Percival praised them as a 'valuable' class: 'And as they are the guardians of health through large districts, no opportunities should be neglected of promoting their improvement, or contributing to their stock of knowledge.'[21]

The new general practitioners proved popular with their clients; yet they themselves did not prove exempt from competition from below. In particular, 'chemists' and 'druggists' mushroomed. These shopkeepers, without a medical education, sold medicaments and often made up drugs to practitioners' or patients' prescriptions, their growth in numbers evidently being a response to perceived or potential demand. All kinds of tradesmen – chandlers, grocers, general dealers etc., – had long sold drugs as part of their trade; and the bigger towns had had specialist chemists at least from the close of the seventeenth century, making up paints, dyes, polishes, solvents and so forth. But from the mid-eighteenth century, and especially in the nineteenth century, specialist druggists' shops proliferated, proving that there was money to be made out of medicines, toiletries and cosmetics, and offering to the public one further ready *entrée* into medical supplies and services.[22]

MEDICAL ENTERPRISE

Sometimes the outcome was fiery rivalry. The protests from surgeon-apothecaries against the druggists' encroachments echoed earlier groans from physicians petitioning against competition from the apothecaries themselves.[23] Yet such competition itself bespeaks an expanding demand for multifarious medical services, in which it was relatively easy for the enterprising to create new business niches. Ambitious young provincial general practitioners angling for advancement developed expertise in new specialities such as man-midwifery (obstetrics)[24] or smallpox inoculation.[25] The humble Suffolk surgeon, Robert Sutton, and his dynasty of sons, made fortunes out of variolation, setting up private nursing homes for wealthier inoculees and organizing mass inoculations for entire parishes. Parson Woodforde's brother-in-law, Dr Clarke, was a noted inoculator.[26]

At least among the more affluent, the emergent accoucheur or man-midwife elbowed out the traditional female midwife during the course of the eighteenth century.[27] Dentists likewise secured for themselves a more polished and remunerative trade. Tooth-pulling had always been a service to which all sorts of people had turned their hands, from barber-surgeons to blacksmiths: one recalls Parson Woodforde's horrendous experience with a superannuated tooth-drawing farrier:

> My tooth pained me all night, got up a little after 5 this morning, & sent for one Reeves a man who draws teeth in this parish and about 7 he came and drew my tooth, but shockingly bad indeed, he broke away a great piece of my gum and broke one of the fangs of the tooth, it gave me exquisite pain all the day after, and my Face was swelled prodigiously in the evening and much pain. Very bad and in much pain the whole day long. Gave the old man that drew it however 0.2.6. he is too old, I think, to draw teeth, can't see very well.[28]

But the new breed of itinerant dentists, while, of course, keeping up the bread-and-butter business of tooth-drawing, pioneered conservation work, and specialized in dentures and cosmetic effects. 'The celebrated Mrs BERNARD and Mr DAVY, DENTISTS from Berlin', fanfared the publicity for one such team of operators, astutely aware of the importance of looks rather than mere pain-relief to the *ton*, 'are just arrived again at Mr Sturdy's Glass-Shop, at the Corner of Goodramgate,

YORK, and respectfully acquaint the Public' of their operations. What did they do?

> Transplant Human Teeth, or fix artificial Teeth from one to an entire Sett, in a much easier and by a far superior Method than practised hitherto in this Kingdom. – Their Pearl Lotion is particularly recommended for restoring the Teeth to their native Whiteness and Beauty; (although ever so tarnished) without injuring the Enamel. The Efficacy of their admirable Preparations for eradicating the Scurvy, in causing the Gums to adhere close to the Teeth, in fastening such as are loose, in preserving them from future Decay, and in removing all offensive smell from the Breath, (the natural Consequence of Disease, and Fowlness in the Teeth and Gums) has been honoured with the Approbation of all foreign Universities, and all the principal cities of these three Kingdoms.
>   They have also a peculiar Mode (more preferable than ever practised), extracting Stumps, ever so difficult, with no more Pain than Bleeding; also Children's first Teeth, to cause the second Sett to grow regular and even.
> *** *The Tooth-Ach* cured without drawing.[29]

During the Georgian century, provincial dentists commonly rose to positions of public esteem and financial reward.[30]

Another way forward was through authorship. Many practitioners published books targeted at the laity, or inserted letters and articles in newspapers and periodicals, giving their addresses and puffing their powers.[31] Other perfectly reputable practitioners marketed their own nostrums. The most famous of all, James's Powders, was made to a formula patented by Dr Robert James, the friend of Samuel Johnson. Similarly, the eminent John Radcliffe advertised his 'Dr Radcliffe's Royal Tincture, or the General Rectifier of the Nerves, Head and Stomach', which was claimed to correct 'all irregularities of the Head and Stomach by hard drinking or otherwise'.[32] What would have been denounced as unprofessional conduct in 1870 was praised as enterprise a century earlier.[33]

As can be seen, the divide between reputable, regular practitioners with an eye for business and those often branded as quacks, might seem fluid and elusive, depending more upon rhetoric than reality. Regular practitioners were not ashamed to present themselves as good business-men; for this reason it is probably not very helpful to conceive of quack doctors as a breed apart from the regulars. Being largely itinerant, quacks traded heavily upon razzmatazz, and typically made their living out of sales of pre-packaged medicaments, in person or by post, rather than, as with the physician or general practitioner, through cultivating a long-term clientele.[34] But it would be as false to imply that all quacks were cheats or incompetents as it would be to suggest that all regulars were above consideration of gain.

It is noteworthy that the swelling ranks of regular practitioners did not squeeze irregulars out of business. Even the traditional mountebank, setting up his stage in the market square, seems to have survived, and new-style irregulars, pioneers in modern techniques of salesmanship and newspaper advertising, clearly made big profits.[35] In the first half of the eighteenth century, Joshua Ward, proprietor of Ward's Pill and Drop, was able to enjoy the company of top physicians and high society, just as, the better part of a century later, Samuel Solomon made a fortune and secured fashionable entrée. Whereas traditional *ciarlatani* had made a comic appeal to the vulgar, during the eighteenth century such fringe practitioners as the sex-therapist, James Graham, adopted more refined airs and graces, directing their appeal to a genteel, or aspirant, clientele.[36]

Wherever money was to be made out of medicine, the opportunity was seized. Shoals of shopkeepers sold drugs,[37] not least opiates and the score or two of nostrums advertised non-stop in the columns of provincial newspapers, newsagents providing the main retail outlet for them.[38] Certain individuals specialized in bone-setting and manipulation, sometimes doubling as vets.[39] Many women were employed as nurses, not in hospitals, as today, but in the home as the need arose. The parochial poor relief system often drew upon the services of nurses. People were paid to 'watch' the critically ill, particularly through the night, or to lay out and dress corpses and attend funerals.[40] In 1698 the Verney family, faced by a sudden smallpox emergency when a maid fell sick, searched around locally for a nurse:

> gett her [instructed Sir John Verney] an honest and good nurse, one that hath been used to be with people that have the Small Pox, & doubtless such a one you may hear of at Aylesbury or at Buckingham, for at such large Towns the Small Pox is very frequently, & I believe the Apothecaries can best provide you with a nurse . . . she must wash all that sick body's linnen at Holmes' house, for none of it must come to my house to be wash't that being dangerous, nor anything that is used about the sick body until the maid be recovered and the things well aired.[41]

Regulars, of course, deplored recourse to all manner of irregular healers and medical hucksters. The Stafford apothecary, William Westmacott, informed Henry Oldenburg in 1676:

> A poore Woman aged 50 upwards (the post master of Stafford his letter carrier), being tormented with a dolorous paine of her head, did make her Complainte, to a Confident petticoate docteress her Neighbour; Who (whether out of Experience of the thing I know not,) made a small tent with some Cotton, or some such like thing, & suffered it to Imbibe as much *spir. Castordj* as it would, & put it up her Nosthrill, about six of

the Clock on a Munday Evening; upon which she fell a sleep, & never awaked, as she affirmeth, (for she dwelt by herself alone) till her Neighbours through her long Absence were Invited to breake downe her dore upon her, On the Wensday evening following; & then was with great difficulty raised, lying for some time after in somnolento Comate, & att last would hardly be perswaded, but that it was but Tuesday morning . . . her paine did returne.[42]

Rather in the manner of that near-lethal 'petticoate docteress', many friends and neighbours dispensed medical advice and remedies free, or as part of the complex networks of reciprocity integral to parish-pump society. Gentry, ladies bountiful and clergymen commonly laid claims to pharmaceutical knowledge and kept a medicine chest open to the parish poor.[43] Richard Baxter, the Nonconformist minister, recorded how he built up a medical practice in Kidderminster in the 1670s, without even seeking it – 'no Physician being near': 'I was troubled this year with multitudes of melancholy persons from several parts of the land, some of high quality, some of low, some very exquisitely learned, some unlearned . . . I know not how it came to pass, but if men fell melancholy, I must hear from them or see them (more than any physician that I know).'[44]

Someone would commonly make a name as a local adept – as a dab hand with herbs, as one who had inherited a knack or a calling from his forebears or as the proverbial wise woman. One never knew who might fancy his or her medical skills. John Aubrey told of the wondrous wife of the Revd William Holder, Canon of St Paul's: 'Amongst many other Guifts she haz a strange sagacity as to curing of wounds, which she does not doe so much by presedents and Reciept bookes, as by her owne excogitancy, considering the causes, effects, and circumstances.'[45] She had even succeeded – where all others failed – in curing the King:

His Majestie King Charles II had hurt his hand, which he intrusted his Chirurgians to make well; but they ordered him so that they made it much worse, so that it swoll, and pained him up to his shoulder; and pained him so extremely he could not sleep, and began to be feaverish. Then one told the King what a rare shee-surgeon he had in his house; she was presently sent for at eleven clock at night. She presently made ready a Pultisse, and applyed it, and gave his Majestie sudden ease, and he slept well; next day she dressed him, and in a short time perfectly cured him, to the great griefe of all the Surgeons, who envy and hate her.[46]

The recipe books commonly kept in gentry kitchens typically included tips from such local notables.[47]

Thus a multiplicity of people in pre-modern England claimed to possess some special medical aptitude, and many gained a livelihood, or at least some reward or repute – notoriety even – out of plying their skills.[48] Medicine was far from exclusive; its practice stretched in a spectrum from the self-patching everyone performed (as when Parson Woodforde cut himself shaving and stopped the bleeding by applying a hapless moth providentially flying too close) to the exquisite skills of the surgeon, William Cheselden, who could extract a bladder-stone in two minutes flat.[49]

THE OPEN WORLD OF MEDICINE

Several features of this pluralist medical scene deserve special notice. First, there was almost complete freedom of practice. Anybody could try his hand – even on the monarch! – without let or hindrance. Pukka physicians jostled for custom alongside unorthodox practitioners such as Sally Mapp, the bone-setter from Epsom, or Gustavus Katterfelto, the Prussian quack with his talking black cats who blamed epidemics on insects.[50] Admittedly, certain forms of practice were regulated: above all, midwifery. The bishop's licence required by midwives testified not primarily to their medical skill but to their good morals and character. But licensing could, ironically, serve to legitimate, rather than exclude, irregular practice; for example, the issuing of royal mandates to foreign mountebanks and royal patents for proprietary medicines.[51] There was no equivalent in England to the drumming of Mesmer out of Vienna and Paris by the conjoint action of the medical faculty and the crown. In England, regulars denouncing charlatans were mainly limited to exposing them in pamphlets and the press.[52] This was a strategy that could backfire: John Coakley Lettsom's attempts to expose the urine-gazer, Theodor Myersbach, merely provided him with massive free publicity. *Ancien régime* society, the world of Old Corruption, is often characterized by historians as a closed world of oligarchy (Cobbett's 'THING'). But medically speaking, it operated, *de facto* at least, as an open market, whose watchword was *caveat emptor*. Cobbett himself published medical advice.[53]

Second, this open medical world presented genuine alternatives to sufferers, rather than services exclusively appropriate only for those within particular income, social or gender brackets.[54] Genteel families drew without compunction on the know-how of social inferiors such as housekeepers and grooms – hardly surprising in a society in which many still put their babies out to lower-class wet-nurses. At Bath, the upper classes were 'rubbed' and 'dipped' by strapping peasant women. So there was nothing anomalous about their drawing upon folk remedies or occasionally visiting a flashy quack. In the mid-seventeenth century,

Anne, Viscountess Conway, suffered appalling migraines. She was first treated by the world's most eminent physician, William Harvey; but when he failed, she passed to mountebanks' drinks and unorthodox healers such as Valentine Greatrakes, the Irish 'stroker'.[55] Family recipe books are an extraordinary collage of remedies emanating from the nobility, from eminent doctors, from nursemaids and from newspapers.[56]

Why was medicine such a hotch-potch at precisely the time when, in other aspects of social life, divides were solidifying between distinct cultures, high and low, patrician and plebeian, polite and popular? The answer, in part at least, lies in the fact that its therapeutic efficacy remained hopelessly hit-and-miss. It would be a mistake to make too much of the lurid incompetence of practitioners in the so-called 'age of agony'.[57] There were some areas of genuine advance – a broad improvement in surgical skills, the increasing use of opiates as analgesics and, of epochal importance, the introduction of smallpox inoculation (itself a folk remedy) and, later, vaccination.[58] Yet everyone recognized that the medical art was difficult and the empire of pain and death unshaken; because no single group of doctors could reliably cure, patients inevitably shopped around. At a time of innovation, sick people would seek out improvements wherever they might be found, possibly outside the mainstream in the grey area of the 'fringe', for as William Buchan reflected, 'very few of the valuable discoveries in Medicine have been made by physicians'.[59] That patients might consult a multitude of doctors and dabble with their favourite quack nostrums, were facts of life, acknowledged, if mildly deplored, in Thomas Percival's influential *Medical Ethics* (1803).[60]

The sick shopped around because there was no monopoly, and no single, unequivocal 'best buy', no scientific medicine palpably effective in restoring the ailing and failing to the pink of health. They took whatever medicine was to hand. Urgently needing medical help on a journey, William Pulteney was told 'that there was no one could do it, but a Man that lived three miles off, who was a good Physician, bled every Man, and Calf, in the neighbourhood, and was a pretty good Surgeon, for he had been originally a Sowgelder.'[61]

The sick also shopped around, one suspects, because they enjoyed it. The laity took it as their privilege and prerogative to sample distinct medicines and various practitioners, and exercise their own critical judgement. As we shall see below, questions of which doctor to choose for which condition greatly exercised those with time, information and money enough to deliberate. Undergoing medication was not a matter of abandoning oneself blindly to professional authority. It involved active decision-making and negotiation, equivalent to buying an estate or selecting an education for one's children. We shall repeatedly see the sick personally, energetically, and tenaciously insisting upon managing their medical affairs. All this 'meddling' was often deplored by the regulars, as when Thomas Trotter complained against self-dosing run wild. Parents find their children have some skin infection, he noted. What do such ignoramuses do?

> It is immediately decided that these spots are owing to bad humours and foulness of the blood, and must be carried off by a purge. Such reasoning as this formerly prevailed among medical people; we cannot therefore be surprized that persons not in the profession should still retain a little of the old leaven. Purgative medicines differ extremely from one another; and if it is a nice point in medical practice to suit the purge to the nature of the complaint and peculiarity of constitution, it must be often dangerous to trust them in common hands. I was once called to visit a farmer who had taken two ounces of saltpetre, instead of Glauber's salt. I found him in extreme pain about the stomach, with ghastly looks, an intermitting pulse, and cold sweats. A few minutes longer would have been too late to save him: by drinking plentifully of warm milk and water, and a brisk emetic, he was recovered. But I have known similar cases prove fatal.[62]

But despite all the grisly warnings, the self-dosing went on.

Thus medicine was relatively open to patient power. The Civil War undermined the monopolistic dreams of the medical colleges; in the eighteenth century, the mobilization of the market enfranchised the consumer. It was not until 1858 that the regular profession reasserted its control over medical services through the setting up of the Medical Register, which demarcated the regular profession from its competitors, and gave it important privileges. The situation in England was significantly different from that obtaining on the Continent. In *ancien régime* France, for instance, each major provincial centre had its own faculty of medicine, regulating entry into practice, and the Société Royale de Médecine was charged with licensing proprietary medicines.[63]

The establishment of the medical market-place had momentous consequences for the uptake of medical services. For it enshrined a system, one face of which spelt out a freedom, the other side of which was radical uncertainty. Those who could afford to do so, chose their own form of medicine, practitioner and mode of treatment. They were tenacious of their rights. Yet anxieties constantly arose as to the wisdom of their choices. Constant vigilance was demanded.

Faced with such life-and-death choices, laymen informed themselves about the state of medicine, about which practitioners were believed to be rising or falling, about the experiences of their acquaintances with this therapy or that surgeon. Eighteenth-century letters, and no doubt even more so, its tea-table chitchat, teemed with talk of courses of physic, operations and the 'fortunes of physicians'. A full flow of reliable information was of overriding importance in a system fraught with uncertainty. There was no substitute for self-help. Sometimes it took collective forms. Thus it was reported that, in Plymouth, prostitutes 'kept up a sort of police', inspecting each other for venereal infections.[64]

Above all, it was a matter of moment to decide correctly whether and when to place oneself under medical care at all, to turn from being a *sufferer* or a *self-treater* into a *patient* – because to do so was to some degree to abandon independence, albeit in the hope of gaining confidence in the authority of another.

The micro-history of bedside medicine at this time is thus the story of innumerable decisions made in times of crises, in matters of life and death. The 'New Disease' broke out across the Home Counties in 1658. Many perished. A Mr Wakefield chose to turn to the local 'Horse-Smithe' for treatment, yet, not surprisingly, needed to justify this singular choice to himself and to his betters, the Verneys. 'I have had my two youngest Children, 4 Maydes & 2 men, downe at a tyme of this new Disease, & yett through God's mercy are all recovered againe', he explained:

> I impute it under God, to a meanes that some people would have scrupled to have made use of his Phisicke; Hee being by profession a Horse-Smithe and keepes a shoppe in our Towne. Butt hee having practised upon many others about us, before we made use of him, the successe his Phisicke hath had in our Family, hath much encreased his fame, and really I thinke nott without desart; for he gives you as rationall an Accompte for what hee doth, as any Phisitian that I ever yett mette withall.[65]

Wakefield evidently feared he was speaking out of turn, for he concluded:

> What I write is nott to derogate from the honour due to many Phisitians of quality, but in the country, such cannott spend any tyme with us; and the trouble of sending soe farre too & againe, besides often tymes the mistakes and miscarriages of thinges, forces us to doe that which if we were in London, we should hardly venture upon.

PART II

Patients

3

Self-medication

Middlemarch society was sitting at tea. Conversation turned to Lady Chettam's 'remarkable health'. She herself attributed it to her 'home made bitters', slighting, by contrast, Mrs Renfrew's advocacy of 'strengthening medicines'. Everyone took up the subject:

'It strengthens the disease', said the Rector's wife, much too well-born not to be an amateur in medicine. 'Everything depends on the constitution; some people make fat, some blood, some bile – that's my view of the matter; and whatever they take is a sort of grist to the mill'.

'Then she ought to take medicines that would reduce – reduce the disease, you know, if you are right, my dear. And I think what you say is reasonable'.

'Certainly it is reasonable. You have two sorts of potatoes, fed on the same soil. One of them grows more and more watery – '

'Ah! like this poor Mrs Renfrew – that is what I think. Dropsy! There is no swelling yet – it is inward. I should say she ought to take drying medicines, shouldn't you? – or a dry hot-air bath. Many things may be tried, of a drying nature'.[1]

George Eliot had a fine ear. All responsible lay people believed it was up to them to look after their own and their dependants' health, not to mention dishing out some gratuitous crumbs of advice for poor dears such as Mrs Renfrew. It was a self-evident duty, accepted automatically, without elaborate rigmarole.[2] But if people needed any reminding of their responsibilities, scores of self-help, health-care books (for example, Tissot's *Essay on the Disorders of People of Fashion*, 1766) were pouring off the presses. These books recommended simple rules for diet, exercise, fresh air, cleanliness etc., and showed how to treat pains, sprains and strains with home-made remedies.[3] Health manuals were commonly shelved next to the family Bible in a body-and-soul bedside care package – the Revd Patrick Brontë, for example, swore by

John Graham's popular *Modern Domestic Medicine*. Home health care was necessary, argued Hugh Smythson's weighty digest of family medicine, so as to 'enable the diseased to have immediate recourse to proper remedies, without the delays occasioned by sending many miles for a physician or apothecary, and without incurring an expence which in many cases they are ill able to bear.' Yet in matters of healing, native wit and first aid needed to be supplemented by expert advice, in order 'to bring men of common capacities so well acquainted with the *symptoms*, *nature*, and the *origin* of their disorders, that they may not be in danger of using improper medicines and unsafe methods of cure; and to direct them to the administration of simple, easy, and cheap ones.'[4]

People sometimes did, and sometimes did not, heal by the book. But they certainly took energetic action on their own initiative to protect their health. William Wordsworth, whom Coleridge diagnosed as a hypochondriac, was so concerned that he inspected his boils under a microscope.[5] Benjamin Franklin was recommended cold baths for his health; he tried them, but found 'air baths' preferable: 'I rise almost every morning, and sit in my chamber without any clothes whatever, half an hour or an hour, according to the season, either reading or writing. This practice is not in the least painful, but, on the contrary, agreeable.'[6]

Not everyone had Franklin's success in following catechisms of health (few had such easy rules to follow). In September 1743, Thomas Cooke decided it was high time to grapple with his own drinking problems. He pored over the *English Physician's Guide*, with a view to following its rules for temperance, scribbling rather woozily in the margin: 'whereas for about 6 years past I have been grievously tormented by drinking strong liquors therefore for the future I intend by God's assistance to drink nothing but to lead a temperate life.'[7] A subsequent morale-booster a few pages on reads: 'after December ye 14th 1743 drink nothing strong'. But Cooke's next piece of marginalia records the first set-back in his crusade: 'after March ye 28th 1744 drink nothing strong'. After that, reverses followed thick and fast: 'after April ye 12th 1744 Drink Water and Drink Nothing Strong'. And then: 'from May ye 19th 1744 Drink nothing strong but water'. And finally: 'after June ye 17th 1744 never drink anything strong'. Self-control was easier said than done.

People tried to keep checks on their health in various ways. Some weighed themselves regularly. Some took up faddish new gadgets – the Georgian precursors of exercise bikes – to tone themselves up. Lybbe Powys was fetched by the idea of a 'portable hygeian chair, by which persons may swing themselves with safety'.[8]

Granted that energetic steps were taken to keep healthy, it will come as no surprise that, when these measures failed, and people fell sick, they equally took sickness management into their own hands. 'I have had a headache for these last four or five days', groaned Lord Herbert to his friend, Archdeacon Coxe, in March 1783, 'to remedy which I am going to take an emetick when this [letter] is sealed.'[9] His confidence ebbed with events. Next day he wrote, somewhat impiously, that he had spent the night 'vomiting up my soul'.[10] The day after brought 'Nothing new, except that I have been obliged to take some more physick today.'[11] His head was still thumping a week later; the next day he swallowed twenty grains of 'Epicicuana, which made me very miserable till one this morning', yet even this heroic dose of a trusted emetic failed to relieve his head.[12] At length, he approached his apothecary, who recommended tartar emetic, yet another vomit. But still it produced no effect.[13] Self-medication did not always work, but it was not necessarily any worse than other courses to hand.

The practice of what was variously called 'domestic medicine', 'family medicine' or 'kitchen physic' was utterly standard. All took it for granted that there were everyday ills and spills with which a resourceful lay person should cope, that emergencies would occur which could not wait for the arrival of a practitioner perhaps several hours distant (first aid was needed) and that some complaints were so trivial that no one would countenance incurring a practitioner's bill for them, or risk being thought hypochondriacal.[14]

A person ignorant of self-care would have been equivalent to a woman unable to bake, stitch and manage the servants, or a gentleman who could not ride. Cotton Mather had a trio of daughters. Enamoured, apparently, by the division of female labour, he wanted one to grow up good at cooking, one at sewing and one at home physic.[15] Some even gloried – maybe with a touch of self-mockery – in the name of 'physician'. 'When you go to Dublin [from the country] you will lie abed, play at loo, and keep bad hours, which heats the blood and hurts your nerves', Caroline Fox warned her sister, the Marchioness of Kildare, adding with a smile, 'great physician as you are you must know that tho'.'[16] It was a compliment she liked paying. When the Marchioness's husband was sick, Caroline wrote, hinting what action to take: 'Don't you as a physician think bathing in the sea would do him good?'[17] 'I have played the physician myself', beamed Fanny Burney, having just successfully nursed her children through bad coughs.[18]

Such self-help activities had their place within a historical mythology of the development of knowledge and power. John Wesley, no less a champion of self-healing in medicine than of conversion experience in faith, argued that in the good old days of patriarchy, heads of households had assumed responsibility for health as well as for godliness. The advent of commercial society, with all its attendant corruptions, encouraged doctors – that ambitious professional priesthood – to arrogate such basic human responsibilities to themselves. This was, Wesley believed, both needless and harmful.[19] Each man should take health, as well as salvation, into his own hands.

Wesley practised what he preached. His journal shows that his invariable response to illness was to medicate himself. It always worked. His face became swollen; he cured it with nettles. He had lumbago; it went when he applied garlic to his feet. He was believed to be wasting with consumption: 'A thought came into my mind to make an experiment. So I ordered some brimstone to be powdered, mixed with the white of an egg, and spread on brown paper, which I applied to my side. The pain ceased in five minutes, the fever in half an hour; and from this hour I began to recover strength.'[20] When fellow Methodists fell sick, Wesley played doctor to them, and was eager to give them electrical treatment: 'I prepared and gave them physic myself'.

Despite Wesley's drift, self-medication and professional care were not generally seen as rivals, but as allies within the larger enterprise of healing. Hence self-help was commonly endorsed by doctors themselves, though some decried the bandying around of phrases such as 'home doctor' or 'every man his own doctor', lest they give the laity ideas above their station.[21] For doctors recognized that to a large degree health must inevitably lie in the sick person's own orbit: 'three good physicians – air, water, exercise', advised the great Thomas Sydenham.[22] Health had to begin at home. And it would continue there too, in that medical prescriptions would be implemented only with active lay co-operation.[23]

That is why practitioners themselves contributed medical tips and recipes to the magazine culture which played no small role in broadcasting practical knowledge during the Georgian era.[24] 'Read part of *The Universal Magazine* for June', recorded the Sussex grocer, Thomas Turner, in summer 1757,[25]

> wherein I find the following receipt recommended (in an extract from Dr. Lind's Essay on the most effectual means of preserving health of the seamen in the Royal Navy) as a specific against all epidemical and bilious fevers and also against endemic disorders. He first recommends a regular course of life and to abstain as much as possible from animal food, and to confine as much as possible to a vegetable diet. Then he orders about 2 ounces of the following tincture to be taken every day upon an empty stomach (and better if taken at twice):
> 8 ounces of bark
> 4 ounces dried orange peel, which infuse in a gallon of spirits.[25]

In the spirit of the age, which did not kowtow to the printed word or to supposed expertise, the tradesman could not resist adding his own improvement: 'But in my opinion it might be rendered a more grateful bitter if instead of the 4 ounces of dried orange peel there was put 1½ ounces of it and 3 ounces of undried lemon peel cleared from the white.'[26]

Of course, self-help manuals urged that in serious cases a practitioner should be summoned; but that very piece of advice presupposed that it would be within the lay person's powers – indeed it would inevitably fall to his lot – to size up such a situation.

PHYSICKING ONESELF

The young nonconformist law student, Dudley Ryder, had such distressing experiences with physicians (he feared they cynically over-dosed him) that he recorded in 1716, 'this had made me almost resolve to be my own physician'.[27] Such disillusionment with the professionals was not uncommon. Roger North thought the illnesses of his brother, John, had largely been brought on by over-eager professional inter-vention, when some plain, old-fashioned home-nursing would have done the trick. This was a verdict which, he feared, 'may offend the medical faculty': 'But I am not free to suppress or palliate matters of fact which were of the last concern to my subject. If one may be so free to interpose a censure, their fault (if any was) lay in meddling at all, and not sending the good man home to his mother to be nursed.'[28] North did not merely suspect the doctors' motives, but felt sure he knew enough medicine to expose their incompetence: 'But instead of that, partly as I guess to humour him, and partly to put in practice their university learning, fell in pell-mell with their prescriptions to divert this flow of rheum from discharging at his throat and mouth and to send it another way.'[29] Here the doctors could not win: in Roger North's eyes, they erred both by humouring the patient and when laying down the law.

Many complained about medical mistakes, deeming it dangerous to vest unconditional trust in doctors or to use their services beyond necessity. When his business partner, Thomas Bentley, poured out his worries about his wife's health, Josiah Wedgwood slipped in a word of reassurance: 'Let the Doctors say what they will, don't place too implicit a faith in them. They are often deceiv'd, & look graver than they need to do.'[30] Yet Wedgwood was no enemy to doctors, counting physicians such as Erasmus Darwin amongst his bosom friends.[31]

David Garrick, too, was a man well disposed towards practitioners as individuals. The great actor used William Cadogan to dose his whole troupe when they fell sick. Yet he entertained no great faith in their healing powers, and reserved the right to follow his nose. When his kidney complaints worsened, he called upon Myersbach, the quack uroscopist. Likewise, he recommended the Revd Joseph Smith to take

'Adams's Solvent' (a proprietary remedy) to cure his stomach disorders – 'be a little careful of yr Food, & drink', he advised, 'I will answer for your cure'. The distinguished physician, Richard Brocklesby, was not amused: such medicines, he warned, will be 'the death of you'. Yet Garrick was not abashed: 'I have taken all your medicines', he rebuked Brocklesby, 'and from this solvent only I think I feel some relief, and I had rather die than suffer as I do.'[32]

Samuel Johnson took a rather similar view. Doctors deserved respect, and medicine was a means to an end. On occasion, Johnson delivered himself to the doctors. Labouring with dropsy, he told the surgeon, William Cruickshank, 'I am going to put myself into your hands'.[33] Yet medicine must not, in his view, be allowed to usurp life. Keep taking the bark (that is, quinine) so long as it was really needed, Johnson instructed his friend, Mrs Thrale, 'and then, *throw physick to the dogs*'.[34]

Some went one step further and excluded the doctor altogether. They were, it was often said, quite unnecessary; people held the key to health themselves. 'If you are *ill* at this season', barked William Hone's *Table Book* for January 1827, 'there is no occasion to send for the doctor – *only stop eating*.'[35] Sometimes higher principles seemed at stake. Thus the sturdy radical, William Cobbett, argued (rather in the manner of his arch-enemy, Wesley) that the new-fangled men-midwives were an unnecessary interference, because, throughout history, women had always given birth perfectly well on their own, aided by friends and familiars:

> Who can perform this office like women? who have for these occasions a language and sentiments which seem to have been invented for the purpose; and . . . they have all, upon these occasions, one common feeling, and that so amiable, so excellent, as to admit of no adequate description. They completely forget, for the time, all rivalships, all squabbles, all animosities, all hatred even; every one feels as if it were her own particular concern.[36]

Here medical self-help dovetailed with a 'separate spheres' view of the natural domestic duties of women.[37]

We have already seen Dudley Ryder disillusioned with doctors. He tried dosing himself with made-up nostrums. 'Rose at 7. Began to take my quack medicine again in order . . . to see whether it will do me any good or no', he wrote in 1716. He thereby displayed a blend of experimentalism and scepticism, enthusiasm and self-exculpation, typical of the laity when self-dosing.[38] 'I would not see a physician at the worst', was Horace Walpole's hard line to Thomas Gray, 'but have quacked myself as boldly, as Quacks treat others.'[39]

Within a highly health-conscious milieu, the sick commonly took remedial action on their own initiative. They scrutinized the severity of their symptoms and the source of their distemper before deciding whether they themselves had the skill and means to act, or should seek professional advice. Many then continued to exercise independent judgement. Sick in 1756, Samuel Johnson summoned the trusted Dr Lawrence, but in the end overrode him; Lawrence 'would have given some oil and sugar, but I took Rhenish and water, and recovered my voice . . . I have been visited by another Doctor today, but I laughed at his Balsam of Peru.'[40]

Many went in for standard forms of self-medication almost as a routine or a reflex response. People purged and vomited themselves, rather as this century they take aspirin for everyday aches and pains. Such evacuations presumably had a cleansing effect, upon both body and mind, and self-dosers were relieved to see evidence of their 'working', for diarists regularly quantified their bowel motions in minute detail. Such self-physicking also offered a secondary gain by providing perfect justification for withdrawal – usually for a day – from normal social demands, and a legitimation of complete rest. The self-penalization involved in taking a vomit or a purge vindicated limited social irresponsibility.

FAMILY PHYSIC

'The Queen is my physician', exclaimed George III when trying to shake off the doctors dogging him when he grew delirious in 1788.[41] Not everyone had a queen to count on, but someone in the family circle was typically on hand, happy to dabble, for, as Keith Thomas has put it, 'medicine began at home'.[42] Classically, mothers looked after their ailing children, calling themselves their offsprings' 'physicians'. John Clare wrote of Richard Turnill that 'his mother was skilld in huswife phisic and Culpeppers Herbal and he usd to be up gathering herbs at the proper time of the planets'.[43] Mothers often consulted practitioners for advice, but administered the treatments themselves; they clearly saw this as their duty, but also had the psychological insight to recognize that nasty medicines coming from themselves were more likely to be acceptable to their children. (A pair of Verney children in the late seventeenth century refused point-blank to see the doctor at all.)[44] When the Duke of Beaufort fell ill of smallpox early in the eighteenth century, it was his grandmother who took charge, implementing the time-honoured folk procedures (closed windows, drawn curtains, a well-stoked fire, etc.). It was only later that Dr Radcliffe was called in.[45]

Fanny Burney wrote to her husband on 6 October 1804 about their son, Alex, sick with cough and fever: 'I have not mentioned, I believe, that on Saturday, finding he had no more fever, I omitted the saline draughts, & gave him sulphur, cream de Tartre, & Honey, for his worms, as the most cooling medicine I dared administer, for I fear rhubarb with his Cough, & Bark & Garlick & Wine are hors de question.'[46] She clearly knew her medicines. She had summoned the physician:

> M. Bourdois was all kindness & friendliness; I told him in full detail the illness, in its progress, of Cold, Fever, Worms, & Cough, & all my management, of James's powder, analeptic, etc. To the two first he could say nothing, as he knows not their properties [she preened herself]; but all the rest he approved, & after examining the dear Child, must be taken care of: & finally said I had succeeded & done so well, he saw *nothing to change* in my present procès, as the sulphur & creme de Tartre with Honey were as good for his *rhume* as for worms: he should therefore only *add* one prescription, which was Turnip juice. He told me how to make it; recommended that he should take as little drink & as much solid [food, as] not further to relax his stomach, to *garder* him from W[orms] & to give him the Turnip Juice by *spoonfuls* frequently but [not] by draughts; nor Tisans, etc. He left me amazingly contented, & more for *you* still than for myself, as you now see how much confidence you may have in your household apothecary.[47]

The letter reveals mixed emotions: Burney congratulated herself for her display of competence – the doctor had given her his blessing, surely her husband would too – but she also needed to keep detailed minutes in case anything untoward befell. Children's ailments posed parents agonizing problems of responsibility; they had to deal with the doctors, yet also retain overriding control.

When Sarah Lennox's daughter, Louisa, fell sick, she felt sure neither of the disorder nor of the treatment. She was not even convinced that much was wrong at all ('people laugh at me sometimes for fancying she is not well; at others, people can scarce refrain from alarming me about her looks'), but concern was clearly in order. Her elder sister, the Duchess of Leinster, sent her own medicines along, but Sarah was evidently not too happy with such interference, wishing to appear competent and in charge: 'I shall not try this medicine, although I am very much obliged to you for telling me of it. But I think you will agree with me it is better not when I tell you the state of her health. She grows very fast, very thin and very weak, her stomack is disordered, and upon the whole, she has the appearance of worms.'[48] Hers was the classic dilemma. She did not want to appear guilty of inaction; but the action hitherto taken seemed worthless: 'She has taken several medicines for [the suspected worms], and none appear (although two years ago she had them). I fear this variety of things hurts her stomach, and if no worms come what is to be done? My own opinion is by nourishment, and gentle bathing twice a week in the sea to strengthen her constitution and battle against her growth, which perhaps is her only complaint.'[49] In the plan of self-help, she had secured medical approval: 'This I am now going to try, and if it agrees with her, as the doctors tell me it will, I shall be satisfied that by care and patience we may prevent the bad effects of her growing too fast; but if she don't mend in a month's time I shall be alarmed.'[50] She concluded with an expression of proprietorship over her own child: 'You see, my dear sister, that it would not be wise to try any medicine *à l'aventure* without knowing precisely what her complaint is; besides I dare say she could not keep it a moment on her stomach.'[51] Overall, she had clearly formulated her own notion of the complaint (nothing serious; growing pains; bathing would help), and in this had co-opted the agreement of the doctors. She trusted to events to bear her out: 'In short, I hope a short time will decide her complaint to be weakness which bathing and great attention will recover before winter.'

Thus family medicine involved all the regular ploys of power and prestige, and the sick easily became pawns in domestic politics. In 1640 Lady Brilliana Harley informed her son, Edward, that his brother, Tom, was sick of an ague. Things had nearly turned out disastrously because the nurse watching him 'made so much fier' (the classic 'hot' treatment) that it 'allmost burnt the clothes of the beed, and put him into a violent heate'. Fortunately, Lady Brilliana had taken complete control in good time: 'now I haue him lye in the chamber by me, which pleases him very well'.[52] Sometimes we seem to catch the sick person's weary response to being subjected to family manipulation played out in the name of medicine. 'My Father', Betsy Sheridan complained, 'was for dosing me with James's powders but as my disorder arose entirely from fatigue, I can not think such violent medicines necessary or indeed safe.'[53]

PHYSICKING THE COMMUNITY

The master or mistress of the household – men and women were equally active in this role – commonly took responsibility for physicking servants and employees, and indeed the wider village circle. Lady Byron boasted she once saved a maid's life, 'by a timely dose of Castor Oil when she was in danger of an inflammation in her bowels'.[54] Of course, physicking servants also saved the master a practitioner's bill. Moreover, servants were presumably forbidden to treat themselves; that would have offered far too many opportunities for them to exploit the sick role, and given them undesirable access to the family medicine chest. Servants cannot have had much say in their own treatment. Parson Woodforde tried out some pretty robust treatments upon his household, including giving a man with malaria a ducking in a pond.[55] Doctoring parishioners was part of *noblesse oblige*. 'Poor Neighbour Downing very bad indeed this evening', wrote Woodforde, 'the Small Pox being upon the turn. They sent to me to desire me to come and see him they all thinking that he was dying. I went to him and saw him, his Pulse was very high owing to drinking some Beer etc. to-day. He was quite light though not in a dying way, tho' he laid as if he was. I ordered them to give him some electuary in warm water, and when I came away he seemed a little better.'[56] Woodforde took the usual nursing action: 'My man Ben I ordered to sit up with him to-night'.

Often it was the parson who became the village Hippocrates, but not always so. 'Agues are much about', wrote the Revd George Woodward in the mid-eighteenth century, 'and my wife being a professed Sangrado for that distemper, has multitude of patients, that come to her three or four miles round, and great success she has with her powders.'[57] Neither did village physic stop with servants and labourers; it was offered to sick animals too. Woodforde performed surgery on his pets and livestock, once operating on his cat, sewing it up and making good with Friar's Balsam.[58] The Duke of Montagu even ran 'a hospital for old cows and horses'. It was said that 'none of his tenants near Boughton dare kill a broken-winded horse: they must bring them all to the Reservoir'.[59]

SELF-DOSING CIRCLES

People thus dosed themselves, and treated inferiors and dependants. They also made extremely free with medical advice amongst friends and fellows. Everyone seemed to be telling everyone else how to be healthy (self-physician, heal thyself). In 1771 David Garrick commiserated with his friend, John Moody, 'I am sorry that you have been plagu'd with yt cursed Distemper, the Piles'. The advice inevitably poured out: 'live abstemiously for a little time, & take Every Night a large tea spoonfull of flower of Brimstone (night & morning) mix'd up with honey or treacle, & you will be ye better for it – You should make up a Gallipot of it & take it by way of Sweetmeat.'[60] Every cloud had its silver lining, Garrick thought, alluding to the traditional belief that one disease drove out another: 'thank ye Stars for ye Piles – if you had not them, you would have gout, or Stone or both & ye Devil and all – While I had ye Piles, I had Nothing Else, now I am quit of them, I have Every other disorder.'[61]

When her niece, Amelia, was ill of suspected worms, Fanny Burney was told, evidently in great detail, about a heroic technique which her friend, Lydia Huber, had used to expel worms from her own adolescent niece. In hopes of being helpful, Fanny passed on the advice to Amelia's mother, Esther Burney: 'Mrs Hube[r] tells me she has not only cured her Lydia of this malady, but strengthened her to a stoutness & health quite astonishing, by giving her a glass of red port every morning fasting, taken from a Bottle in which a clove of garlick had been soaked for 24 hours. When a pint of this has been taken, she stops it for a dose of rhubarb & senna, & then resumes the wine till it is finished.'[62] It had worked wonders: 'Her Lydia was a poor pale thin green yellow Girl for many years till she tried this, & succeeded. She is now about 12 years old, I fancy. I wish you to make the essay with Amelia.'[63]

Samuel Johnson, too, was always dishing out medical advice. On hearing his acquaintance, John Perkins, was about to travel for his health, Johnson said (in a somewhat ambiguous phrase), 'I am much pleased that You are going on a very long Journey . . . by proper conduct it may restore your health and prolong your life':

Observe these rules
1　Turn all care out of your head as soon as you mount the chaise.
2　Do not think about frugality, your health is worth more than it can cost.
3　Do not continue any day's journey to fatigue.
4　Take now and then a day's rest.
5　Get a smart seasickness if you can.
6　Cast away all anxiety, and keep your mind easy.
This last direction is the principal; with an unquiet mind neither exercise, nor diet, nor physick can be of much use.[64]

Self-dosers of the world united in discussing each others' cases and doling out advice. For nearly thirty years around the mid-seventeenth century, the large correspondence network surrounding Lady Anne Conway was seemingly preoccupied by her appalling headaches and how to assuage them.[65] Often the motives must have been purely philanthropic, but sometimes something more was surely at stake: covert disapproval (sickness betrayed bad family management) and the exercise of control through medical know-how. For many, there were no inhibitions about ostentatiously airing one's ailments and self-treatments in public. Joseph Farington filled his diary with the health-care habits of his companions. Underlying this tireless inquisitiveness, one imagines, lay worries about his own health – anxieties that occasionally surfaced, as when he recorded an exchange with the Revd William Barclay, the classic doctor *manqué*: 'Rev. Mr Barclay I called on, and had a long conversation with him. He considers my inconveniences of feeling as arising from supressed gouty humours. He advises a disuse of wine – particularly Port Wine – and to substitute a little Brandy & Water.'[66] This was just the beginning of an avalanche of advice that descended upon Farington! Once Parson Barclay mounted the health pulpit, there was no stopping him: 'To eat roasted Apples for supper [he told

Farington], – White Biscuits instead of Bread – to avoid eating web-footed Animals – Salmon, Mackrell. To eat in preference Venison, all game, Fowls; Beef & Mutton are less to be preferred than the former. *Large* Cod, – whitings, Soles, Haddocks – Turbot, all good. To avoid Pork entirely.'[67] Barclay warmed to the doctor's role, taking the patient's history:

> He asked me if I had warm feet, I said, Yes, *that* He replied was a good sign. To regulate the Bile ought to be the great object of life – the oppressions caused by it when in a vitiated state destroy mankind. Avoid Milk. I remarked on it being the natural food of Children, and what, said He, is so bilious as a young Child. Sea bathing would be bad for me – Those constitutions only can stand sea bathing which perspire very freely. Do you start in your sleep sometimes – that is irritation from Bile. When you wake in the night or in the morning, are you instantly broad awake? No; then you have not *that* Symptom of irritation. Are you much troubled with Phlegm collecting in the Stomach? Not to be sensible of it. That is a bilious symptom. (I observe Sir George often labours with Phlegm). Avoid vegetables.[68]

Barclay continued the peroration:

> Take my Pills at night, going to rest – one, two or three as you find necessary – if in the morning they have no effect, take one two or three more. An hour after breakfast, an Hour after Dinner, and an Hour after Supper take two tea spoons full of the *Specific*, in a third of pint of *soft* water. At any time of the day that you may find yourself uneasy take of the *Volatile Cordial* 4 or 6 tea spoons full in water as above.[69]

Whatever did Farington make of this? Did he find it helpful, officious or utterly preposterous?

Though not always with such passionate zeal, people were for ever sounding out symptoms and passing on tips. When Mrs Thrale's daughter, Sophie, was diagnosed by her doctors as possessing a 'nervous constitution', Samuel Johnson took it upon himself to reassure the frightened mother, brushing the physicians aside: 'I received yesterday from your Physicians a note from which I received no information, they put their heads together to tell me nothing.' He continued, 'Do not let them fill your mind with terrours which perhaps they have not in their own'; the doctors were bandying around such terms as 'hystericks', but 'they are the bugbears of disease of great terrour but little danger'.[70]

People did not merely seek, or receive, advice. The self-medicating circle also worked through the exchange of actual medicaments. When Parson Woodforde's niece fell sick ('in a decline, on Account of her lately having had the Measles and catching cold after, which affected her Lungs'), he reacted by popping a prescription in the post: 'I sent a very long letter to my Sister Pounsett by Ben and in it a Recipe from

Dr. Buchan for Julia Woodforde, Nancys Sister, for her bad Cough.'[71] Buchan's *Domestic Medicine* (1769) was Woodforde's vade-mecum in time of sickness. Nicholas Blundell did not restrict himself to prescriptions; he actually pounded and ground the medicines himself for friends and neighbours. 'I mixed up a dose for William Abbot's Wife who has the Ague Fits', he wrote on 24 January 1712 (Abbot was one of his tenants).[72]

Sometimes lay medical help was by way of emergency first aid. Henry Yeonge records an exciting rescue from drowning. A boat overturned at Deal. A man was trapped beneath it, eventually released, but left on the beach for dead: 'A traveller, in very poor clothes (coming to look on, as many more did), presently pulled out his knife and sheath, cuts off the nether end of his sheath, and thrust his sheath into the fundament of the said Thomas Boules, and blew with all his force till he himself was weary; then desired some others to blow also; and in half an hour's time brought him to life again. I drank with him at his house.'[73] In the second half of the eighteenth century, the humane movement was set up to instruct people in the techniques of resuscitation in cases of apparent drownings.[74]

Occasionally, blood-letting and other minor operations were performed by a family member or a servant. 'My brother came over in the even in order to have 2 blisters laid on behind the ears', wrote Thomas Turner, who rather fancied his medical expertise (artificial blisters were meant to draw out peccant humours in the pus).[75] Indeed, some people acquired a notoriety for their eagerness to medicate their circle. Blood-letting was a well-known foible of Lord Radnor. Needing his political support, Lord Chesterfield pandered to that whim:

> Lord Chesterfield, wanting an additional vote for a coming division in the House of Peers, called on Lord Radnor, and, after a little introductory conversation, complained of a distressing headache.
>
> 'You ought to lose blood then', said Lord Radnor.
>
> 'Gad – do you indeed think so? Then, my dear lord, do add to the service of your advice by performing the operation. I know you are a skilful surgeon'.
>
> Delighted at the compliment, Lord Radnor in a trice pulled out his lancet-case, and opened a vein in his friend's arm.
>
> 'By-the-by', asked the patient, as his arm was being adroitly bound up, 'do you go down to the House to-day?'
>
> 'I had not intended going' answered the noble operator, 'not being sufficiently informed on the question which is to debated; but you, that have considered it, which side will you vote on?'
>
> In reply, Lord Chesterfield unfolded his view of the case; and Lord Radnor was so delighted with the reasoning of the man (who held his surgical powers in such high estimation), that he forthwith promised to support the wily earl's side in the division.

'I have shed my blood for the good of my country', said Lord Chesterfield that evening to a party of friends.[76]

Concern for health and self-medicating sometimes reached a suffocating and even health-threatening pitch. Pope wrote of a claustrophobic visit to Sir William Codrington: 'All his sisters . . . insisted I should take physic'. He could not get away from this Macbethian scene: 'My Lady Cox, the first night I lay there, mixed my electuary, Lady Codrington pounded sulphur, Mrs Bridget Bethel ordered broth. Lady Cox marched first up-stairs with the physic in a gallipot; Lady Codrington next, with the vial of oyle; Mrs Bridget third, with pills; the fourth sister, with spoons and tea-cups.'[77] Did Pope secretly enjoy all that female cosseting? It could, indeed, all be a bit much. For his part, Thomas Gray complained to Horace Walpole, he was sick of endless talk of sickness and of 'quality receipts': 'There is not a Man or Woman here that is not a perfect old Nurse, & who does not talk gruel & anatomy with equal fluency and ignorance. One instance shall serve; Madame de Bouzols, Marshal Berwick's daughter, assured me there was nothing so good for the gout as to preserve the parings of my nails in a bottle close-stopped. When I try any illustrious Nostrum, I shall give the preference to this.'[78]

HOME THERAPEUTICS

If Georgian salons trembled with people agitated about their health, eagerly exchanging information, pills and potions, what exactly did these self-medicators do and take? An astonishing range of procedures and preparations was tried. 'Dear Sister', opened Lady Fermanagh to Mrs Stone in 1737, 'I was most extreamly concerned to hear that Mrs. Jackman has been so ill and if it is anything of her fitts, and she will take anything of the Drops I had from Mr. Middelton before he was out of order, which did me a great deal of good, I'll send her some with all my heart.'[79] When the son of her friend, Mrs Dewes, fell sick with ague, Mrs Delany despatched two infallible recipes, one a plaster made of ginger and brandy, and the other a spider put into a goose quill, to be hung round the child's neck.[80]

Sometimes the simplest of remedies was recommended. Thus Ben Franklin, like John Wesley, believed in self-dosing with water. 'In the evening I found myself very feverish, and went into bed', wrote Franklin on his travels: 'but, having read somewhere that cold water drank plentifully was good for a fever, follow'd the prescription, sweat plentiful most of the night, my fever left me, and in the morning, crossing the ferry, I proceeded on my journey on foot.'[81]

Everyone had his favourite remedy, and boasted of it until it achieved some public fame. Joseph Spence enjoyed recording the recipes he had obviously heard on the grapevine. Did you have a chill? Then: 'For a cold that seems to begin to affect the lungs; two handfuls of bran boiled in two quarts of water till the bran is all sunk, put into it a pound of raisins and half a pound of figs, and sweeten it with sugar-candy.'[82] Sometimes Spence listed proprietary medicines worth a try ('The diet drink against the scurvy at Mr. Hartley's Marylebone Street'). But above all he enjoyed copying down recommendations picked up from noblemen no less anxious to get their names on to medicines than on to streets, squares and ships – for example, 'Lord Northumberland's cure for an ague': 'gromwell seed, pounded quite fine, the weight of 18d in silver a dose, to be taken in half a pint of ale, blood warm, when the fit is coming on. Lord Northumberland says three doses never fail of curing.'[83] The sly old Earl of Howth confided to the attentive Spence his own 'never-failing recipe for a sore throat':

> his directions were – just before going to bed to get scalding water, and the finest double-refined sugar, with two juicy lemons, and above all some old Jamaican rum, and when in bed take a good jar of it as hot as possible.
> 'Why, my lord', said I, 'your prescription seems to be nothing more than punch'.
> 'And what is better sir for a sore throat than a good punch?' asked his lordship. 'Good punch at night and copious gargles of old Port by day, would cure any mortal disease in life'.[84]

One-half of John Baker's recourse when sick was less appetizing: 'Took caster oil – read Tristram Shandy'.[85]

Some people's penchants in self-medication wear a slightly bizarre look. For example, Sir Samuel Romilly kept his own pair of pet leeches, which had been used to let his blood when he was taken dangerously ill at Portsmouth: 'they had saved his life, and he had brought them with him to town; had ever since kept them in a glass; had himself every day given them fresh water; and had formed a friendship with them. He said he was sure they both knew him, and were grateful to him. He had given them different names, Home and Cline (the names of two celebrated surgeons).'[86] But most home cures were far more familiar, as can be seen from surviving family recipe books. These reveal a self-help medicine that was thoroughly eclectic. Recipes involving native roots and herbs, collected from the hedgerows or the kitchen garden, jostle alongside what was clearly the growing use of exotic spices and medicaments imported from the Old and New Worlds.[87]

During the course of the century, people had increasing recourse to shop-bought medicines. Assisted by the emergence of druggists' shops, they stocked up with a widening range of strong minerals and chemicals, including calomel (for purging) and antimony (a febrifuge). Patent and proprietary medicines caught the eye. 'English ladies always keep a regular chemists' shop in their dressing rooms', snarled Dorothea Lieven.[88] Not least, they made full use of the latest convenience, ready-made medicine chests. Advertised in newspapers and pamphlets, these could contain up to a hundred different preparations, keyed to an instruction pamphlet. William Buchan thought a good home medicine chest should contain the following ingredients:

> Adhesive Plaster, Agaric of Oak, Ash coloured Ground liverwort, Burgundy pitch, Cinnamon water, Crabs claw prepared, Cream of Tartar, Elixir of Vitriol, Flowers of sulphur, Gentian root, Glauber's salts, Gum ammoniac, Gum arabic, Gum asafoetida, Gum Camphor, Ipecacuanha, Jalap, Jesuit's Bark, Liquid laudanum, Liquorice root, Magnesia alba, Manna, Nitre or Salt peter, Oil of almonds, Olive oil, Pennyroyal water, Peppermint water, Rhubarb, Sal amoniac, Sal prunell, Seneka root, Senna, Snake root, Spirits of hartshorn, Spirits of wine, Sweet spirits of nitrate, Sweet spirits of vitriol, Syrup of lemons, Syrup of oranges, Syrup of poppies, Tamarind, Turner's cerate, Vinegar of squills, Wax plaster, White ointment, Wild Valerian root, and Yellow basilicum ointment.[89]

Stocks of such medicaments became an important part of people's domestic necessities. 'Rode thro' Stowey, got some Physick for the great horse and some camomile flowers for myself as I have been troubled with bile more than usual of late', wrote Parson William Holland.[90] The Countess of Kildare began a letter to her husband on 10 May 1759 with news about her own health ('I am rather better today'), and with a loaded question about her husband's condition (what did the doctor think? – 'I am sure he don't approve of the vomits', which were presumably self-inflicted). She concluded by reminding him that he was to obtain some medicines for her: 'of all my commissions, don't forget Ward's drop, for I have finished my bottle'. Ward's Pill and Drop was one of the most popular nostrums, widely taken for stomach complaints.[91]

Commercial nostrums gained ground amongst self-medicators. They had a twofold appeal. One was to the imagination, to day-dreams about health, longevity, fitness and beauty. Many preparations, such as Solomon's 'Balm of Gilead', promised the impossible – to restore youth, ensure fertility, recover potency.[92] Resort to such nostrums left little mark in letters and diaries, presumably because people were ashamed to admit to their vanity or gullibility. Yet 'wonder drugs' of this kind, pandering to dreams, clearly sold well.

Second, shop-counter preparations rose in appeal because their effects could be particularly dramatic. Many nostrums, for example, contained potent mixtures of alcohol and opiates which would dull pain, reduce fever, soothe stomachs, quell diarrhoea, produce relaxation and induce sleep.[93] Opium found ardent advocates, none more so than the eccentric lay writer, Philip Thicknesse, who extolled it as little less than the elixir of life. The drug was not, he reassured friends and readers, seriously habit-forming; more than once, he had weaned himself off it. Thicknesse recommended twenty drops of laudanum a day to those wanting their 'days to be lengthened'.[94]

Other relative newcomers to the medicine chest were bark (quinine), dramatically successful as a specific against ague (malaria), and ipecacuanha, which featured in many popular emetics, above all, Dover's Powders.[95] But the most widely used patent medicine was Dr James's Powders, a powerful febrifuge, built upon an antimony base.[96] Some treated it as a cure-all, to be tried in any serious bout. 'James' Powder is my panacea', Horace Walpole confided to Sir Thomas Mann in 1764, 'I have such faith in these powders that I believe I should take them if the house were on fire.'[97]

During the eighteenth century, for the first time ever, anyone with a couple of pounds to spare could arm himself with a battery of standardized, brand-name, prominently advertised nostrums, readily available through thousands of retail outlets. John Newbery, who doubled in the mid-eighteenth century as newspaper proprietor and medical entrepreneur, ran a 'medicinal warehouse' which tempted self-dosers with such delights as:[98]

Dr James's Powder	Arquebusade Water
Dr Steer's Oil for Convulsions	Hungary Balsam
Dr Hooper's Female Pills	Rowley's Herb Snuff
Glass's Magnesia	English Coffee
Henry's Calcined Magnesia	Cephalic Snuff
Mrs Norton's Mordant Drops	Kennedy's Corn Plaister
Beaume de Vie	Issue Plaister
Greenough's Lozenges	Hemmet's Dentifrice
Stomachic Lozenges	Hemmet's Essence
Grant's Drops	Greenough's Tincture
Hill's Balsam of Honey	Ormskirk Medicine
English's Scots Pills	Dr Bateman's Drops
Dicey's Scots Pills	Dr Norris's Pills
Cook's Rheumatic Powder	Dalby's Carminative Mixture

Purchasers of a handful of these would have the means (so the flyers claimed) to reduce fevers, numb rheumatic pains, settle stomachs, cure hangovers, clear up skin complaints, deal with menstrual problems (or, for those choosing to read between the lines, procure abortions), and many other wonders, not to mention the potential to make himself extremely ill! Such proprietary medicines did not simply appeal to the naïve and the credulous. The elite dabbled as well. The poet, William Cowper, reported that Mrs Unwin, with whom he lodged, believed 'Opodeldoc' – a proprietary camphorated ointment – worked wonders

for her 'nervous rheumatism': 'she had it rubb'd into her back at bed-
time, and it seems to have been of prodigious use to her. We can easily,
I believe, get more of it at Northampton. She wishes much for an
aperient electuary, and if Dr. Austen can prescribe one that will be
effectual, will hold it a great additional obligation.'[99]

A market also developed for medical gadgets for use at home. In the
1790s, Cowper was converted by his friend, the poet William Hayley,
to the virtues of an 'electrical machine' borrowed from 'neighbour
Socket'. It was a cylinder for producing sparks; one person turned the
handle, another assistant directed the spark on to the sufferer's tongue
or teeth. Cowper studied its properties in Tiberius Cavallo's monograph
on medical electricity. He admired Hayley's devotion to domestic
medicine, 'which at our great distance from a physician made him
particularly useful'. From time to time Hayley was in the habit of
sending Cowper a 'basket of medicine'.[100]

Another vogue was for cold-bath self-treatment. Francis Place made
a sustained clinical trial when his bronchial problems became oppressive:

> with a fit of heavy coughing and expectorating I went to my bedroom,
> stripped myself naked, stepped into a large hip bath, dipped a large
> spunge into cold water and squeezed it on the top of my head, this I did
> three times dried myself as rapidly as I could dressed and came down
> stairs. There was great reaction I was in a glow all over and somewhat
> relieved. I went up early to bed and again repeated the ablution. Next
> morning after my wife had left the bedroom I repeated the experiment,
> and thus I proceeded during the nine following days when all my bad
> symptoms had departed.[101]

As was common with diarists, Place felt such a strange mixture of
exhilaration and embarrassment at instigating his own medication that
he was obliged to vindicate himself on paper:

> It seemed to me to be a desperate attempt in which I could not expect
> any one to concur, and was ashamed also to let any one know how I
> was proceeding but when I found myself comparatively well I told my
> wife how I had been acting. I then borrowed a shower bath which I used
> three times a day for a week, then night and morning for another week,
> then once a day as soon as I rose in the morning during the whole winter
> and had no return of the complaint.[102]

More dramatic still was the practice of minor domestic surgery. As
mentioned above, people commonly bled themselves. 'Att my awaeking
in much paine in many of my joynts', wrote William Tyldesley, on
14 April 1713, 'I tuck 12 ounces of blood from my right arm, wch
abated ye paine.'[103] Charles Waterton, the early nineteenth-century
Yorkshire naturalist squire, recorded, near the close of his life, that he
had bled himself 136 times.[104] William Cowper recounted, with some

self-satisfaction, how he succeeded in yanking out an aching tooth over the dinner table, without interrupting the meal.[105] The eccentric physician, Messenger Monsey, extracted his own teeth in a more spectacular manner:

> Round the tooth sentenced to be drawn he fastened securely a strong piece of catgut, to the opposite end of which he affixed a bullet. With this bullet and a full measure of powder a pistol was charged. On the trigger being pulled, the operation was performed effectually and speedily. The doctor could only rarely prevail on his friends to permit him to remove their teeth by this original process.[106]

DANGERS

'To talk of making all men physicians, is the extreme of folly', commented William Buchan, himself the staunchest advocat of domestic medicine, so long as it were contained within proper limits.[107] His caution is not surprising, for the records abound with reports of self-medicators dosing themselves into dire straits – one of the most notable instances possibly being Charles Darwin, whose self-instigated use of arsenic for a skin infection may well have precipitated his long-standing stomach disorder.[108] Maria Edgeworth reported in 1813 that a certain Mrs Cholmondeley and her sister Laetitia 'injured their health irreparably by the means they have taken to preserve their complexion and beauty – starving – and *taking medicines* perpetually'.[109]

The dangers of rampant self-medication were much reiterated. Farington wrote of the painter, Daniel Gardner, who died in 1806, that 'he had been much accustomed to *quack Himself* and did not know his disorder'.[110] Lady Sarah Napier commented similarly on her own brother's sickness: 'by Henriette's account it is all owing to his own mismanagement. . . . Only think what he does! He gets wet, he takes laudanum, he takes salts, he takes emetics, all out of his Grace's own head!'[111]

It might be surmised that, as professional medical provision expanded during the eighteenth century, self-medication would have correspondingly diminished, because more people would consult a doctor instead. But the opposite was probably the case. The more sick people came into contact with doctors, the greater their own preoccupation with health, their hunger for medical knowledge, and their consequent tendency to tamper with the powerful drugs increasingly advertised in newspapers and available in shops.

Doctors sometimes read the riot act. 'Contrary to my advice', reported Edward Jenner, 'an old woman rubbed over a scalded head with snuff; next day little Tommy died.'[112] Time and again they wearily recorded how a patient had taken 'remedies of his own prescription', with disastrous results – prior to summoning the doctor.[113] 'Poor Sir Francis Burdett died this morning', wept Lady Holland in 1844, 'a victim to the cold water practice. He was warned by Pennington, his apothecary, not to venture upon it; but too late.'[114]

Not least, habitual self-examination and dosing could lead to hypochondria.[115] As eighteenth-century opinion tended to construe it, hypochondria was health-consciousness taken to the point of tragicomical self-parody, a virtue turned vice. Hypochondria was not the rejection of orthodox physic, but the enthronement of a full-time physician within. 'Formerly, people were not accustomed to think of the physical state of their body, until it began to be afflicted with pain or debility', argued the diet-specialist doctor, Willich, 'in which case, they entrusted it to the practitioner in Physic, as we deliver a time-piece to a watchmaker, who repairs it according to the best of his knowledge, without apprehending, that its owner will be at the trouble of thinking or reasoning upon the method which he judged to be the most proper.'[116] All that had changed, however, and changed utterly for the worse:

> In our times, we frequently undertake the charge of prescribing medicines for ourselves: and the natural consequence is, that we seldom are able to tell, whether we are healthy or diseased; that we cannot conceive him to be perfectly free from the systems of the schools, from self-interest, or professional motives. Thus, by an acquaintance with medical subjects, which of itself is laudable, not only the skill of the physician is frequently thwarted, but the recovery of the patient unhappily retarded, or at least rendered more difficult.[117]

Willich's moralizing pointed to the ironical dynamics of an individualism which was no less ambiguous in health than it was within England's market economy at large. Georgian self-help did not give rise to a primitive, autarkic health economy, in which everyone was king over his own pains, but formed one facet of an integrated economy in which individualism fuelled market demand. (One might almost compare Do-It-Yourself *house*-maintenance nowadays.) In the extreme case, hypochondriacism formed the indispensable middle term, the ideological articulator of the market. If the sick were not their own grave-diggers, they at least turned themselves into patients.

4

Attitudes towards Doctors

'Never for God's sake see a d——d D–ct–r again as long as you live', was the advice given Lord Herbert in 1786, after he had done with the services of 'butcher Pott', the surgeon. To withstand the doctors' onslaughts, he was told, required 'a full quota of patience & no bad constitution'.[1]

We have argued so far that when people fell sick, they initially took responsibility for their own illness. In this, practicality joined with duty. A certain sturdy self-help was expected. He who bothered doctors over every little ailment became ridiculed as a hypochondriac – not least by the doctors profiting hand over fist from him. With many complaints, in any case, the sick thought they knew perfectly well what was wrong and what needed to be done. 'We have been detained here by one of my bilious headaches', wrote Viscount Palmerston from Brussels in 1818: 'brought on by being overheated in travelling & perhaps by partaking too copiously of the good things given us by our royal entertainers. There is a very good English physician here, a Dr Doratt, whom I have fee'd for telling me what I knew before, & for giving me some calomel which I should have taken without his advice.'[2] Yet the fact is that Palmerston actually called the doctor. For even though the sick commonly thought they knew best, they wanted the blessing of the professionals, reassuring them they were doing the right thing. Often, they called the physician precisely because they were in doubt about their complaints. Some distempers failed to respond to self-treatment, and others were so severe as to require expert help. Doctors grumbled about being called in to pick up the pieces after disastrous auto-medication. Moreover, self-help could never replace the skilled surgical hand. However self-reliant the laity appeared, very few entirely avoided doctors' ministrations. Indeed, as argued above, the signs are that the sick were drawing ever more heavily upon their services.

So what did the sick think of their doctors? How did the medical profession stand in the public eye?[3]

DOCTORS DIAGNOSED

'If the world knew the villainy and knavery (beside ignorance) of the physicians and apothecaries, the people would throw stones at 'em as they walked in the streets', was the verdict of Dr Ridgeley (himself a medical doctor) as recorded by John Aubrey.[4] Scepticism – cynicism even – towards doctors was as old as the profession itself. The New Testament told physicians to heal themselves. That was, according to Ben Franklin, the last thing they could do: 'God heals and the Doctors take the Fee', was his verdict.[5] A peck of proverbs warned the public that death and the doctors were as thick as thieves. 'Apollo was held the god of physick and sender of diseases', ventured Swift, 'Both were originally the same trade, and so continue.'[6]

Doctors were even considered as beyond the pale of Christendom. 'Ubi tres medici, ibi duo Athei, hath been an old though a false calumnie', bemoaned Dr John Ward.[7] The gibe continued to stick. As late as the turn of the nineteenth century, Coleridge was affirming to Charles Lloyd: 'A Physician who should be even a Theist, still more a *Christian*, would be a rarity indeed. I do not know *one* – and I know a *great many* Physicians. They are *shallow* Animals: having always employed their minds about Body and Gut, they imagine that in the whole system of things there is nothing but Gut and Body.'[8]

Professions at large came under the lash in Georgian England, being seen, in Shaw's later formula, as conspiracies against the laity. Medicine suffered more than most, for doctors, it was alleged, fleeced the public first and killed them afterwards. 'When a Nation abounds in Physicians', the *Spectator* commented, 'it grows thin of people.'[9] Doctors themselves developed a line in self-abuse, occasionally making merry over their own incompetence, mercenariness and indifference. The mid-eighteenth-century physician, Messenger Monsey, imagined a sick-bed scene:

> Seven wise physicians lately met,
>   To save a wretched sinner;
> Come, Tom, said Jack, pray let's be quick,
>   Or I shall lose my dinner.
> Some roared for rhubarb, jalap some,
>   And some cried out for Dover;
> Let's give him something, each man said –
>   Why e'en let's give him – over.[10]

The ancient accusation that doctors cared not a fig for their patients but only for their fees was frequently levelled. It was put specially succinctly by Bernard Mandeville – another practitioner – in his *Fable of the Bees*:

Physicians valued Fame and Wealth,
Above the drooping Patient's Health,
Or their own Skill: The greatest Part
Study'd, instead of Rules of Art,
Grave pensive looks, and dull Behaviour;
To gain th' Apothecary's Favour,
The Praise of Mid-wives, Priests and all,
That served at Birth, or Funeral;
To bear with th'ever-talking Tribe,
And hear my Lady's Aunt Prescribe;
With formal Smile, and kind How d'ye,
To fawn on all the Family;[11]

Medicine itself was envisaged as both the cause and the symptom of the Fall by William Blake in his 'Island in the Moon'. He imagined 'Old Corruption's' child, a kind of epitome of the human race, growing up:

She soon got pregnant & brought forth
  Scurvy & spott'd fever.
The father grin'd & skipt about,
  And said, 'I'm made for ever

For now I have procur'd these imps
  'I'll try experiments.'
With that he tied poor scurvy down
  & stopt up all its vents.

And when the child began to swell,
  He shouted out aloud,
'I've found the dropsy out, & soon
  Shall do the world more good.'

He took up fever by the neck
  And cut out all its spots,
And thro' the holes which he had made
  He first discovered guts.[12]

Thus in the Blakean vision, disease and the doctors were blood brothers, partners in crime, the marks of fallen man.

It would be foolish to take such jibes and quips *au pied de la lettre*, or to imply they were uniquely Georgian. Yet certain diatribes against doctors were repeated so frequently as to suggest that the disquiet they voiced was heartfelt and not limp cliché. Gravest of all was the charge – often hinted at in cartoons (see plate 1) – that doctors were utterly inept: they did not know what to do. 'While the doctors consult', John Heywood claimed, the patient dies'; or in Pope's couplet: 'Who shall decide when doctors disagree, / And soundest casuists doubt, like you and me?'[13] Some hinted, however, that vacillation might be a mercy, for when doctors did act, it proved lethal. Endless barbs caricatured

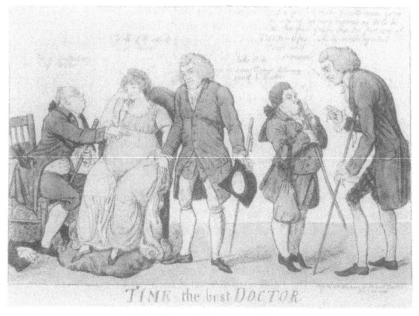

PLATE 1 Patient scepticism

doctors as far more likely to kill than to cure (Byron dubbed them 'assassins').[14] In case of sickness, the anatomist Frank Nichols was asked, should one consult a young or an old physician? 'The difference', replied the doctor, is this: 'The former will kill you, the other will let you die.'[15]

Regular doctors warned the public against quacks. But it was a common *tu quoque!* that the profession itself was the fringe's mirror image. Doctors seized every opportunity for commercial exploitation. Patients resented what they saw as verbal sleight of hand. 'My complaints', complained Colonel Ellison in 1744, 'are what the Modern Physicians term nervous, a cant word the Gentlemen of the Faculty are pleased to make use of when a distemper proves obstinate and does not yield to their medicines.'[16] Even members of the profession sometimes confessed to dressing up the naked truth in obscure 'cramp terms' which had the effect, if not the intention, of leaving the public befogged. 'It would . . . be no difficult matter to prove', contended William Buchan, 'that every thing valuable in the practical part of Medicine is within the reach of common sense, and that the Art would lose nothing by being stripped of all that any person endued with ordinary abilities cannot comprehend.'[17] (Except, critics carped, the art would then lose its whopping profits.) Indeed, many saw doctors as men on the make, a professional ramp, conspiring, as John Wesley suggested, to exploit people at the very moment when they were most vulnerable.[18] Matthew

Prior summed it all up: 'You tell your doctor, that y'are ill / And what does he, but write a bill.'[19] In his engraving, 'The Company of Undertakers', Hogarth juxtaposed leading faculty physicians against the most notorious contemporary quacks of London – 'Spot' Ward, Sally Mapp, John ('Chevalier') Taylor – and many turned this vision of the two as terrible twins into words. 'They rail mightily in their writings against the ignorance of quacks and mountebanks', sneered the journalist, Ned Ward, *à propos* of the Royal College of Physicians, 'yet for the sake of lucre they license all the cozening pretenders about town.'[20]

Patients were always complaining about doctors' exorbitancies. 'After being four weeks in the very essence of misery with being stewed in hot water, physicked, leeched and butchered', grumbled Colonel Hawker, 'I this day went with Macilwain to consult this most extraordinary old bear that ever appeared in a civilised country, the celebrated Dr. Abernethy.'[21] Abernethy, possibly the most famous surgeon in London, was notorious for his curtness. Fanny Burney encountered another Hawker-like grumbletonian, who apparently retailed this bit of conversation some three or four times a day, rather as one might take medicine:

> 'Some years ago', he says, 'let's see, how many? in the year luck, I was persuaded to ask advice of one of these Dr. Gallipots: – oh, how I hate them all! Sir, they are the vilest pick-pockets – know nothing in the world! poor ignorant mortals! and then they pretend – In short, sir, I hate them all; I have suffered so much by them, sir – lost four years of the happiness of my life – let's see, '71, '72, '73, '74 – ay, four years, sir! – mistook my case! – and all that kind of thing. Why, sir, my feet swelled as big as two horses' heads! I vow I will never consult one of these Dr. Gallipot fellows again! lost, me sir four years of the happiness of my life! – why I grew quite an object! – you would hardly have known me! – lost all the calves of my legs! – had not an ounce of flesh left! – and as to the rouge – why, my face was the colour of that candle! – those —— Gallipot fellows! – why they robbed me of four years – let me see, ay, '71, '72 – [and so forth]'.[22]

The point of the yarn, Burney thought, was to exploit every 'opportunity of inveighing against the whole faculty'.

Yet all this bile needs to be taken with a grain of salt. It was an understandable response to inevitable tensions between customers and clients. Distrust and suspicion against doctors were bound to boil up in a culture in which more people were putting themselves more frequently into the power of doctors – indeed, of professionals in general. They *saw* doctors getting richer and more prestigious, thanks to their own custom. Georgian doctors were never shy in displaying their worldly success, without the decorous fig-leaf of genteel respectability assumed by Victorian professionals. What clients could not see for certain was whether they were any healthier as a result. If promise so far exceeded performance, how could they be sure they were not being imposed upon?[23]

The Georgian public thus vested no automatic trust in the powers, or even the good faith, of the medical profession as a corporate body blessed with scientific expertise. If doctors were to be respected, they had to earn that respect as individuals. To get to the heart of the matter, it is necessary to examine estimations of individual practitioners. As one would expect, these were rarely cut and dried. People liked some doctors and not others, depending upon demeanour, character and the power to please.

DISTRUST OF DOCTORS

Some Georgians were allergic to doctors. 'The sight only of her Physician disorders her extremely & throws her into convulsions', wrote Mary Heber about her friend, Miss Fanshawe.[24] The poet, Thomas Gray, was hostile almost to the point of implacability. Commiserating with his friend, Mason, about the health of his consumptive wife, Gray railed on as usual: 'I will not trouble you to enquire into the opinions of her Physicians: as you are silent on that head, I doubt you are grown weary of the inutility of their applications.'[25] Gray recommended instead that the Masons should take treatment into their own hands by travelling to the south coast for the better air.

Some claimed to know better than the doctors. Whereas Lady Mary Coke recorded, *à propos* of a sick friend, "twould be ridiculous for me to set up my opinion against so many of the faculty',[26] many were prepared to do just that. Farington recorded the sad story of the decline and fall of Lord Macartney, who 'was subject to a *periodical strangury*', as well as suffering from gout and a general failure of spirits: 'He had much thirst which was believed to be owing to something formed in the stomach. To alleviate his thirst & from an opinion of its quality He drank largely of *Lemonade*, acting in opposition to the advice of Sir Walter Farquhar who recommended to Him to live more generously. But He had little confidence in medicine or medical advice.'[27] Alas, poor Macartney! 'He gradually sunk into such weakness as to have fainting fits till He expired.'

But if some had no confidence whatsoever in the doctors, others criticized them on particular points. Many found the upper echelons of the London physicians too busy, too superior to take enough trouble over individual cases. Lord Pembroke's daughter, Charlotte, fell ill in 1783, apparently with a consumptive complaint. She was treated by Richard Warren, then perhaps the most glamorous of the younger generation of metropolitan physicians. He first tried routine treatments, until Pembroke chid him that he would jog 'her on to the grave, without thinking any more of her'. Pembroke was disgusted: 'the indifference of London Physicians, when once a patient is out of their sight, is terrible & dishonest.'[28] Charlotte was then transferred to Sir Lucas Pepys, in whom Pembroke felt greater confidence. 'I had much conversation with Pepys yesterday', he wrote: '& he openly & fairly said that what had been done, & was doing with Charlotte, could only *palliate* & never *cure*. Moreover he was clear in recommending what happens to be exactly what Glass & Hunter [other eminent practitioners] said at first. He will write to Warren, & he has, he says, no doubt but that he shall be able to give him such reasons as will convince & make him acquiesce.'[29] A week later, Pembroke was pleased to report that 'the method of treating her has been changed, & that recommended by Glass and Hunter adopted exactly by the advice of Dr Pepys, to which Warren has at last agreed.' Thus patients had a potential for playing off one doctor against another in the shaping of therapies.

Sometimes patients found their doctors both inhumane and inept. In 1775 David Hume fell into a rapid decline and required protracted contact with the medicos. Physicians' obscurantism, and their inveterate differences of opinion – those time-honoured subjects – filled his genial chatter. 'You have frequently heard me complain of my physical Friends that they allowed me to die in the midst of them without so much as giving a Greek Name to my Disorder', he bantered to his friend, the Revd Hugh Blair: 'a Consolation which was the least I had reason to expect from them. Dr Black, hearing this Complaint, told me, that I shou'd be satisfy'd in that particular, and that my Disorder was a Haemorrhage, a word which it was easy to decompose into αιμοσ and ρηγνυμι. But Sir John Pringle says, that I have no Haemorrhage; but a Spincture in the Colon, which it will be easy to cure.'[30] For that relief, much thanks, was Hume's response: 'This Disorder, as it both contained two Greek Appellations and was remediable, I was much inclined to prefer.'[31] But his delight in his disease was shortlived: 'when behold! Dr Gusthart tells me that he sees no Symptoms of the former Disorder, and as to the latter, he never met with it and scarcely ever heard of it. He assures me, that my Case is the most common of all Bath Cases, to wit, a bilious Complaint, which the Waters scarcely ever fail of curing; and he never had a Patient of whose Recovery he had better hopes.'[32]

Pace Gusthart, and in defiance of all their diagnoses, Hume proved to have just two months to live. His account of subsequent treatment by his physicians for the terminal cancer which they had failed to diagnose makes pitiful reading. He tried the waters at Bath, which 'did not agree with me'. Nevertheless, 'Since that time, I have been prevailed on by Importunity and Teazing, contrary to my Reason, and very much contrary to my Inclination, to delay my Departure some time.'[33] This was because the optimistic Dr Gusthart, perhaps disingenuously, wanted a second chance:

It seems Dr Gusthart, whom I consult here, had suspected from the first
that all my Disorder proceeded from a Vice in my Liver; but not caring
directly to oppose Sir John Pringle, he said nothing of the Matter, to me
at least. But John Hunter . . . coming accidently to Town, and expressing
a very friendly Concern about me, Dr Gusthart proposed that I shoud
be inspected by him: He felt very sensibly, as he said, a Tumor or
Swelling in my Liver.[34]

Hume was true to his philosophical stance as an anti-rationalist empiricist,
and placed his trust in Hunter's fingers: 'this Fact, not drawn by
Reasoning, but obvious to the Senses, and perceived by the greatest
Anatomist in Europe [that is, Hunter], must be admitted as unquestion-
able, and will alone account for my Situation.'[35] As if Hume had not
suffered enough from overweening physicians, there was worse to come.
'They kept, very foolishly, this Opinion of Mr Hunter's a secret from
me till Yesterday': what an insult to a philosopher! Worse still, they
still seemed to the sufferer to be advancing a fatuous prognosis: 'and
now they pretend, that the Tumor, being small, may be discussed [*sic*]
by Medicines and Regimen: A very silly Expectation, that an inveterate
Disease of long Standing and in a vital Part, will yield to their feeble
Remedies, in a man of my Years.'[36] *Le bon David*, however, showed
his habitual good grace: 'To avoid, however, the Reproach of Obstinacy,
I delayed my Journey.'

Hume was terminally ill, and he knew it. The doctors exasperated
him, but could do no measurable damage. But the public feared that
the ineptitude of the doctors would often destroy health or even life.
'Sir George [Beaumont] called on the Duchess of Gordon yesterday',
recorded Joseph Farington: 'She has humour & entertainment like that
of Foote the Comedian. – "Our Physician, said she, has lately been
confined by indisposition, & sent to know how we did. I returned him
an answer that since He was ill, our family had been very well".'[37]

The public was thus alert to the power doctors had, through surgical
interventions and potent drugs, to endanger, rather than enhance health.
It was widely complained that doctors were too lavish with their
medications. 'Papa's health is quite ruined with the *millions* of medicines
he has always taken', complained Elizabeth Wynne in 1798.[38] 'Why
take the bark, pray, my dear Lord?', Lord Pembroke chid Lord
Carmarthen in 1781: 'Ne vous droguez pas, I beg; & remember that
your last illness was meerly ideal [that is, imaginary], & that physick
will create a real one. You will be swamped if you take in so much
medicine.'[39]

But attitudes towards pharmaceutical interventions were complex and
often confused. For the sick equally distrusted what Samuel Johnson
derided as 'popgun batteries' (weak medicines taken in small doses): a

waste both of time and money. Johnson, likewise, had no high opinion of 'alterative medicines', that is, those administered supposedly to strengthen the system without producing any tangible effects at all: he suspected that these were just a swindle.[40] Patients preferred to feel that medicines were working. But one could easily be physicked too far, even to death. Boswell was on a course of medicine prescribed for gonorrhoea: 'This afternoon, by taking too much physic, I felt myself very ill. I was weak. I shivered, and I had flushes of heat. I began to be apprehensive that I was taking a nervous fever . . . I was quite sunk. I looked with a degree of horror upon death.'[41] Illness had moral meanings, and the moral was not lost on the lecher in him, at least for the moment: 'Some of my intrigues which in high health and spirits I valued myself upon now seemed to be deviations from the sacred road of virtue.'[42]

Physicians such as Erasmus Darwin rationalized their *blitzkrieg* preference for heavy medication. But the sick commonly believed they were being recklessly overdosed solely to inflate physicians' fees and apothecaries' profits. Some suggested that physicians had cynically entered into conspiracies with apothecaries to fleece the public. Dudley Ryder was, he believed, apprised of such tricks at first hand, for his cousin, Watkins the apothecary, was just such a double-dealing drug-seller. Standing around in Watkins's shop one day, Ryder heard it all: 'Mr. Budget came in who talked with my cousin about the course of physic he put him in and how much harm he had done him, and rallied him upon his pressing physic upon him.'[43] Ryder blamed his unscrupulous relative: 'indeed this seems to be very much his fault', for it was his practice to 'overload his patients with medicines, and besides, the doctors themselves are privy to it and act in concert with them.' This was a common accusation. Country surgeon-apothecaries, who both prescribed and dispensed, had even more incentives for overdosing.

Sydney Smith expressed doubt about the outcome of all this physicking: '"If I take this dose of calomel, shall I be well immediately?", the patient would ask. "Certainly not", replies the physician. "You have been in bed these six weeks; how can you expect such a sudden cure? But I can tell you you will never be well without it, and that it will tend materially to the establishment of your health."'[44]

Overdosing was thus a worry. So was the doctors' apparent penchant for stringent therapeutics, 'heroic' almost to the point of punitiveness. The rationale offered for violent medication was that desperate diseases typically required desperate remedies. Fevers were signs of lethal toxins and inflammation. The overheating system required extreme counter-active depletion, above all energetic blood-letting and purging. Eager or resigned, many sick people accepted these rationales. But others resisted, perturbed that the further weakening induced by the doctors would administer the *coup de grâce* to patients already debilitated by disease.

Boswell was no stranger to the clap. He tried both the regular cures and quack treatments. The former typically involved a 'lowering' course, which he feared would inflict permanent damage upon his system – a case of the cure being worse than the disease. 'Venereal disorders', he surmised, 'do not hurt the constitution. Only severe cures do.' Yet he was not inflexible. At other times he judged that an 'imperfect cure' by a quack would be worse than useless, because it would merely mean 'having the distemper thrown into my blood'.[45]

Thus people were suspicious of the favourite therapeutics of 'depletion', or, as Horace Walpole put it, 'the nonsensical notion of weakening', which sought to 'hoodwink common sense'.[46] Precisely here lay the thrust of Arthur Young's complaint against the profession when his daughter, Bobbin, was failing with consumption. Her physician, John Turton, 'purged and physicked her until she was little more than skin and bone'. The dying Bobbin's letters to her father, complaining of the endless medicines being poured down her throat, make pathetic reading: 'My dear Papa, – I received your letter yesterday. Thank you for your advice; I had taken the *steel* and *draughts* long before I received it, besides which I take some more stuff . . . and ask him likewise how long the steel, etc. must be taken before you feel any effect from it, for one might take physic for ever without receiving any benefit.'[47] The underlying philosophy with Bobbin's consumption was to lower and cool the system to the point where the fever would be overcome – one rationale for later open-air tuberculosis treatment in the sanatorium.[48] But patients often rebelled against being weakened still further in their weakness. Doctors seemed too hasty with dire remedies. In 1777, Mary Curzon was laid up with a 'dreadfull Cough', for which she was treated by the ebullient Erasmus Darwin, notorious for laying on medicines with a trowel: 'I have got a great Burgundy pitch plaister upon my back; I have a hundred things to take &, if they don't do, I am to be bled & blister'd. Only think what a deal one has to go through,'[49] she reflected stoically. Was it not all unnecessary and counter-productive? – 'I flatter myself my cough will get better without those severe remedies.'

Yet doctors would hardly have been able to sustain the philosophy of hefty and heroic remedies unless enough customers were convinced, or at least open to persuasion, that herein lay the best way. Some patients were just bluffly dismissive. The Revd Edmund Pyle poohpoohed the 'senseless notion' that people were too delicate to survive 'two or three doses of doctor's stuff'. Were it really harmful, the body would expel it smartly enough. His own constitution was 'apt to throw out whatever it dislikes, very vigorously'.[50]

In the public mind, overdosing went with overcharging, a gnawing bone of contention during the Georgian age. Falling sick in Exeter, Farington was treated by Dr Daniell. The regular Exeter fee was apparently one guinea for two visits. Daniell evidently wanted to turn this relatively trivial complaint into a money-spinner: 'While we were talking Dr. Daniell came & saw me, what I professed to be, well in every respect, but a little relaxed from the operation I had undergone. He recommended to me to keep in the house, & on going away sd. He wd. *call again in the even'g.*'[51] Farington thought this too much, and so sent him a note cancelling the arrangement, thereby preventing 'his further visits for *fees*, which I was soon after informed He perseveres in obtaining to the utmost extent of the opportunity afforded him.'

Patients resented 'exorbitant' bills. Parson William Holland growled against Forbes, his local surgeon-apothecary: 'Paid Myster Forbes Bill which he made as much as he could for he is a terrible man for a Bill'.[52] Berating Forbes got to be a habit with Holland. 'Mr Forbe's Physick has not, I thank God, made me worse', he sighed with relief in 1809, pleasantly surprised after the surgeon had grudgingly agreed to see him late the previous evening, though Forbes had, as usual, 'muddled and hummd and hawd'. A few days later, being no better, 'I called on Mr Anstiss and he says I have the Rheumatism and that he will send me some Guaicum Pills.' It proved a busy and doubtless costly day of physicking for Holland, for his 'wife has seen Dr Dunning about her leg'. There was no satisfaction there either, for 'nothing more can be done. She takes Bark and he has prescribed Brimstone twice a day.'[53]

Surviving doctors' ledgers suggest that country practitioners such as Forbes did not, in fact, overcharge for each individual item or visit. People found doctors' bills steep because they were consulting them more frequently, often over complaints – as perhaps Holland's 'rheumatism' – that once would have been thought either trivial or simply beyond the powers of medicine. It was only the London practitioners who charged astronomical fees (even early in the eighteenth century, William Cheselden was allegedly getting £500 for performing a lithotomy).[54] Patients had to weigh up the relative advantages of London and country practice. In 1721 Lady Fermanagh congratulated herself that, by using country doctors, she was in pocket: 'The doctor said he woud give me no more physick, so I have dispatcht him, he had seven ginnes of me and I gave his man a crown, and I have paid Mr. Turner's bill for all the things that I and the children had so I thank God I've got all of under 10 pd.'[55] Ten pounds, even so, was a lot of money. Nevertheless, she concluded triumphantly: 'I daresay if I had gon to London it would have cost me fivety.'

TRUSTING DOCTORS

One could build a mountainous indictment out of the suspicions expressed by the sick against the medical profession in general, and their own practitioners in particular. It is no surprise such anxieties existed: within *ancien régime* medicine, the doctor was inevitably tarred with failure and identified as the accomplice of disease and death. Yet it would be a mistake to set this mountain in the foreground. For what is more striking is the abundance of highly positive attitudes developing towards doctors: 'I'll do what Mead and Cheselden advise / To keep these limbs, and to preserve these eyes':[56] Pope could thus respect his physicians as well as mocking them; and he could pen his couplet, assured that readers would know the names of the top physician and surgeon of the times and share his generous tribute to their qualities.[57] Indeed, as Joan Lane has demonstrated, the correspondence of the Georgian age rings with recommendations of practitioners for their skill and sympathy.[58]

Especially conspicuous is a collective eagerness to extol the virtues of a roll-call of the elite figures of the profession. From Sir Hans Sloane and Richard Mead, through John Fothergill, John Coakley Lettsom and the Hunter brothers, to such figures, in Regency days, as Matthew Baillie and Astley Cooper, a corps of doctors emerged as luminous public celebrities. These names, and perhaps a couple of dozen others, crop up time and again in letters and journals, in journalism high and low, serious and satirical, in anecdotes, literary allusions and so forth. They became the 'stars' of medicine; their company was sought and their deeds became news. Linking one's name with theirs, as patient or patron, assumed a certain quality of glamour. Richard Cumberland wrote a paean in praise of Dr Robert James, the patentee of the best-selling fever powders, in gratitude for the recovery of his son from a dangerous fever.[59] William Cowper, one of Heberden's patients, celebrated him in verse: 'Virtuous and faithful HEBERDEN! whose skill / Attempts no task it cannot well fulfill, / Gives melancholy up to nature's care, / And sends the patient into purer air.'[60] Fashionable and literary London clamoured for Heberden's services. Why? As Cowper implied, it was not because he possessed wonder drugs or the magic touch, but because he was recognized as an expert bedside doctor, whose clinical judgement was as reliable as his integrity was unimpeachable. Patients trusted him: that was of paramount importance.

One of the reasons why Boswell moved to London in the 1780s lay in the hope of finding a cure for his wife, Margaret, wasting with consumption. Boswell sought a physician in whom both he and his wife felt confidence. Initially they looked to the ultra-fashionable Sir Richard Warren; but they concluded he was a 'coxcomb', and availed themselves instead of the services of the stalwart Sir George Baker, whom Margaret admired.[61]

Then as now, ancestral stereotypes flourished about the ineptitude of old-style physicians and the blood-thirstiness of the traditional surgeon. But these are outweighed and belied by what may seem surprisingly frequent testimonials to medical skill. The otherwise unknown W. Hayward Winstone, Esq., inserted in the *Gentleman's Magazine* a set of 'Lines addressed to Dr Fraser at Bath . . . on his Recovery from a Dangerous Illness':

> Next to the Almighty's gracious will,
>   Which guides each sick-bed hour,
> I owe my life to human skill,
>   And Fraser's matchless power.
> The Fever siez'd my shatter'd frame,
>   Each limb refus'd my will;
> But Fraser came, saw, overcame
>   Each complicated ill.
> Disease, as he advanc'd, retir'd
>   Within a narrower sphere,
> The pain's remov'd, as if inspir'd
>   With more than common fear.
> Oh may Hygeia e'er attend
>   Around thy genial bed,
> And all the blessings fate can send,
>   On all thy household shed.
> That thus, defended from distress
>   Of body, as of mind,
> You still may rear while still you bless,
>   And renovate Mankind![62]

The implicit assumption is that publication of such verses reflects credit simultaneously upon the mighty practitioner and upon the grateful and gracious patient-poet blessed with judgement to discern the expert doctor. Praise of individual doctors raised esteem for the profession as a whole.

It is not easy to gauge the typical practitioner of Stuart England: common practitioners are a fairly anonymous bunch. But abundant evidence suggests that a century later, the emergent provincial general practitioner was becoming, and was perceived as becoming, more polite, poised and possessed of social accomplishments. He was good company and a valued member of the community. 'I was called down to Dr. Kerr who came to pay me a voluntary visit', wrote William Cowper in 1786, 'were I sick, his cheerful, friendly manner would almost restore me' (note how the local doctor has become an integral link in the social chain).[63] Parson Woodforde felt much the same about Mr Thorne.

Respect for doctors was advantageous in many ways. 'To have a good opinion of the Physitian', it was thought, 'doth contribute much to the cure.'[64] Late eighteenth-century discussions of the duties and role of the doctor pay notably more attention to medical 'etiquette' than to 'ethics', and set a premium upon mutually gentlemanly intercourse between doctor and patient.[65]

Time out of mind, damning the doctors had come easily. The eighteenth century enlarged these opportunities. The emergent specialities of madhouse keeper and man-midwife, for example, appeared to many disgusting and demeaning, through their association with 'dirty' objects such as lunacy and parturition, and their obvious potential for abuse and exploitation.[66] Yet alongside such ridicule, we may discern a growing public respect and sympathy. Early in the nineteenth century, Princess Charlotte died after an especially protracted labour. A whispering campaign followed against her obstetrician, Sir Richard Croft. Riddled with guilt, Croft finally shot himself. The affair produced vibrations in rural Hertfordshire. 'All the sympathies of the human heart were, indeed, called into activity by Sir Richard Croft's having destroyed himself', commented the Revd William Jones: 'Poor man! he seems to have fallen a sacrifice to popular prejudice, which, to the last, occasioned his being pestered with anonymous & abusive letters, & to the acuteness of his own feelings, which, it is said, were always "tremblingly alive" at the appearance of danger.'[67] The reaction of Jones's wife is instructive. She did not berate the use of a male rather than a female midwife or aver that men had no business to be interfering in such female preserves. Quite the contrary: 'When my dear wife heard of the sad influence of the anonymous letters on Dr. Croft's mind, she wished all such scribbling vermin to be *soused* in the New River. I thought her very moderate, & wondered that she had not wished them to have a *scorching* in Hell; for their malignant spirits & tongues seem ready "to set on fire the course of nature, & are set on fire of Hell;" (James 3.6) – & their pens seem to be dipped in the blackest gall.'[68] Thus Croft had his critics and calumniators; but he also drew a sympathetic response.

SURGEONS AND APOTHECARIES

A gravestone epitaph crystallizes satire against the surgeons:

> Long was my pain, great was my grief
> Surgeons I'd many, but no relief;
> I trust in Christ to rise with the just
> My leg and thigh was buried fust.[69]

Surgery lent itself to horror stories. As with tightrope-walkers, their failures made a splash. The Georgian age produced its crop of surgical disasters. Lady Mary Coke noted that the Princess Amelia, George II's daughter, was 'not well'. Why? Finding herself under the weather, she had thought it 'proper to be blooded'. Hence 'She sent for a surgeon

Mrs Middleton, H.R.H. bedchamber woman, had recommended. The Man tyed up her Arm, attempted to bleed her, but fail'd.'[70] The response was witheringly *de haut en bas*:

> The Princess said to him. 'I believe you had better go down stairs & drink a glass of wine', but he declined the offer & begged She wou'd allow him to try again, to which the Princess consented, but desired he wou'd take care to do it effectually: fright however, or awkwardness, occasion'd his missing the second time, yet the Princess had the resolution to say to him he shou'd try once more; & upon failing the third time, She said, 'Now, my friend, you shall go home'.[71]

It is not surprising, then, that many people, happy enough to swallow physic and follow regimen, quailed before the 'terrors of the surgeon's knife' and feared the cut direct.[72] 'I am no friend to Surgeons', Thomas Gray confided to Mary Antrobus. But even Gray was measured in his suspicions, and believed the surgeon's skills were sometimes required. Considering the case of Mrs Antrobus's daughter, Dolly, he advised her that the knife might indeed be needed; in which case: 'let her not be frighted at the sight of steel, for I can tell her upon some experience, that one half-hour of the pain she undergoes from her illness is much more, than all she will suffer from Mr Thackeray's hand.'[73]

Gray had similar doubts about apothecaries. 'I am extremely sorry to hear of your poor Mr Bentley's illness', he consoled Horace Walpole: 'What I can not account for is, that You or He should trust such a Dog of an Apothecary, after he had shew'd himself, to do any thing, even to sell medicines; when it is just as easy for him to put in a grain of slow poison, as to administer a dose of pure & innocent brown-Paper.'[74] Apothecaries were widely suspected, as all their financial interest lay in maximizing dosing. In his *Valetudinarian's Bath Guide*, Philip Thicknesse averred that 'many patients are killed by ignorant [apothecaries'] apprentices', left in charge of the shop.[75]

PEOPLE AND PROFESSIONALS

Patients recognized that there was a certain professional persona. A doctor might be their physician or their friend, but the two might not sit well together. Boswell discovered this when he consulted his friend, surgeon Andrew Douglas. He clearly hoped that he would be treated in a friendly manner, perhaps at a reduced price, but was soon disabused:

> I opened my sad case to Douglas, who upon examining the parts, declared I had got an evident infection and that the woman who gave it me could not but know of it. I joked with my friend about the expense, asked him if he would take a draught on my arrears, and bid him visit me seldom that I might have the less to pay. To these jokes he seemed to give little heed, but talked seriously in the way of his business. And here let me

make a just and true observation, which is that the same man as a friend and as a surgeon exhibits two very opposite characters. Douglas as a friend is most kind, most anxious.[76]

Many found themselves confronted by able doctors who were not particularly kind. Mrs Thrale notoriously disliked Fothergill, finding him cold and officious. Fanny Burney had precisely the same reaction. 'Dr. Fothergill, the celebrated Quaker, is mama's physician', she wrote when her mother was gravely ill:

> I doubt not his being a man of great skill; but his manners are stiff, set, and unpleasant. His conversation consists of sentences spoken with the utmost solemnity, conciseness, and importance. He is an upright, stern, formal-looking old man. He enters the room, and makes his address with his hat always on, and lest that mark of his sect should pass unnoticed, the hat which he wears, is of the most enormous size I ever beheld.[77]

The bustling, prosperous, career-minded practitioner, who became such a familiar type in the eighteenth century, struck many clients as excessively businesslike and successful, and lacking sufficient charity towards the sick. 'We have lost our doctor as you have heard long no doubt . . . He has dyed immensely rich considering his father's estate was not more than one hundred and 50 a year', Mrs Huntback snarled *à propos* of the late Dr Wilkes: 'he is little lamented but for his judgment in physick. He was without all dispute a good physician but no charity.'[78] Greed got him: 'I thought you might like to know some thing of ye maner of his death you knew him so well.' He met an appropriate end: 'It was very suden. He was at Wolverhampton ye day he dyed and took several fees, and ye week before he rode 50 miles; so ye love of mony held him to ye end.'

Indeed, with rising expectations about doctors, their public performances became increasingly the subject of scrutiny. They needed to tread a delicate middle path. They could no longer afford to appear boorish and disputatious, and their squabbles brought them into disrepute. When George III went mad in 1788, all the doctors fell out. Betsy Sheridan reported 'Great Wars and Rumours of War among the medical Tribe'.[79] Politeness was at a premium. Yet they could not afford to adorn themselves with too many airs and graces, too much self-importance. Richard Sheridan encountered one such coxcomb, whose patients: 'found themselves on the first visit (an effect which Doctors often produce) worse than they were before – with this difference only in the Process that instead of hearing his Patient's Case, He related his own.'[80]

Overall, what counted most for patients was character and temperament. They did not expect miracles from their doctors. 'A physician can sometimes parry the scythe of death', opined Mrs Thrale, 'but has no power over the sand in the hourglass.'[81] But they did seek physicians with a sound judgement. And they themselves were prepared to judge such a man. Patients were concerned to keep ultimate control of the relationship, avoiding placing themselves utterly in the physician's hands. William Cobbett was no lover of doctors, but he believed in their usefulness on occasions. He advocated inoculation (in contradistinction to vaccination), but insisted that in his family, 'We always took particular care about the source from which the infectious matter came. We employed medical men, in whom we could place perfect confidence: we had their solemn word for the matter coming from some healthy child.'[82]

'Professionalization' theorists have emphasized the importance of the creation of a collective ideological carapace, so as to set an idealized moral distance between occupations such as medicine and the public: such a 'halo' is allegedly vital for conferring dignity, respect and authority. Models of this kind may be illuminating for the nineteenth and the present centuries. But, as this chapter has abundantly shown, Georgian patients had little conception of the medical profession as a comprehensive entity, as a collective abstraction. It was individual, face-to-face encounters that tipped the balance between distrust and confidence. *Pace* the physician, George Cheyne, Georgian patients did not necessarily treat their doctors as they treated their laundresses; but the personal idiom his image evokes is entirely appropriate.

5

Consultations

Many bouts of illness were handled, from beginning to end, personally by the sick individual or within his affective group of family, friends and neighbours. Sometimes, however, a doctor was summoned, albeit occasionally after a tussle. Writing from Goodwood in 1779, Lady Sarah Lennox commiserated with her sister's report about 'poor Eddy's eyes', before going on to offer a more depressing account of her own 'dear brother's health': 'He has caught colds upon cold, and is by no means well. He has permitted the Duchess at last to send for Doctor Brocklesby, who will be here to-morrow.'[1] Brocklesby was one of the cream of the London physicians: fees of noble proportions could evidently lure him down to rural Sussex to treat aristocratic colds.

Some people called the doctor once in a blue moon. Living in rural Essex in the mid-seventeenth century, Ralph Josselin, vicar of Earl's Colne, hardly ever summoned a regular practitioner over the course of some forty years, even when his children were dying. Was this because there were few close at hand? Or did Josselin have faith enough in his own medical powers, in the healing power of Nature and in the guiding hand of Providence?[2] By the eighteenth century at least, living in the depths of the countryside did not preclude families from professional medical attendance. Parson Woodforde habitually called upon the services of the surgeon-apothecary, Mr Thorne, who became a family friend.[3]

Some patients felt that their lives were being taken over by doctors. 'After a confinement of three Months without seeing any Creatures except Doctors & Apothecaries and a probability of it continueing as much longer', confessed Eliza Pierce, 'I have not Phylosophy enough to keep up my Spirits.'[4]

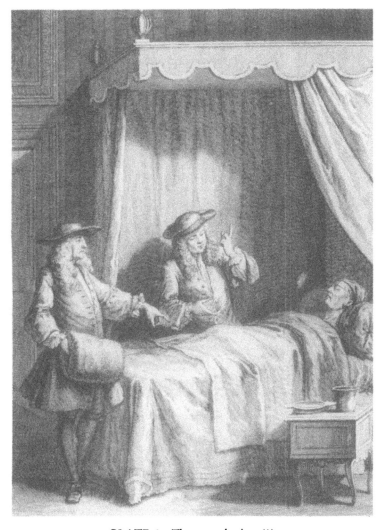

PLATE 2   The consultation (1)

This chapter aims to survey clinical interactions between patients and their doctors. Obviously there were as many different styles of interaction as consultations themselves, for the variables – the state of the disease, the patient's demands, the doctor's disposition – were infinite; some are indicated in plates 2–4.[5] Some patients doubtless terrorized their doctors, rather as Hazlitt could contrariwise speak of himself and his fellow human beings as 'resigned to our fate, like patients to the physician or

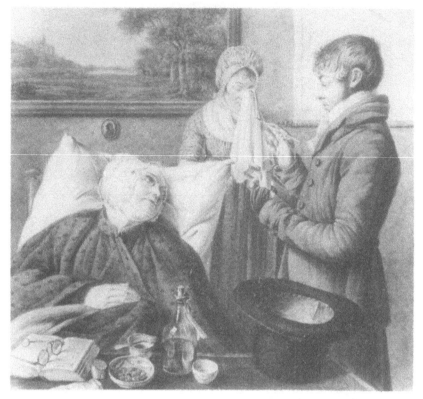

PLATE 3   The consultation (2)

prisoners in the condemned cell'.[6] But there are patterns enough to
permit some tentative reconstruction of the social protocols of face-to-
face practice. The patient possessed urgent needs (to be healed), vital
information (on his condition) and the activator (money). The physician
was in a secondary position; he was to execute procedures initiated by
the patient, yet he alone had the expertise, and thus the authority, to
achieve success.[7]

CALLING THE DOCTOR AND TAKING THE HISTORY

In the Georgian age, the doctor typically visited the affluent patient,
rather than the patient calling upon him. Wealthy clients, enjoying a
well-established relationship with their practitioners, expected house-
calls as of right. On first making contact with a doctor, a sick person
might, however, make the journey himself, being mindful of his pocket
and worried about the cost of a riding call. Charity patients would
queue up outside a doctor's door early in the morning.

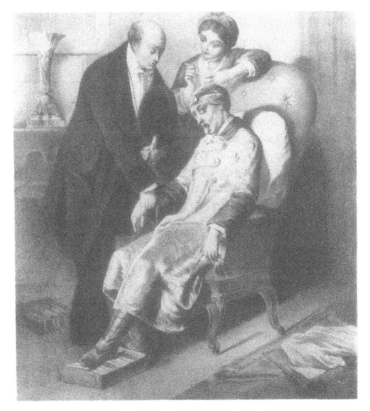

PLATE 4   The consultation (3)

Doctors not infrequently travelled vast distances to see patients. It was expected of them, although they might resent the vast expenditure of time. Having been summoned by the Galtons all the way from Derby to Margate, Erasmus Darwin was given a fee of 100 guineas, but fretted how he thereby ran the risk of losing 'the custom of families' locally.[8] Darwin maintained a practice far-flung all over the Midlands (something made possible by improvements in turnpiking), and was always on the move. Whereas the old-fashioned doctor had been noted for ambling side-saddle on a nag, the smart and successful new physician bustled around in his coach. It was a status-symbol, the very best of advertisements. But it was also what made long hours waiting upon patients bearable. Darwin fitted out his carriage with a larder, a library and a writing-desk; he did his reading, and wrote most of his verse, *en route* for consultations.[9]

Doctors such as Darwin made calls 365 days a year.[10] There were times, however, when some practitioners would not come out. In 1720

Ralph Palmer's wife was taken ill with 'Hysterick Cholick'. At midnight he sent for the fashionable Sir Richard Blackmore, 'but he would not come out of his bed'. Instead, Palmer managed to secure the attendance of his apothecary, of Dr Smart and of Dr Chamberlain. With three for the price of one, Palmer was not outraged at Blackmore's negligence.[11]

Once contact was made between sick person and physician, the first requisite was that the physician should be put into the picture. This was chiefly achieved through the sick person telling the doctor what was wrong: when and how the complaint had started, what antecedent events might have precipitated it, the characteristic pains and symptoms, its periodicity. The patient would also recite, perhaps spontaneously, perhaps on demand, the main features of his life-style: his eating habits, the quality of his sleep, his bowel motions, details of recent emotional traumas and so forth, not to mention the perhaps slightly indelicate matter of his indulgence in home-made, quack or patent medicines.[12]

The practitioner would absorb this history, assessing it in the light of prior experience of the patient. He would also conduct some kind of physical scrutiny. By today's standards, the physician's examination would be slight. It would be conducted primarily by the eye – not by touch – paying attention to skin colour and lesions (for example, the rash or spots of fever), signs of swelling or inflammation and so forth. Doctors would commonly take the pulse, although mainly making a qualitative assessment (was it languid or racing, regular or erratic?) rather than timing its beats. They would, of course, perforce listen to coughs, wheezings and eructations, just as they would sniff the odour of putrefaction.[13]

Thus the physical examination was quite perfunctory, as is suggested by plate 5. For one thing, Georgian medicine had no diagnostic technology to augment the senses. Stethoscopes, ophthalmoscopes and so forth were not introduced until the nineteenth century, and then only after overcoming considerable resistance to new-fangled contraptions from patients and practitioners alike.[14] For another, systematic and disciplined use of the senses, apart from the eye, for diagnostic purposes had not advanced far. As late as 1800, it was exceptional for a doctor to tap the body with his finger (percussion), or listen for tell-tale evidence as to the condition of the internal organs (auscultation).[15]

During the nineteenth century, the physical examination became the *pièce de résistance* of the bedside encounter. Why, then, were earlier physicians apparently so reluctant to get closely to grips with the body? To some degree it was probably a function of professional demarcations: the physician, whose province by definition was internal medicine, wished to differentiate himself from the surgeon, whose terrain comprised

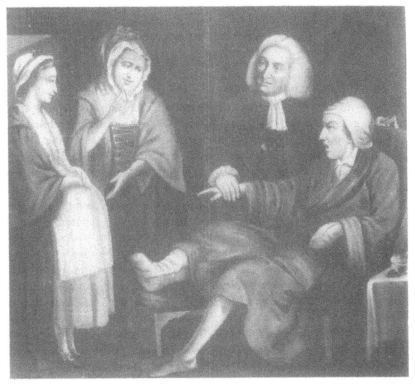

PLATE 5   The examination. The physician is thought to be William Cullen

the externals of the body, and whose skill lay in his fingertips, not in his mind. The physician, by contrast, was a thinker, not a toucher. To some degree, it may register deeply felt notions of decency. There were unspoken taboos as to which parts of the body might be seen or touched by which medical practitioners under which conditions, and the baring of the body to outsiders was not unnecessarily to be multiplied.[16] But it is probably primarily a mark of the confidence felt by the expert clinician in his ability to assess a case from the patient's story and the visible signs; or, put more negatively, an index of how little the Georgian physician believed physical examination would provide an *entrée* into events beneath the skin.

The rudimentary state of intimate physical examination clearly resulted in such misdiagnosis. As we have seen, when David Hume was dying of cancer of the liver, his physicians offered a profusion of quite erroneous diagnoses. It was only when the surgeon, John Hunter, actually felt the tumour that these errors were dispelled.[17]

PRESCRIBING BY POST

One popular form of patient/doctor relations definitionally precluded direct physical examination: the practice of postal treatment. A sick person would write to an eminent physician enclosing his own medical history; the physician's reply would include a diagnosis, directions for a regimen and a prescription to be made up by the local apothecary or druggist, or, if simple, at home. In following this procedure, the patient was expected, as it were, to internalize the doctor. With conscientiousness on both sides, the arrangement could be highly satisfactory.[18]

On 20 February 1726, Hallett Turner wrote from Cambridge to the respected London physician, James Jurin, to seek advice about a 'dizziness in my head which is commonly attended with a pain in my neck & shoulder & back part of my head'. Turner informed Jurin that he had already had the complaint for some six months, 'in which time I have taken a vomit once or twice & frequently ye tinctura sacra, both which I think did me service' (it sounds as though he had been dosing himself). But his friends were not satisfied, thinking his case was 'nervous' (that is, more than merely local), and advising him 'to consult a Physician in time for fear of an ill consequence, a Palsy or Apoplexy &c. But', Turner concluded, with an appropriately deferential bow, 'you will be ye best Judge.'[19] Jurin evidently sent a diagnosis and a prescription. Turner replied on 21 April, indicating that he had taken the medicines, but had not yet applied the recommended blister. 'What also you will think fit to order for me, or what rules to observe in eating or drinking &c I desire you will be pleased to let me know by ye next Post.' Should he, Turner concluded, try the Bath waters?

Jurin's reply is not extant, but a week later Turner wrote yet again. Though he had been continuing with Jurin's medicines, he feared these might prove 'too hot for me', for he was suffering night sweats: Turner evidently thought he was within his rights gently to query the doctor. Further letters followed from Turner over the next months, in particular stating his wish to travel: where would be good for his health? Scarborough? He promised to obey Jurin's instructions, especially in preference to any of the local doctors: 'I am now determed to go out of College this week, to try what change of Air & a long journey will do in my case. I therefore beg y\e favour of a line from you next Post, w\th any directions you think proper. If I take Scarbrough in my way, may I drink y\e waters?'[20] Turner appears to have believed he was consumptive, a condition he gathered was grave. He had clearly consulted numerous Cambridge doctors, but had received contradictory advice:

Since I saw you S^r I have used y^e cold Bath, & y^e medicines you prescribed, & have rode out every day; but I think my illness grows upon me, & I observe my self to waste & fall away flesh very much wch is the thing that discourages me ye most, & makes me think my case dangerous.

You may be sure S^r I have great many Doctors here, some will have me go to Montpelier, & others to Edinborough; the latter place I may perhaps reach within the next month, but shall not think of ye former unless you advise it. You will be so good as to be very particular in y^r directions & I shall punctually observe & follow them. I need not repeat any of my symptoms they continue much ye same . . . I shall only beg leave to ask you whether my blister may not run too much. I have it dressed twice a day & it makes a great discharge.

I must ask pardon for the great trouble I give you, & hope you will give me leave to make some return.[21]

Here the correspondence ends. Turner doubtless disappeared for the vacation. It is clear that postal consultation was not forced upon this patient by lack of access to doctors. Either Turner had a special faith in Jurin, or he rather enjoyed the elbow-room afforded him by keeping a doctor at a distance (while also, it seems, consulting those on his doorstep).

Not surprisingly, when the sick solicited doctors to prescribe by post, their tone was properly humble. But the deference was based upon a confident conviction that they might address the doctor, if not on equal terms, at least as one with a right to an opinion. When Elizabeth Yonge found a walnut-sized tumour in her left cheek, she was sufficiently perturbed to appeal to John Locke for advice, while adding, soothingly, 'I am willing to flatter my self its nothing of that nature [scrofula], our Family having never been subject to it'. She was obviously proud of her own medical understanding, yet in this particular case she was, she told Locke, 'a little causeous how I tamper with it for fear of the worst, therefore beg you to give me your opinion in it at your first leasure, whither a dissolving plaister will be proper, or inward medicins.' Clearly Elizabeth Yonge did not believe her sex debarred her from expressing medical opinions; indeed it was she, not Locke, who recited the alternative therapies.[22]

The flourishing traffic in postal diagnosis simply serves to underline the prime importance of the history and the marginal nature of 'hands-on' examination in Georgian medicine. A certain Mr Webster was 'troubled with Dizzyness in his Head'. His friend, Matthew Dixie, contacted Erasmus Darwin to ascertain what should be done. Darwin did not ask to see his patient, but felt confident enough about what was needed, replying that 'it would be of service to Him to have Issues [that is, artificial scarifications] made on his Back', and various other treatments besides.[23] The Midlands physician often carried out consultation by post, in his later years referring patients to passages in his own books for ampler diagnosis and possible therapies.[24]

What did patients expect from postal consultations?[25] Sometimes it was better medication than that already being used. Thus Mrs Elinor Hawkshaw wrote to John Locke on 10 July 1690, about various matters, including her health: 'My distemper proceeds from the stoon in the Blather yett no violence of fitts. but ill effects as collects and vomittings if you know what will dissolve and doe me good add that Kindness to the rest: and let me heer once more from you.'[26] More often, perhaps, it was a better diagnosis – which might mean a more favourable one, or simply one upon which the sick person felt he could rely. As Samuel Johnson sank with asthma and dropsy in 1784, Boswell, with his consent, sought help by writing to all the top Edinburgh physicians: 'Drs. Cullen, Monro, and Hope for advice upon Dr. Johnson's case. The letter to each was verbatim the same. Dr. Johnson had desired me to talk to our physicians. I thought writing would do better; and this writing I thought a good employment for Sunday.'[27]

As noted above, in postal diagnosis, the physician would give the condition a name, recommend a regimen and supply a prescription. For his pains, he would expect double the normal fee.[28] Physicians were understandably cautious when advancing postal diagnoses; but the fact that they happily acquiesced in this rather lucrative practice – itself the fruit of the swelling reputations of a successful coterie – further indicates the relatively low importance attached to physical examination, by contrast to the patient's story.

NEGOTIATING A DIAGNOSIS

It was probably rare for an educated seventeenth- or eighteenth-century patient simply to go before a doctor, present his symptoms and passively await the diagnosis. All the signs are that patients at least hazarded guesses as to their own diagnoses.[29] Indeed, the many consultations we have recorded of Samuel Johnson's illnesses show that he typically diagnosed himself. The doctor's task would be to *confirm* the diagnosis, and then recommend treatment. In fact, Johnson himself often outlined the treatment which he believed should be initiated. Sometimes he sought authorization from his physician; sometimes he instructed his attendant what to perform. In 1783, he told Mrs Thrale that he had just 'bullied, and bounced . . . and compelled the apothecary to make his salve according to the Edinburgh dispensatory [that is, a leading pharmacological manual] that it might adhere better.'[30]

Patient and doctor often engaged in energetic discussion over the diagnosis. In his *Treatise of the Hypochondriack and Hysterick Diseases*, a fictional dialogue between a doctor and a patient, Mandeville makes his sick character, Misomedon, stipulate that he expected from his physician a 'rational Account' of his condition. He wished not merely to be treated, but to understand the theory underlying his treatment; such was, after all, the privilege of the liberally educated gentleman. The ironist in Mandeville perceived, however, that exercise of this privilege could prove disastrous, because the sick person would thereby fall 'in love with the Reasoning physician', and so become a hypochondriac.[31] Mandeville was surely right to imply that patients played active roles in therapeutic decision-making. When Nicholas Blundell wrote, 'I advised with the Doctor about going to the Spaws', his form of words indicated that he was soliciting advice and not taking orders.[32]

MULTIPLE CONSULTATION

Often a patient would seek a second opinion; either at the outset of an illness, particularly if the diagnosis offered were depressing and the treatment hazardous, or at some later stage, if the illness did not respond to treatment.

A certain Mrs Dare's son had 'long been under Dr German's care for a Rheumatism'. She was not satisfied, and called in Dr Claver Morris, the Wells physician. Morris had certain qualms about what may have seemed an attempt to play off one physician against another: 'I persuaded her not to leave his old Physician who was near him: But she would not be satisfied.' She got her way. Seeing nothing professionally improper in her request, Morris did see the patient, subsequently instructing his fellow practitioner what to do: 'I verbally directed the Dr to give him first the Vitriolick Vomit; Then Antimonial Medicines, Purging him frequently & gently with Alford Water; And afterwards to entertain and strengthen him with Calybate.'[33] That was certainly an energetic treatment.

On occasions, whole tribes of doctors were called in, thereby giving the customer elbow-room to accept whatever diagnostic suggestions most gratified the ears. Fearing her son, Stephen, had St Vitus's dance, Caroline Fox smothered him with physicians: 'Wilmot, Duncan, Truesdale, Ranby and a Doctor Reeves out of the city attend him; he is now taking tin, as yet nothing seems to have any effect. We called in this city doctor as one who attends the hospitals, and sees numbers of these disorders. All say he will do well, except Truesdale, who says nothing and I fear thinks ill of it.'[34] 'He has not', she added, to quell her anxieties, 'great experience in this disorder.' Nor were these five doctors enough! 'To-morrow we are to see Doctor Barry, one of your famous Irish physicians; he is in vast repute here. Indeed my dear sister, I wonder I keep up my spirits so well as I do, but my trust in Providence is great.'[35] Out of all these, Caroline Fox preferred Duncan because he gave fewest medicines.

Multiple consultations were perfectly normal. David Garrick, recovering from a malignant fever, recorded in a letter from Paris in 1765 that he 'had no less than Eight Physicians' – slily adding, 'yet I am alive and in Spirits, tho' somewhat ye Worse for Wear and Tear'.[36] In his latter years, Samuel Johnson drew upon the services of a cabinet of physicians – Heberden, Brocklesby, Lawrence and others. Some gave the great man their services gratis; none took offence.[37] Multiple consultation might even go on by post. 'My sister in law', Andrew Fletcher told John Locke, 'did luckely incline rather to follow your advice than that of two other phisitians that wer sent her at the same time.'[38] It was thus a practice that all parties accepted, when conducted upon rules that did not impugn professional dignity.

How could this be achieved? In his *Medical Ethics* (1803), Thomas Percival set out guidelines for multiple consultation.[39] He assumed there was no stopping the paying patient consulting whoever he liked. It would be improper, however, for the sick person to play 'divide and rule' with his physicians, no less than it would be improper for practitioners to poach patients, or to vilify their brethren. When several physicians were actually assembled around a bedside, they should keep disagreements out of the patient's earshot, and offer their opinions in rising order of seniority – a device to prevent the eldest physician from losing face.[40]

All assumed that certain practitioners possessed specialized expertise, and so would attract a particular clientele. Similarly, it was accepted that, in case of especially serious conditions, eminent London physicians would be consulted by those normally drawing upon local services. Practitioners themselves were often not unhappy to act as a team, finding safety in numbers when dealing with very precious lives. When George III grew delirious in 1788, Fanny Burney diagnosed a paralytic crisis in the royal bedchamber, with none of the court physicians being prepared to take responsibility for action: 'Dr Heberden and Sir George [Baker] would now decide upon nothing till Dr Warren came'.[41] Of course, rifts soon appeared amongst the court physicians themselves, leading to the entry of yet another doctor upon the scene: the Revd Dr Francis Willis, a provincial madhouse keeper whose abrasive presence was hard for courtly physicians-in-ordinary to stomach.

Of course, multiple consultations and encroachments by one physician upon another's territory could lead to fierce dispute. The ensuing divisive politics was well caught by the physician, John Arbuthnot, in his 'John Bull' satire. Arbuthnot imagined a woman falling sick (she serves as an emblem of the state): 'Physicians were sent for in haste; Sir *Roger*, with great difficulty, brought R[adcli]ff; G[ar]th came upon the first Message. There were several others call'd in; but, as usual upon such Occasions, they differ'd strangely at the Consultation.'[42] The upshot was that the physicians split into quasi-political factions, analogues of Whigs and Tories: 'one sided with G[ar]th, and the other with R[adcli]ff'. Arbuthnot then evoked the infighting over diagnosis and therapy.

> G[ar]th: *This Case seems to me to be plainly Hysterical; the Old Woman is Whimsical; it is a common thing for you Old Women to be so: I'll pawn my Life, Blisters, with the Steel Diet, will recover her.*
>
> Others suggested strong Purging and Letting of Blood because she was Plethorick. Some went so far as to say the Old Woman was mad, and nothing would do better than a little Corporal Correction.

If doctors perforce tolerated above-board multiple consultation, they were nevertheless furious if they caught others fishing in their ponds. As David Harley has shown, such territorial violations commonly led to vituperation, pamphlet wars and even to duels.[43] Typically, doctors blamed fatal results on such underhand meddling. Defending himself to John Locke, Dr John Hutton thus denounced a certain Dr Andrew Broune, who (he alleged) had been responsible for the death of Lord Crichton:

> He payed a visit to my Lord Chrighton who was then ill off a continued fever, and who askd Dr Brown any Remedy might Help Him out off a fever Had continued severe upon some 17 days; Brown without the Knowledge of my Lords physiciens gave Him a dose off purging medicinne which gave Him upwards of 20 stooles, and in a few dayes after died; Some physiciens made use off this opportunitie to Reproch both Brown and His practise.[44]

DOCTORS DISAGREE

Multiple consultation brought out the disagreements of doctors into broad daylight. John Opie, the painter, was sick. Joseph Farington ran into his apothecary, 'who said Opie's pulse was better this morn'g, but that He had yet no *passage through Him*, & was partly delirious, & partly dozing, but did not appear to entertain any expectation of his recovery. – Prince Hoare told me that it had not at last been ascertained what His complaint was. It was thought to be in the *bladder*, but was not so; the physicians who first attended him judged it to be *inflammatory*, & bled him & purged him.'[45] (This was another case in which the almost automatic recourse to phlebotomy and purging looked a blunder.) Further help was then sought from Opie's father-in-law, Dr Alderson, who was brought in from Norwich, '& gave a different opinion. He thought it arose out of a *morbid habit* & tended to *putridity*.'[46] This further difference in opinion seemed to require yet another bench of medical adjudicators: 'Mrs Opie, distracted at this difference of opinion, called in Dr. Vaughn, who agreed with those who first judged the case, & Dr. Pitcairne & Dr. Bailie being also consulted differed from Dr. Alderson. Such was the sad uncertainty.'[47]

Sometimes it was not a case of the doctors disagreeing, but of their advice conflicting with other opinions being bandied around. Only the patient could decide whom to believe and follow. Travelling through France in 1654, John Finch grew asthmatic, feverish and colicky. He called in the local doctors. The French physicians, it seemed, were true to their reputation: they would 'never prescribe any thing, be the disease what it will, but letting of bloud'.[48] This did not please his travelling companion, Francis Baines, 'who objected that my Asthma being a cold distemper and my body no whit pletherick, to take away blood was to hinder the maturing of that distillation the concoction of which was my cure. That my feavourish distemper came from the want of free inspiration and the cholick which by riding and fasting was heightened.'[49] Not for the first time, or the last, Finch listened to Baines and took his medical advice: 'thereupon he himself prescribed me a clyster one night and a purge the Day following which after I had stopt made me in health to a miracle. I professe I never found so visible an effect in my life of a Medicine: and I am at this present in as good health if not better than ever I enjoyed.'[50]

The quarrels of doctors were particularly galling to Gideon Mantell, the eminent Sussex geologist, when he developed appalling back pain in the 1840s; for he was a practitioner himself. He travelled up to London to consult the metropolitan top brass, such as Sir Benjamin Brodie: 'Well may the unmedical sufferer exclaim 'Who shall decide when doctors disagree?' – when I am at a loss to decide upon the conflicting opinions upon my case!'[51] The doctors differed profoundly. Brodie and Thomas Lawrence diagnosed 'periostitis', believing there was a bone disease, and that 'an abscess has formed and will probably require to be opened'. Thus far accord: 'But the one recommends entire rest in a horizontal position, and blisters, moxa, or some other external stimulant; while the latter advises no external application, gentle carriage exercise, and sarsaparilla.[52] Other surgeons, however, formed quite opposite diagnoses. 'Liston and Coulson think there has not been nor is any disease of the bone, but simply the formation of an abscess, which will be discharged and get well.' For his part, Mantell suspected cancer. He was to die nearly a decade later of this same complaint (or perhaps of the opiates he took to quell the pain) without having reached any more conclusive notion of its precise nature.

'How strangely the greatest Physicians have disagreed in the most essential Points of their art', bewailed Mandeville's fictional character, Misomedon.[53] The disagreement over Mantell probably did no harm; he was past help anyway. Yet sometimes the outcome of doctors disagreeing appeared to the public bystander to be fatal. What of the sad end of Mr Hope? 'He caught cold', recorded Maria Edgeworth: 'felt very ill. Sir Henry Halford insisted contrary to the advice of 2 other physicians on his taking a dose of James's powder. The 2 other physicians said he had not strength to bear it. He died the day after swallowing that dose.'[54] *Q.E.D.*

REGIMEN

It was the aim and claim of traditional physicians to commend comprehensive courses of action to their patients, touching upon the regulation of all aspects of life-style, habit and health management. Diet, exercise, work, rest, leisure and travel were all to play their parts in schemes of recovery.[55] Sick people and their doctors were in accord on the desirability of such regimens. Patients might like the idea of following a regimen because it promised less vile-tasting and debilitating medication. Regimen, by contrast, was 'a cours of gentell fisek', according to Brilliana Harley, or, as Robert Burton's dictum had it, 'a wise Physician will not give Physick but upon necessity, & first try medicinal diet, before he proceed to medicinal cure'.[56] When her sick soldier son, Phil, had a 'tedious illness', which needed treatment for no less than 'fifteen weeks', Lybbe Powys fussed him back to health with a regimen: 'On the 15th September we had a letter to say he would come down the next day, as he believed something had flown in his eye as he was walking in the Park, and it gave him great uneasiness. He had shown it to the surgeon of his regiment, who said he would bleed him in the morn, gave him a cooling mixture, and desired him to go into the country.'[57] On the way down, disaster overtook him:

All this was done; but it being a very dark rainy evening, that, tho' the postboy and himself knew the road perfectly through our wood, they lost it, and found themselves in a horse-way of Mr. Freeman's near the root-house, where they put the horses behind, and with much difficulty dragg'd the chaise down again into the coach-road; but he had not gone above ten minutes when he was overturn'd over a stump. The chaise, glasses, etc., were now broke. They did not attempt to raise it, but each took a horse, and at last reach'd home, and found they had been about an hour and a half in the wood, when twenty minutes is the usual time! Poor Phil went immediately to bed, being greatly fatigued, and the pain in his eye vastly increased, as he had lost his bandage, and his arm, too, had bled again; in short, he was a most miserable object, and gave us all infinite anxiety, and for many days the inflammation increased.

What was to be done?

He was in too much pain to return to London, but fortunately a Mr. Davenport, an eminent surgeon, has bought an estate near Marlow, and retired from town, and he was so kind as to come immediately, and has order'd our surgeon here how to proceed, and is so good as to come to him every two or three days. He now mends amazingly, as all the faculty tell us. Time and warm weather only can make a perfect cure; but as for many weeks we were apprehensive for the sight, we are most thankful . . . It is hardly possible to imagine with what fortitude he bears the sufferings he has gone through, though he has not since the *accident tasted a bit of meat or drunk a drop of wine, had a perpetual blister ever since, and blooded every three or four days for many weeks.* His health is certainly better than even I knew it, most probably from the *discipline,* some of which might be necessary for a young man in full health with a good appetite, and who never minds over-heating himself in shooting, cricket, etc.

Patients could see the wisdom in pursuing regimens not just to recover health but to stay healthy. Thus the ailing and failing Samuel Richardson grew preoccupied with death after the deaths of his two brothers and a whole succession of other fatalities ('No less than Eleven concerning Deaths attacked me in two Years').[58] He found he needed medical advice: 'My Nerves were so affected with these repeated Blows, that I have been for seven Years past forced, after repeated labouring thro the whole Medical Process by Direction of eminent Physicians, to go into a Regimen, not a Cure to be expected, but merely as a Palliative; and for Seven Years past, have forborn Wine, Flesh, and Fish.'[59]

The faculty claimed that physician-directed pursuit of regimen was precisely what distinguished true medicine from mere quackery, with its quasi-magical faith in specific nostrums.[60] If diseases were constitutional – as best medical and lay opinion allowed – then cures must not merely strike at superficial features (that is, suppress symptoms) but must go to the root, ridding the constitution of its corruptions and strengthening it for the future.[61]

The recovery of health through regimen was necessarily time-consuming and often nerve-fraying. Patients might cavil at the petty regulation of day-to-day minutiae and at the sheer cost in time, effort, and patience.[62] (For instance, the ailing Parson Woodforde objected when Thorne, his physician, instructed him to take his meat boiled rather than roasted.) Yet patients themselves often became wedded to their own regimens, believing that survival itself might hinge upon some minute item of diet or a change in the weather. Physicians grew exasperated when sent messages from patients asking precisely which foodstuffs it was safe to eat, etc. – but what was this but their own chickens coming home to roost?[63]

Such pursuit of regimen was not an alternative, but a supplement, to the prescribing of materia medica. The role of prescribing within patient/doctor relations will be considered below in chapter 8.

POWER

The establishment of an unwritten contract between patient and doctor obviously initiated a micro-politics of power. The sick person's state of illness was itself both a source of weakness and dependency (he needed help) and a bargaining counter (it commanded attention and sympathy). It always remained to be seen whether the patient, or the doctor, possessed the ultimate power of healing.

The physician's situation was likewise highly ambiguous. Notionally, he professed the healer's art, but all too often that power was, and was known to be, illusory. When patient and doctor met, their relation was putatively one of mutual accord – they shared the goal of restoring health and needed each other's co-operation. But the number of issues upon which they could fall out was legion: interpretation of the classification of the illness, obedience to the doctor's instructions (see plate 6) and the question of payment. Power politics are never very far from the surface in the interplay of the sick and their physicians.[64]

An early eighteenth-century clergyman, Robert Leake, ensnared himself in the maze of medical authority; where lay its source? 'Falling into a valetudinarian state', he took to reading medical books with a view to mending his health. He became a zealot for the 'low diet' and vegetarian teachings of the celebrated Dr George Cheyne, the fashionable author of best-selling regimen books targeted at the laity. The result was that Leake grew 'greatly emaciated, in course of time, by keeping too strictly to that gentleman's regimen'. In the end, 'his friends advised him to apply to Dr. Mead', then perhaps the leading physician in the capital. Leake went 'directly to London to wait on the doctor', telling him 'that he had hitherto observed Cheyne's directions, as laid down

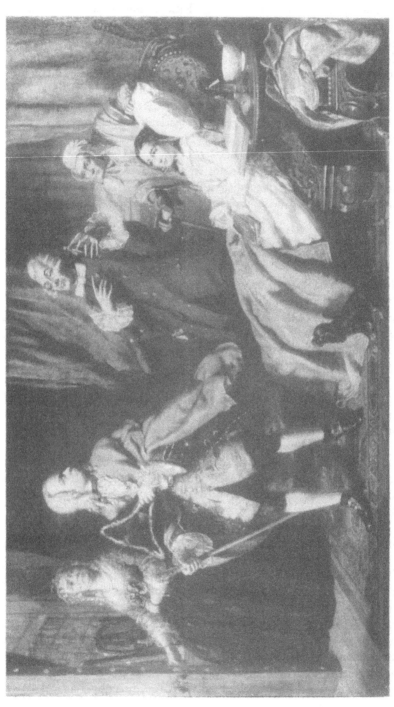

PLATE 6 Patient power. Goldsmith, the physician, leaves in a huff because the patient prefers to follow the advice of the apothecary

in his printed book'. An honest but insouciant remark, which sparked deep professional jealousies: 'Mead, a proud man, and passionate, spoke with contempt of Cheyne and his regimen. "Follow my prescriptions", said he, "and I will get you up again".'[65] Leake, however, did not accept that being under Mead automatically suspended the use of his own independent medical judgement:

> Mr. Leake asked the doctor, every now and then, whether it might not be proper for him to follow, at the same time, such and such prescription of Cheyne, which Mead took ill. When the well-meaning patient was got pretty well again, he asked the doctor what fees he desired or expected from him. 'Sir', said the physician, 'I have never yet, in the whole course of my practise, taken or demanded the least from any clergyman; but, since you have been pleased, contrary to what I have met with in any other gentleman of your profession, to prescribe to me, rather than follow my prescriptions, when you had committed the care of your recovery to my skill and trust, you must not take it amiss, nor will, I hope, think it unfair, if I demand ten guineas of you'.[66]

The story is revealing. It shows, for one thing, the delicacies of etiquette as to whether automatic obedience was expected of a patient. But it also reveals the role played by the exchange of money as an earnest of harmony or a weapon of war. The customary waiving of fees between fellow professionals – physician and clergyman – would be a mutual salutation: both were above the filthy lucre of trade. Normally it would have demeaned the physician to request fees of a cleric (it would have been insulting and preposterous to *demand* fees of any gentleman); in this case, charging a fee was a way of humiliating the payer.[67]

Patients expected to be allowed their say. They would not necessarily expect to get their way. Lady Mary Wortley Montagu recorded her struggles: 'Mr Mason has ordered me blooding, to which I have submitted after long contestation.'[68] They did, however, expect a right of veto. When Sir Ralph Verney fell sick in 1686, the much-loved family physician, Denton, wanted to 'let blood under his tongue'. Sir Ralph, however – weary of being 'Blooded, Vomited, Blistered, Cupt & Scarifyed, & hath 3 Physicians with him, besides Apothecary & Chirurgien' – understandably had 'noe mind to'.[69] In certain circumstances, lay authority was pitted against professional. As a parson, William Jones commonly had to deal with the apparently dying. He regretted the habit, common amongst doctors, of 'giving them over'. 'In the case of Mr Lewin & some others' he wrote, pondering one such instance, 'I have opposed the opinion of the medical men who have thought the complaint hopeless' – and rightly so – 'the event has justified my opinion'.[70]

As argued in the previous chapter, patients, above all, required physicians they could trust. When William Cowper spoke of Lady Hesketh engaging Sir Walter Farquhar as her 'Aesculapius', he clearly implied such a physician.[71] The trustworthy doctor had tact and a certain pliancy; patients hated feeling bullied, and expected at least to have their wishes respected. Thus Thomas Percival noted in his *Medical Ethics* that, much as regular practitioners must abominate quack remedies, if patients obstinately wished to use them, doctors should acquiesce with good grace ('some indulgence seems to be required to a credulity that is unsurmountable').[72]

Yet patients did not want servile, sycophantic yes-men; they sought physicians who spoke plainly and would be prepared to lay down the law when appropriate. With a bear such as John Abernethy, the client knew where he stood. By contrast, patients occasionally voiced their disquiet at the ultra-fashionable silver-tongued physician intent upon ingratiating himself and pandering to what he thought the patient wished to hear. 'Never listen to any Doctors' of that kind, Sara Hutchinson admonished Thomas Monkhouse in 1824, 'London Doctors are, in general, too *polite*, to say disagreeable things – all except Abernethy, & I wish you would consult him.'[73] She likewise sang the praises of 'Mr Knight', who treated a Mrs Q and 'never flattered her that anything but the most rigorous confinement to the couch would be of the least use'. Sara approved of this rigour: 'and to me . . .it appears as plain that this is the *only* remedy – as that 2 & 2 make 4 – Mrs Q had tried the half measures – Sara Coleridge has done so for years – & Miss Fleming received no benefit while she pursued them.'[74]

OBEDIENCE

'We must obey Dr Warren's orders', Lord Duncannon ordered his wife in 1791.[75] This platitude fell frequently from patients' mouths. The alternative might be dire: 'Here enclosed I have sent you two letters', Lady Brilliana Harley told her son, Ned, 'by wch you may know Mr Hibbons tooke a vomit contrary to all counsell, and thereupon died.'[76] The records of the sick divide into those who obeyed, and those who rebelled against what the doctor ordered. One of the classic medical stereotypes was the disobedient patient. 'This morning died my Lord Sackville in the 71st year of his age', Betsy Sheridan recorded: 'I think I told you he has a house in this neighbourhood where he has been ill some time, but his disorder was not apprehended to be dangerous, 'till he chose to indulge in eating a pine Apple and drinking Champaigne expressly against the advice of his Physician.'[77] Silly man! The dénouement was inevitable: 'his complaint was in his bowels, and this imprudence it is supposed has hasten'd his end.' The 'it is supposed' perhaps hints that Betsy did not believe all the doctors put around.

Indeed, a genre of warning literature developed, advising patients in all but trivial cases not to dabble in self-medication but to call the physician, and then obey him to the letter. J.M.'s *Letters to a Sick Friend* (1682) considered the case of the typical imprudent sick person who would insist on neglecting 'advice until it be too late': 'then the Physician is sent for, to share with the Patient in the infamy of the miscarriage: the time for Purgation and Bleeding being over, nothing now remains but to toll the Bell.'[78] The patient, continued the lugubrious author, will typically claim hardly anything is wrong: 'nothing but leaving off a Coat, or putting on a Damp Shift, or eating a Dish of meat that did not agree with the Stomach, or Drinking a Glass of Bad Wine, or over-walked, or a little frighted, or the like.'[79] But that was the way the sick typically deceived themselves about their condition: 'when it may be all the time the Stomach is disordered with a Quagmire of corrupt humors, the Blood inflamed, the Liver obstructed, the Lungs perish and all these not taken notice of: as if a man whose House is on fire, because it only happened by a Boyes throwing a Squib.'[80] Worse still, the author claimed, the sick would never automatically obey the therapeutics prescribed by the physician: 'when the distemper requires a Sweat, they'l bring cooling *Juleps* . . . If the Physician throw water to extinguish the fire of a Fever, and the Patient throws on more fuel, how can it be put out?'[81]

Of course, it was self-serving of doctors to paint such a caricature of the delinquent, defaulting patient. Yet the problem was real. Deciding just when to obey, and how far, could be a torment. When Dorothea Herbert's mother fell sick with a 'dreadful Fever', the 'Doctors' applied 'burning Blisters' (caustics attached to the skin to draw toxic material to the surface where it would disperse). She was in appalling pain: 'After the Doctors and Attendants had left her She supplicated me in the most piteous Manner to get her a little Mutton Suet to cool her Back – Her Face was like a Coal of Fire with Agony and her frantic Vehemence and Screams made Me run down for her own Remedy contrary to Orders.'[82] Dorothea began to obey her mother, but halfway through was interrupted in her 'Surgical Operations' by 'Mr Carshore . . . who attended her'; the doctor rebuked her, saying that 'her Life depended on the torment of the Blisters'.[83] The outcome of this clash of authorities is not known.

Implicit obedience to doctors' orders was no easy matter. Henry Liddell, suffering from some kind of palsy, was put on a severe, restrictive regime. He tried, but could not always keep it up: 'If I did not trespass sometimes on my Doctor's Rules I should never have an opportunity of the least correspondence with any friend and when I am drove to that extremity, farewell to one of ye comforts of life. I can barely keep on foot tho' have followed pretty strictly my Doctor's prescriptions.'[84] As Liddell complained, recommendations for regimen were often costly and disruptive: 'He [the doctor] ordered me to take a new house wch is just on the back of where we are, called East Street. We have a little more room, a better neighbourhood but I can't say so much of the air.'[85]

Obeying the doctor was often a wearisome business, smacking of finical ritual. The Revd John Penrose came up from Cornwall to take the waters in Bath; he found them beneficial, but the time-tabling was quite confusing: 'The Doctor has altered my Regimen: I am now to take Water from the Cross Bath at 7 and 8 o'clock mornings, and from the King's Bath at 12, quarter a Pint each time.'[86] Was such an extraordinary meticulousness really necessary? 'Every one, who comes in, tells me this exactness as to Time and Quantity is a mere Farce, notwithstanding the Doctors so gravely prescribe.'[87] Yet, Penrose was willing to give it all a try: 'it may be so for ought I know; but as it may not be so. I'll try strictly adhere to Rule.'

Overall, what is most striking is how far patients actually co-operated. Lord Pembroke was a cantankerous railer against doctors at large. In reality, however, he respected the advice of those he personally consulted. He commented upon the dilemma he faced as a parent when his daughter, Charlotte, was sick: 'I do not yet know what the Doctors have finally determined. If they all agreed, I should not dream of having an opinion.'[88] This notion of medical harmony was, however, a pipedream, as Pembroke knew, and so decision-making – following one physician in preference to others – would necessarily fall upon his own shoulders: 'If they differ, & I fear they do, something must be determined from their pro's & con's. For my own part, I should not hesitate one moment to follow the opinions of Dr Glass, & Mr John Hunter. They seem to be the most reasonable, & I am the more led to a partiality to them from seeing, that little, the other Physicians have given in to them, though they rather reprobated them at first.'[89]

Some patients were exemplary. 'He is an excellent patient' – thus Lady Holland complimented Lord Melbourne – 'abiding entirely by his doctor.'[90] Jane Austen awarded her brother a similar accolade, though not without a sting in the tail: 'Henry is an excellent patient, lies quietly in bed and is ready to swallow anything.'[91] Elizabeth Iremonger was racked with pain. She went to Bath to consult the eminent Dr William Falconer, and then strictly 'adhered to the Plan he advised of using the Warm Bath three times a week & drinking plentifully of the Waters, and presently found my advantage in this course'. Falconer, she made sure to add, 'is a very sensibly informed, philosophical man & his Conversations on all Subjects were pleasant & improving'.[92]

Certainly many made it their business to obey. 'You may imagine I am willing to submit to the orders of one that I must acknowledge the instrument of saving my life, though they are not entirely conformable to my will and pleasure', Lady Mary Wortley Montagu informed her daughter, the Countess of Bute, concerning the virtues of her physician:

> He has sentenced me to a long continuance here [at Lovere, Italy], which, he says, is absolutely necessary to the confirmation of my health, and would persuade me that my illness has been wholly owing to my omission of drinking the waters these two years past. I dare not contradict him, and must own he deserves (from the various surprising cures I have seen) the name given to him in this country of the miraculous man.[93]

Lady Mary was entirely taken with this physician:

> Both his Character and practice are so singular, I cannot forbear giving you some account of them. He will not permit his patients to have either surgeon or apothecary: he performs all the operations of the first with great dexterity; and whatever compounds he gives, he makes in his own house: those are very few; the juice of herbs, and these waters, being commonly his sole prescriptions.[94]

Some patients appear to have taken obedience to extremes. Mrs Delany, for example, followed doctors' orders, while being convinced they would be the death of her. A friend, Mrs Astley, reported that she suffered 'an inflammation of the lungs':

> After three days' illness, the fever began to intermit, and she was thought better, then it was that the doctors ordered bark to be administered. When I told Mrs Delany, she looked so distressed, and said, 'I have always had a presentiment that if bark were given, it would be my death. You know I have at times a great defluxion on my lungs; it will stop that, and my breath with it.'[95]

The doctors were informed of her view, but they declared 'there was no alternative': 'it was [the] only medicine they could depend on to remove the fever; but seeing the dear lady so averse to taking it, I offered to keep her secret, and put it away. "Oh no", she said, "I never was reckoned obstinate, and I will not die so." The effect was what she had foretold.'[96]

DID THE DOCTOR PLEASE?

In the Georgian age, the public grew intrigued by the medical profession, clutching at every scrap of information about their skills and trying to evaluate their successes. The diarist, Joseph Farington, often dined out with the doctors, and the conversation would turn to their comparative merits:

> Carlisle [the surgeon] drank no wine & talked much against the use of it . . . He said, Dr. Baillie who now has a high reputation, has great knowledge of anatomy, & was an excellent Schoolmaster while He gave Lectures in it, but that He had not much *medical knowledge*, & held the power of medicine very cheap. For this Carlisle blamed him, as by attention to the progress of a complaint, medicines may undoubtedly be occasionally employed with great effect.[97]

Anthony Carlisle rattled on – despite his abstinence – vilifying all his colleagues, and Farington was all ears at the flow of scandal:

> He spoke of [Dr] *Reynolds* as being a weak man, & consequently not a man capable of judging in cases where sagacity & penetration are necessary. [Dr] Lettsom, He allowed to be above Reynolds in understanding, but yet an inferior man. — Dr. George Fordyce, He sd. killed himself by drinking . . . Sir Francis Milman He spoke of as being a man of sense, & very capable; but doubted whether He had had sufficient experience. Dr Ash He mentioned as being the best informed man of His profession; with the additional advantage of an extraordinary memory. – Dr. Frazer, who died lately, He sd. had injured his constitution by drinking too much which had hurt some of the Viscera: but He had abstained from it latterly. – Dr. Vaughn He spoke of as being a man amiable in His manners, but one who did not seem to possess any great power of mind.[98]

If the Georgian patient made it his business to keep *au fait* with doctors and medicine, and had decided views about the kind of doctor he wanted, did he receive satisfaction? Can we form any general conclusions about the quality of doctor/patient relations?

The standing of the medical profession was decidedly mixed: some doctors were appreciated and others not. 'Lady Cardigan is brought to bed of a dead child', Catherine Verney informed her husband in 1709: 'Dr. Shadwell gave her a vomit six weeks before her time . . . My Lord threathens to stab him whenever he meets, but the Roman Catholicks all say tis a judgement upon him for turning Herritick . . .'[99] Some seem to have succeeded with certain patients only. Fanny Burney, as we have seen, found the eminent Quaker physician, John Fothergill, a cold fish. But others loved him. Barbara Hoyland enthused about her fellow Quaker:

[The doctor's presence] was never waited for above a minute or two beyond the time fixed for his coming. His gentle though firm demeanour calmed sorrow into silence. His penetrating eye and abstracted thought always inspired confidence in his judgment [even] though there might appear not the least prospect of success. To him . . . my father spoke of his concerns as to a friend, and of his complaints as to a physician of distinguished skill. On being one day asked whether Dr. Heberden should be called, who was the only senior physician, and consequently the only one who could act with the doctor, he replied, 'No; my life is in God's hand and Fothergill's.'[100]

Indeed, the successful doctor was – if only temporarily – the recipient of gladsome thanks. 'A man coming out of a bed by chance', reported John Ward: 'jabbing his bare breech down on ye side of ye bed a needle ran up his breech just by his anus. Hee sent for a surgeon of Abbington to pull itt out and hee catching hold of itt with his forceps but not being able to hold itt but itt slipped and afterwards attempting itt hee thrust itt in further within ye cuticula.'[101] Another surgeon was tried, but the fellow got off to a bad start: 'After wch Mr. Smith, an Oxford Chirurgian, was sent for; but ye fellow had made an incision and cut ye haemorrhoidal veins wch bled abundantly att wch ye fellow, being discouraged, threw down his instruments and ranne away leaving him bleeding.'[102] A woman had to be got in to patch up the mess before Smith could get to work again: 'Smith could see no signe but went and made a great incision 2 inches deep in ye Menbrana adiposa and thrust his finger and turned it about and felt it; then getting an instrument under hee drew itt out cleverly and gave itt him. Ye fellow when he sawe itt, took him in his arms and kisst him and made exceeding much of itt.'[103]

Many doctors were undoubtedly well respected by patients. Garrick appreciated Ralph Schomberg's services ('I am just rising from ye Bed of Death by ye help of our Friend Schomberg').[104] Lady Sarah Lennox reported a happy encounter to her sister, the Duchess of Leinster: she had chanced upon a 'surgeon . . . an old friend of my two brothers'. She consulted him about her daughter Louisa, who 'had, I thought, one breastbone higher than the other'. 'I found him so sensible and attentive to every trifling complaint I mentioned of hers, that it gave me a good opinion of him, and I consulted him for myself . . . I am now following his orders about her', she reported, going into great detail into all his recommendations.[105]

Many patients expressed full confidence in their doctors. Miss Berry was happy with Baillie: 'He is very rational, kind, and sensible – pities my complaints'.[106] Lord Hervey (probably a sufferer from gallstones) waxed positively lyrical about George Cheyne. He read Cheyne's *Essay of Health and Long Life*, became a convert and put himself under the author in person:

> He advised me to take the Bath waters for six weeks (as I had often done before) in order to cleanse and strengthen my stomach; during that time to eat no meat; and at the end of it to go into a total milk diet for two months. He ordered me to take a vomit of thirty grains of Indian root once a week, in which I obeyed him so punctually that I did it every Monday morning without intermission for six months together. He gave me no other medicine but an infusion of the bark (which I left off in a very little time) and a little rhubarb the day after every vomit.[107]

It turned him from a sickly invalid into a pillar of health:

> From the time of my first putting myself into his hands, to this hour, I never had one formed fit of the colic; though for three years together, according to his prescription, I ate neither flesh, fish, nor eggs, but lived entirely upon herbs, root pulse, grains, fruits, legumes and all those sorts of foods, which, before I left off meat and wine, I could never eat of, though in the smallest degree, without feeling a pain at my stomach in half an hour after they were lodged there.[108]

So what were the qualifications requisite for a doctor to be liked or trusted? Probably what was crucial was the right blend of candour and the ability to inspire confidence. When in the late 1770s Henry Thrale suffered seizures, Samuel Johnson tried to assure Mrs Thrale that the fits were 'hysterical' rather than 'apoplectic' (he may simply have been trying to cheer her). He recommended her to 'consult such Physitians as you think you can best trust. Bromfield seems to have done well, and by his practice appears not to suspect an apoplexy.' He thus seemed ideal.[109] The personal touch – the capacity to establish bonds beyond merely medical considerations – was recognized to be of paramount importance in building trust. Thus Charles Darwin recalled with pride how his father, Dr Robert Waring Darwin, had surpassing 'skill in winning confidence', owing to which 'many patients, especially ladies, consulted him when suffering from any misery, as a sort of Father-Confessor'. The old doctor was wise to patients' indirect strategies: 'He told me that they always began by complaining in a vague manner about their health, and by practice he soon guessed what was really the matter. He then suggested that they had been suffering in their minds, and now they would pour out their troubles, and he heard nothing more about the body.'[110]

Georgian medicine may have had the power to cure only rarely; it could not always give relief. But there is much evidence of powerful bonds being forged between patients and doctors on the basis of satisfying mutuality. The theory of the professions has typically stressed the hierarchical inequalities of patient and doctor, either to praise the physician's superior expertise and ethical dignity, or, more cynically, to point to professional dominance and mystification. But Georgian England seems to reveal relations between paying patients and their medical attendants built upon a rough-and-ready parity. In this, the ubiquity of cash-nexus contractual relationships in that commercial, market-place society certainly played its part, as did the uncertain success of the medical help offered.

6

Irregulars

The pre-modern medical world, as we have noted, gave a modicum of formal recognition and prestige to practitioners who met the criteria of being regularly trained. But it did so within a wider politico-legal framework that increasingly proclaimed the sovereignty of market mechanisms. Medicine was viewed as a commodity, and health care a service, freely traded in accordance with the laws of supply and demand.[1] Within this, regular doctors accepted that a legitimate, though limited, sphere existed for medical autarky or barter: the economy of home medicine and the routine exchange of minor medical services within families, households and the local community.[2] However, the faculty reviled root and branch the activities of those professional competitors they stigmatized as 'quacks', that is, 'pretenders' to medical knowledge.[3] Such quacks proliferated in pre-modern England alongside every other form of opportunist commercial enterprise. They ranged from the occasional, part-time healer, to ritzy showmen and large-scale capitalists. Giuseppe Grimaldi, father of the great clown, Joe, made an often precarious living as a dancer, clown, theatre manager, conjuror, dentist and physician. In contrast to such small fry, some grew very rich. Nathaniel Godbold reputedly made a steady £3000 a year (and over £10,000 in a peak year) from his 'Vegetable Balsam', a much-puffed restorative and rejuvenator. Joseph Farington believed Isaac Swainson, the vendor of Velno's Vegetable Syrup, gained some £5000 a year from it. At one stage, the uroscopist, Theodor Myersbach, was said to be raking in some £1000 a month in fees.[4] Figures like this are beyond verification and probably inflated; all the same, the social perception of such operators as highly successful is accurate and itself significant.

Indeed, the air of Georgian England was filled with quackery. It was impossible to step into a coffee-house or open a newspaper without being bombarded by advertisements parading the services of itinerant dentists, oculists, electrifiers, mesmerists and the like; or promoting a welter of nostrums which would restore one's health or youth, cure cancer without need of the knife, purge and cleanse the system, dissolve hangovers, sooth the nerves, remove female obstructions (a euphemism for procuring an abortion) or cure the cholic. Regular doctors themselves often prescribed from the London coffee-houses. Ironically, as the jounalist, Ned Ward, remarked, the walls behind them were commonly plastered with quack bills, advertising such wonders as: 'May Dew, Golden Elixirs, Popular Pills, Liquid Snuff, Beautifying Waters, Dentrifices, Drops, Lozenges, all as infallible as the Pope. "Where", as the famous Saffold has it, "everyone above the rest, Deservedly has gained the name of best"; good in all cases, curing all distempers; every medicine pretends to nothing less than universality.'[5] 'Indeed', Ward banteringly concluded, 'had not my friend told me 'twas a coffee-house I should have took it for the parlor of some eminent mountebank.'[6]

But it was the advent of the newspaper that transformed the coverage available to the medical advertiser. It was a rare copy of a Georgian paper that did not contain at least half a dozen advertisements for patent medicines, taking up perhaps a quarter of the available advertising space. The great bulk of general advertisements were essentially local (notices of property for sale, auctions, dancing lessons, concerts and the like); quack medicines, by contrast, were amongst the very few brand-name commodities advertised nation-wide.[7] If publicity for such nostrums was typically repetitious and uninspired, some advertising copy was tailor-made to catch the eye, often drawing upon testimonials, real or fake, to lend an air of authenticity. 'The following intelligence is well worthy the public's notice', readers of the *General Evening Post* would have spotted in 1784: 'Alderman Pugh, who was afflicted with the Gout upwards of 20 years, and during his last fit, at the age of 67, September 1783, kept his bed ten months, unable to stir hand or foot, is now, to the utter astonishment of his friends, and particularly of the Faculty, who had pronounced him incurable, (indeed an instance of the like nature cannot be found in the annals of medicine) regarded by all who see him as risen from the dead.'[8] To what did he owe this miracle?

for this surprising cure, scarcely to be credited by credulity itself, he is indebted to Mr. Buzaglo, of the Strand, who, in twenty-eight days, at an hour a day only, absolutely effected his cure, *without Medicine*, so that the worthy Alderman is now able to walk the streets, and ride a horse-back, as well as he did at the age of thirty-five; and for that humanity and desire for the general welfare of mankind, for which he is universally distinguished, is willing and desirous to satisfy all enquiries concerning his own late desperate case, and also of many surprising cures of others to which he was witness. This remarkable and uncontrovertible instance of the infallibility of Mr. Buzaglo's method of curing Gout is the strongest and most convincing confirmation of its effect, and must have its due weight on the minds of all those who have been taught to believe that pills, bathing, travelling, flannels, and patience, can cure the Gout.[9]

Regular doctors also advertised their services in the papers, but tended to do so far more discreetly: for example, through announcing removal to new and larger premises.

Newspapers were particularly significant as mouthpieces for proprietary medicines because their owners and agents typically acted as the principal distributors for the medicines. Bookshops and circulating libraries also doubled as medicine stockists. In 1784 the *Coventry Mercury* was telling its readers that an entire alphabet of nostrums could be purchased at the local bookstore, coming to a crescendo with:

Radcliffe's Purging Elixir
Ruston's Pills for the Rheumatism
Royon's Ointment for the Itch
Spilsbury's Drops
Stoughton's Elixir
Swinfen's Electuary for the Stone and Gravel
Spirits of Scurvy Grass
Sans Pareil Powder
Storey's Worm Cakes
Smyth's Scouring Drops
Steel Preservative
Specific Purging Remedy for Venereal Diseases, by Wessels
Tasteless Ague and Fever Drops
Turlington's Balsam
Tincture of Centaury
Tincture of Valerian
Vandour's Pills, for Nervous Complaints
Velnos's Vegetable Syrup
Ward's White Drops
West's Elixir[10]

The Georgian medical consumer was thus enticed, or bemused, by no less a variety of shop-counter medicines than is available nowadays. Many of them, in those unregulated times before the Food and Drugs Acts and prescription-only medicines, were extremely potent brews.[11] We must never underestimate the sheer range of medical treatments on offer in that nation of shopkeepers, or the degree to which advances in distribution and marketing techniques gave a tremendous fillip to all forms of medical entrepreneurship.[12]

IRREGULAR HEALERS

Irregular medicine thus had a high profile in pre-modern times. From the quack *à la mode* down to the village wise woman, it commanded a huge following. 'My Wife took a Doce of Phisick by Advice of Betty Morice', Nicholas Blundell wrote in 1713, ''tis the 3rd time she has taken from her since Lent came in.' This Mrs Morice also dressed and bandaged limbs and gave out purges; her daughter performed small-scale surgery too.[13] Such 'doctoress' figures had long been popular, and not merely with countryfolk or women, partly because, as Lord Fermanagh was informed, they often used 'very safe things'.[14]

Feminists have argued that women healers were being squeezed out of the medical market-place in the eighteenth century; after all, expectations for quasi-formal qualifications were rising – a degree, walking the wards in hospitals – and women were decidedly excluded from these. This claim may prove true, but the records of the sick, and of newspaper insertions themselves, provide abundant evidence that 'surgeonesses' and the like continued prominently in practice. The most eminent 'faith healer' in Georgian England was a woman, Bridget Bostock; and Mrs Joanna Stephens sold her stone-dissolving nostrum to Parliament for a handsome £5000.[15]

It would be anachronistic and distorting to propose a set of categories – historical, sociological, medical or ethical – rigorously demarcating so-called quacks from the regulars, at least before the introduction of the Medical Register in 1858 achieved that very object by legislative *fiat*.[16] Accusations of quackery were flung around in an atmosphere charged with emotion and *ad hominem* abuse. The self-same person could readily appear simultaneously true-blue orthodox and quite quackish to different judges. Thomas Beddoes was an Oxford MD and some-time Reader in Chemistry at the University. He believed quackery ought to be publicly outlawed. Yet he was accused of practising it himself, because of his championship of the use of factitious air for treating consumption. The medical pamphlet literature teems with accusations and counter-accusations of quackery, which are best taken as indexes of mutual mud-slinging and self-publicizing.[17]

The quack was typically accused of being a cheat, yet many so labelled were patently sincere.[18] He tended to be arraigned as being one who dabbled in medical secrets, yet various impeccably orthodox doctors marketed their own nostrums, or, like Robert James (who sported an Oxford MD) patented medicines with formulae expressly designed to mystify imitators.[19] Indeed, it was common practice for regular doctors to be involved in, or to lend their names to nostrum-mongering. The great Sir Hans Sloane vended his own eye-salve; Richard Mead sold an antidote for mad-dog bites[20] and John Radcliffe advertised

> Dr. Radcliff's Royal Tincture, or the General Rectifier of the Nerves, Head and Stomach, It corrects all irregularities of the Head and the Stomach by hard drinking or otherwise. It is also recommended to drinkers as the best purl in the world: in beer, ale or wine, or purl royal in sack. Merchants and shopkeepers may be supplied with these drops with good allowance to sell again, at Lloyd's Coffee House, Lombard Street, London. Price 1/- a bottle.[21]

So-called quacks certainly exploited the opportunities of the market-place, but so did many regulars, albeit not on the same scale.[22] Admittedly, there were certain out-and-out charlatans – authentic frauds – amongst the quacks. But historically it would be unwise to divide regulars and quacks into heroes and villains or saints and sinners. Regulars and irregulars alike were selling medical services, but they were managing their own commercial operations in rather distinct ways. And that is how the medicine-consuming public saw it. They would pick and choose from amongst the range of practitioners and treatments on offer.

DOCTORS AND QUACKS IN CONFRONTATION

Regular practitioners could not, of course, stomach this point of view. Their vilification of quacks, they claimed, was a public duty, to protect the gullible and defenceless consumer against the quacks' fleecing tactics. Alluding perhaps to Hogarth's terrible trinity of 'Credulity, Superstition and Fanaticism', William Buchan described irregular medicine as a sad matter of 'Ignorance, Superstition and Quackery'.[23] And if human nature itself left people ripe for exploitation, the particular resonances of Georgian culture exacerbated the problem, according to physicians such as Thomas Trotter. For the search for sensibility begat hypochon-dria, which in turn led to a passion for medication, typically producing great pain in its wake. Thus 'the acute, but too often false perceptions of nervous people', Trotter contended, left such morbid souls 'easy prey' to 'jugglers and mountebanks'.[24]

The public was particularly vulnerable, moreover, because it was, as a certain Philip Stern MD contended, 'an age when almost every week produces a new medicine'. How could the public decide? For the public good, Stern offered 'a few general rules to the reader', the better to distinguish the *bona fide* healer from the shark medicine vendor: 'The first general rule is, never to pay the least regard to the canting of those who pretend, that the good of mankind is their sole motive for offering their medicine to sale.'[25] His advice continued in the same vein, arguing that the quack accused himself by the grandeur of his pretensions:

> Secondly, disregard all assertions concerning the excellency of a medicine, which are mere assertions, without any foundation in reason and experiment.
>
> Thirdly, conclude the advertizer to be either a knave or a fool, in physick, who pretends, that his medicine will cure several disorders which have not the least analogy to each other.
>
> Fourthly, give no credit to the recital of Cases, as they are generally invented by the doctor.
>
> And lastly, when the doctor writes a pamphlet, with an intention to recommend his medicine, if it betray a manifest ignorance of his subject, of style, and grammar; in short, when his language is evidently that of a potter, conclude him to be some illiterate, ignorant person, whose medicine and opinions deserve no attention.[26]

If the claims of quacks were not to be trusted, how could their medicines possess any authentic virtues? Worse, it was widely maintained, they were positively harmful. They frequently contained high concentrations of opium or alcohol, which temporarily dulled the pain, masked the symptoms of fever or settled the stomach. But the long-term effects were dire, requiring ever heavier doses to reproduce the analgesic effects. Quack remedies might occasionally work, but only through introducing unsafe ingredients in dangerous dosages. Thus proprietary vermifuges, used to treat intestinal worms in children, were said to contain perilously high concentrations of mercury or lead.[27]

Of course, the guardians of orthodoxy were right to argue that quack medicines promised the earth but often delivered next to nothing. They were wrong, however, to contend that the public was simply gullible when exposed to the hyperbole of the charlatans. People were no more willing to take the pufferies of quacks on trust than to believe the faculty or any of that other Babel of politicians, preachers and publicists clamouring for the public ear. Thomas Turner noted dismissively that his wife was patronizing the local mountebank: clearly such credulity was not for the likes of modern males such as himself.[28]

Indeed, adroit Georgian quacks did not primarily go in for 'promise, large promise', but rather appealed to the active, intelligent, seasoned judgement of the public, and exploited widespread public suspicion of regular medicine itself. In that sense, the pitch of the quacks became a mirror image of that of the regulars. Ned Ward noted the evils of the charlatans, but condemned fellows of the College of Physicians for being the pot that called the kettle black:

They rail mightily in their writings against the Ignorance of Quacks and Mountebanks, yet, for the sake of Lucre, they License all the Cozening Pretenders about Town, or they could not practice; which shews it is by their Toleration that the People are Cheated out of their Lives and Money; and yet they think themselves so Honest, as to be no ways answerable for this Publick Injury; as if they could not Kill People fast enough themselves, but must depute all the Physical Knaves in the Town to be Death's Journey-men. Thus do they License, what they ought carefully to Suppress; and Practice themselves, what they Blame and Condemn in others.[29]

If all sorts of medicine were on a par, who had the right to decide? It was a variation of the old conundrum of who should decide when doctors disagreed. The answer lay in user choice. Irregulars made all sorts of high-falutin appeals to authority: to antiquity, to science, to Nature, to divine revelation, to experience, to secret sources of occult wisdom and the like. But they also made an astute appeal to consumer free choice. They denounced the privileges of the regulars as self-serving restrictive practices, mere attempts to monopolize and police the field. Above all, shrugging off the common attack upon themselves as mere empirics, they turned it to advantage by contending that empiricism, in its proper sense, was the foundation of judgement, since it was the philosophy of experience itself, the very life-blood of the 'new science'.[30] They themselves were practitioners of long and varied experience (in contradistinction to the mere paper diplomas and certificates waved around by the regulars). It was, moreover, experience – not reason, books or colleges – that brought new medical truths to light. William Buchan admitted that medical innovations rarely emerged out of orthodoxy, but from the fringe instead.[31] And the irregulars paraded endless testimonials to prove the experience of thousands of satisfied customers.

In the end, quacks claimed, the public must decide on the basis of experience. Thus in the 1770s Theodor Myersbach, the fashionable London uroscopist, defended himself against the attempts of regulars such as John Coakley Lettsom to discredit him. In a free country, Myersbach claimed, everyone should be free to medicate himself as he pleased.[32] In an oblique fashion, the orthodox Buchan agreed. Buchan loathed quacks, whom he saw as rank exploiters. But he could not gainsay the truth of the view that if the faculty appeared to act as self-serving monopolists, hoarding medical knowledge, they would lose all credit, and quacks would be the beneficiaries. Only by laying regular medicine open would the quack menace be overcome.

RESORTING TO IRREGULARS

How was a sick person to determine which forms of medicine to trust? That same Thomas Turner, who, as we saw, mocked his wife for going to a mountebank, was himself eager to cull scraps of medical knowledge from magazines.[33] It might be difficult to discover a single sick person who never stepped outside the magic circle of the regular medical profession in search of a cure.

The continuing, indeed growing, popularity of unofficial medicine of many kinds was undoubtedly connected with its availability in tangible commodity form. During the Georgian age, regular medicine itself leant increasingly upon the prescription of drugs.[34] But that applies all the more so to unorthodox medicine. The paper of powders or jar of ointment purchased from the huckster or over the counter had a symbolic force. It marked the power of the purchaser, the idea that relief or health were things that could be bought. It possessed a reassuring tangibility – it was solid and substantial; it could be swallowed, applied, rubbed in, or whatever. It thereby also symbolized speed and convenience (it was less trouble to gulp a pill than to follow an exacting regimen or diet over many months). Not least, nostrums were medicines of which the patient was totally the master.[35]

In the first consumer society, a greater variety of goods was being purchased ready-made which, in previous centuries, had been made up at home in the kitchen or in the still-room: soaps, varnishes, paints, cosmetics, washes, scented waters and so forth.[36] Shop-bought medicaments were closely associated with such items, as part of a joint appeal to beauty, hygiene and health, all being sold together in the growing number of druggists' shops, grocers and general stores.[37]

We have seen already that the vendors of commercial medicines appealed to patient choice in the free market. The sick enjoyed exercising such choice, being eager to try out all that was new, different and exciting in the way of health. Was there 'any truth in what we had heard concerning her having experienced the effects' of animal magnetism, Betsy Sheridan asked Mrs Sheridan, her mother-in-law?

> She confess'd that she had and entirely confirm'd the account I had heard . . . The first time She went to Dr Maneduke [De Mainauduc], She staid only a short time and found no effect from his experiments. She promised to return to him again and to allow him what time he thought necessary. This she did in the course of a few days in company with Mrs Crewe. She was that time thrown into a state which She describes as very distressing. It was a kind of fainting without absolute insensibility. She could hear and feel but had no power to speak or move. The fit gradually

went off and she told Maneduke She was not even then convinced as She thought such effects might be produced on a nervous person by the effects of imagination.[38]

As this example shows, the public response to unorthodox healing was by no means uncritical. Often it was a matter of 'once bitten, twice shy'. 'Let me beg you not to have anything to say or do with the Magnetizers', warned Lady Bessborough in 1787:

> If they can do nothing it can be of no use, & if they can really affect the human frame it may as well do it harm as good. I am not at all sure that your sister's being so subject to these cramps & spasms may not have been a consequence of that if there is anything in it. At all events I have some reasons, which I cannot well explain by letter, why I wish you to avoid, in as quiet a way as you can, going or even conversing, if you can help it, with any of them.[39]

Similarly, when Boswell's wife, Margaret, was wasting away with consumption, he shopped around the regular London doctors, including Richard Warren and Sir George Baker (as we noted, Margaret had more faith in Baker). But he also called on the nostrum-vendor, Nathaniel Godbold, 'and got a pint bottle of his vegetable balsam' for her ('but she would not try it as yet').[40] Boswell had a try-anything attitude with medicines (as is evident from the mix of quack nostrums and regular physic he took for his gonorrhoea).[41] It upset him that his wife did not approve of his buying her patent medicines: 'I was very miserable. She seemed hurt from a notion that I grudged the expense of a physician because I talked of the difficulty of getting free of them. This distressed me deeply.'[42] Unable to decide between fringe and orthodoxy, the Boswells descended into medical chaos: 'I was sending for Sir George Baker again, but she stopped me. I was for calling Dr. Warren.'[43]

People commonly displayed a 'see if it will work' outlook. In 1767 Sylas Neville had a 'return of the toothache'. He first tried a proprietary medicine, but it did not work ('Mack's Anodyne fluid has done me no service').[44] His next resort was to a woman dentist, Elizabeth Miller, in Whitechapel, 'who said to cure the Tooth-ache. She dressed the tooth which ached last.' (Were there lots of specialist women dentists in the East End? When, some twenty years earlier, Henry Fielding's wife had toothache in Wapping, a woman was summoned.)[45]

Celebration of free consumer choice became linked with the conceit of the 'favourite remedy'. It became almost a point of honour to those in the know to have some special medicine to recommend, perhaps on the basis of a 'miracle cure' which they or their friends had undergone. It gratified their sense of self-importance, making them seem expert in medical matters, no less (for example) than in taste or connoisseurship.

It was flattering to put someone else in one's power or debt through being able to experiment upon them medicinally. Favourite nostrums assumed all the aura of charms. Tar-water was all the rage in the mid-eighteenth century. Some stuck by it, for example, Cowper's friend, Mrs Unwin.[46]

In adopting such favourite remedies, the laity was merely mimicking top-notch doctors, who commonly made much of their own special 'secret weapon', and for whom a 'wonder cure' could make a reputation overnight. In 1737 Queen Caroline was seriously ill with what proved to be a strangulated hernia; each of the royal physicians, Lord Hervey reported, wished to press his own medicine upon her: 'Dr. Broxholme was immediately sent for by Lord Hervey. When he came, Tesier and he agreed to give the Queen immediately some snake-root with Sir Walter Raleigh's cordial.'[47] Well and good, but for some reason, dispensing this prescription proved a slow business, which gave the surgeon, John Ranby, his chance. He informed Hervey that: 'insisting on these occasions upon a cordial with this name or t'other was mere quackery, and that no cordial was better than another in these cases but in proportion to its strength.'[48] Hervey took the hint and got the Queen a glass of whisky, which was 'immediately given to the Queen, who kept it about half an hour, which was about twenty nine minutes longer than she had kept anything else, but then brought it up.'[49] By then it was the original physicians' turn with their favourite preparation:

> Soon after the snake-root, and Sir Walter Raleigh's cordial arrived from the apothecary's; it was taken and thrown up about an hour after. All these strong things, twice Daffy's Elixir, mint-water, usquebaugh, snake-root, and Sir Walter Raleigh's cordial, had without easing the Queen's pain, so increased her fever, that the doctors ordered Ranby to bleed her twelve ounces immediately. She took a glister but it came from her just as it went into her.[50]

When laymen could see the faculty apparently having recourse to such a ragbag of remedies, it is hardly surprising they often reserved their own judgement and experimented for themselves. Some apparently got a narcissistic kick out of such self-experimentation. The Revd Edmund Pyle enjoyed dosing himself and reporting the results to his friends. 'When I took Mrs Stephens' medicines', he noted: 'I swallowed two ounces of soap a day, for six months together. Besides the oyster shell, or egg shell powder, in small beer, to the quanitity that will lie on a half-crown with each dose of soap; I think the doses were 3 or 4 in a day.'[51] Presumably Pyle was taking Mrs Stephens's medicine for bladder-stones, though maybe he was simply testing what effects it would have. He also experimented with 'some tricks for the gout', including 'The

Duke of Portland's Powder', which disagreed with him violently ('thanks to my constitution, am not killed'). Indeed, he concluded, gout was best left alone: 'He that is subject to it, had better bear the fits, as nature throws them out than strive to put her out of her way, which if you do furca licet, usq recurret.'[52]

But if some resorted to quack medicines out of a genuine experimentalism, or even a perverse vanity, the great majority did so out of the 'desperation factor', having already tried everything else in vain. 'People apply to quacks', claimed William Wadd, early in the nineteenth century: 'because, like drowning men, when honest practitioners give no hope, they catch at every twig. Thus, the love of life on the one hand, and the love of gain on the other, create a tolerably good correspondence between the quack and the public.'[53]

Patients would often start with regulars, find no satisfaction, try quacks – and even go back to their original doctors (by then, typically, the latter claimed, ruined by their medical promiscuity). Dr John Moore thus described the hypochondriac's progress of he who initially consulted regulars, but, lacking a cure, worked his way through 'the whole tribe'.[54] He then moved on to quacks, receiving from them an 'appearance of sympathy which the rest of his acquaintances refuse': 'and they possibly relieve or palliate the costiveness, the flatulency, the acidities, and other symptoms which are brought on by the anxiety attendant on this complaint.'[55] What such quacks could never achieve (argued Moore, speaking as a regular physician) was to get to the root of the disease: 'the original cause . . . continuing in spite of all their bitters, and their stomachies, and their purgatives, and analeptics, the same symptoms constantly recur. The wretched patient growing every hour more irritable remedies hurry on the bad symptoms with double rapidity.'[56] So what happens finally? Anything and everything gets tried, out of sheer desperation:

> he returns to physicians, goes back to quacks, and occasionally tries the family nostrums of many an old lady. His constitution being worn by fretfulness and by drugs, he at length despairs of relief, and either sinks into a fixed melancholy, or roused by indignation, his good genius having whispered in his ear, *fuge medicos et medicamina*, he abandons the seat of his disappointments, tries to dissipate his misery by new objects and a different climate, consults no practitioners of any country, sex, or denomination; and forms a fixed resolution to swallow no more drugs.[57]

Despair, one might think. Yet from the depths comes relief: 'from which happy epoch, if the case be not quite desperate, he has the best chance of dating his recovery.'

There were thus plenty of plausible reasons why resort to nostrums and quacks was permissible and popular. Their medicines sometimes tasted better, and might occasionally even be more effective, than those of the faculty. Cost was also important: quacks appealed, William Wadd stressed, because 'health is offered at a reasonable rate'.[58] Mass-produced and mass-distributed medications, not surprisingly, often cost less per unit than pills laboriously rolled individually by the apothecary's apprentice; indeed, commercial nostrums could hardly have captured so much of the market had they not conspicuously undercut the one-off prescription.

Buyers were often aware that nostrums – cheap because made in bulk – contained ingredients essentially identical or comparable to the remedies doctors prescribed: both regular and quack analgesics typically contained opium; emetics contained ipecacuanha; laxatives, senna; stronger purges, mercury or calomel; and so forth.[59] Indeed, regular doctors themselves routinely prescribed certain proprietary nostrums, such as the famous (or notorious) febrifuge, Dr James's Fever Powders. James's Powders were valued because, despite their well-known dangers, they did actually work.[60] Thus Fanny Burney, nursing her sick son, was most grateful to have the powders to hand, recording, almost as if penning a testimonial: 'Our dearest Boy [she told her husband] had so much fever, & so dreadful a Cough, which latter exercised every moment, that, after a second analeptic had failed of cure, though it had procured him, thank God, a good night, I gave him 1 grain of James's powder. This soon operated like magic in relieving his lungs, by stilling his Cough.'[61] The sick child made a splendid recovery, almost from death's door, it seems, thanks to these wonder proprietary powders: 'The whole day, however, his fever was too continual to permit me to let him rise, except to make his Bed, & he suffered so severely from his Cough during that interval, that I repeated the dose when I put him to Bed, & watched by him till midnight, when the soundness of his sleep, & the amendment of his pulse, encouraged me to go to Bed.'[62]

Not only in cases of fever did people find relief through a proprietary nostrum. When suffering from chest complaints, dysentery or simply severe pain, proprietary opiates did the trick. Mixtures such as Godfrey's Cordial or Dover's Powder (opium, saltpetre, tartar, liquorice and ipecacuanha), were widely used – not least for stupefying infants while their mothers worked.[63]

Quack remedies were preferred for other reasons too. Sometimes they were thought to be milder than the draconian mixtures prescribed by the regulars. For example, the dozens of 'cures' for venereal disease marketed by empirics attracted customers by claiming to obviate the protracted, nauseating and extremely painful mercurial treatment favoured by the orthodox.[64]

Overall, in a medical market-place in which doctors of all kinds enjoyed freedom to buy and sell, all manner of medicines proliferated and people habitually shopped around. Probably few sick people restricted themselves solely to regular, or to unorthodox medicine. How choices were struck between them is perhaps best shown by sampling the behaviour of well-documented individuals.

BOSWELL CLAPPED

One of the growth points in unorthodox medicine in the Georgian age was venereal disease. 'Its treatment has fallen into bad hands', lamented William Buchan:

> Not only Quacks of all descriptions undertake to cure it; but every idle fellow who does not chuse to follow some useful employment, sets up for doctor, assumes some well known name, and advertises an infallible remedy for the venereal disease. The apothecary's man, or even the apothecary's man's man, often passes for an adept in curing this malady. Nor is it uncommon, for the fellow who brushed the surgeon's coat, or cleaned his shop, to step into his master's shoes, and sometimes into his chariot, by his pretended skill in curing the lues venerea.[65]

For Buchan, no such treatment had the slightest redeeming virtue: 'These nostrum-mongers not only sell the same medicines to all their patients, however widely their symptoms may differ; but, unfortunately for them, the nostrum often does not contain a single grain of what we know to be absolutely necessary for their cure.'[66] Buchan exaggerated, of course, for effect. But there is no denying that clap-doctors and pox-nostrums mushroomed during the century, perhaps reflecting looser sexual mores. Venereal disease cures were widely advertised in newspapers.[67] Because of the embarrassing and private nature of the condition, many patients patronized all sorts of healers other than their regular practitioners.[68]

James Boswell was clapped on no fewer than nineteen occasions. What did he do? For his youthful bouts of 'Signor Gonorrhea', Boswell religiously went to regular surgeons, such as Andrew Douglas in Pall Mall. Douglas initially treated him with purges, put him on a light diet and ordered bed-rest; many years, many claps, later, having changed his strategies, Douglas was to try injecting fluids into the urethra.[69]

When he was infected in Italy, Boswell went to the very best doctor – James Murray, personal physician to the Old Pretender – and secured an audience with no less eminent a man than Morgagni.[70] On later occasions, he waited upon regular surgeons, such as Peter Adie in Edinburgh and Daniel Johnstone in Ayr. By 1767 Boswell, still only twenty-five, had his seventh attack, and paid a visit to the Edinburgh surgeon, Duncan Forbes. On a later occasion he consulted Percivall Pott, perhaps the most illustrious surgeon in Britain. On the point of marriage, he consulted a whole gaggle of doctors – Douglas, Forbes, Pott, John Gregory and Sir John Pringle – to ensure he was infection-free.

But at the same time, just to make sure, he travelled to London to take Kennedy's Lisbon Diet Drink, a popular nostrum vended by Gilbert Kennedy, graduate of both Rheims and Oxford. It consisted of sarsaparilla, sassafras, licorice and guaiac wood, and cost half a guinea a bottle. Boswell was instructed to drink two bottles a day. Perhaps feeling defensive about making this double check, Boswell mounted a defence of Kennedy's mixture, and was offended when his regular doctors tried to dissuade him from taking it. What could this be but professional sour grapes? 'It is amazing to see a man of Sir John's [Pringle] character so impregnated with partiality as to refuse its just credit to a medicine which has undoubtedly done wonders.' Here, as so often, a layman tried to trump medical authority with 'experience'. Boswell noted Pringle had been equally 'prejudiced' against Keyser's pills, another remedy he had mooted taking for venereal disease.[71]

Was Boswell, with his espousal of a quack remedy, conforming to the stereotypical quack clap-cure customer as delineated by Buchan? 'The most frequent dupes to quackery are the young and unwary. They credit the contents of every puff that is put into their hands as they walk the streets, and swallow with eagerness the drugs it recommends.'[72] To such green young men, to such Boswells, Buchan had sage words of advice: 'I would beg leave just to hint to such inexperienced youths, that the advertising quack, is, ten to one, more ignorant of medicine than themselves, that his sole aim is to take their money, and when he has got that, he cares no more for the patient. I am warranted to say this from daily observation, and am sorry to add, that too many, from woeful experience, know it to be true.'[73]

Boswell thought otherwise: he believed self-interest underlay the doctors' distrust of such proprietary cures. As early as 20 January 1763, when being treated by Douglas, he had voiced his doubts. Douglas was his 'friend'; yet he behaved not as a friend, but in the 'opposite character' of a surgeon. 'Douglas as a surgeon will be as ready to keep me long under his hands, and as desirous to lay hold of my money, as any man.'[74]

Matrimony did not put an end to the clap, and subsequent attacks saw Boswell often consulting Pringle and Douglas. The latter, despite being orthodox, by now had his own personal injection fluid ('a secret known to only a few').[75] But by this stage – maybe less sanguine about the doctors, or simply feeling that intimate familiarity had made him an expert – Boswell also took to self-medication, having read in 1786 John Hunter's *Treatise on the Venereal Disease*.[76] It is noteworthy that near the close of his career, Buchan himself produced a treatise on venereal disease, in which he suggested that most outbreaks could perfectly well be handled by self-medication.[77]

Possibly both Boswell and Buchan modified their views with time. Certainly Boswell's experience showed that evaluating the best course of treatment was difficult, and that all recourses had their advantages and drawbacks. As with whores, so with cures, Boswell tried them all.

QUACKS AND MEN OF LETTERS

It should be no surprise that many of the leading writers of Georgian England were involved in the promotion, use or critique of proprietary medicines. The commercialization of mass-market writing – most notoriously in Grub Street – bears close affinities to the commercialization of medicine.[78] Through their contacts with booksellers, writers mingled with medicine dealers. All were in the business of creating publicity and commanding attention. Christopher Smart, the poet, married into the family of John Newbery, perhaps the largest London dealer in magazines and newspapers, and medicine vendor; his wife was involved in the sale of James's Powders.[79]

Oliver Goldsmith had close publishing connections with the Newberys. He was probably the author of 'Little Goody Two Shoes', the popular children's story that Newbery published. That tale contains a blatant piece of puffery for James's Powders.[80] Goldsmith himself (a doctor by training) was a devotee of the Powders, which apparently precipitated his death in April 1774. Suffering from a multitude of disorders, probably due to kidney failure, Goldsmith became feverish and sent for Dr Hawes. He wished to take the famous febrifuge; his physician advised him against it, as did George Fordyce, who was also called in. Nevertheless, Goldsmith took three powders; he worsened, and despite the attendance of his physicians, died. Many said he died of taking James's Powders; Horace Walpole, their foremost champion, claimed, by contrast, that Goldsmith died for just the opposite reason: 'The republic of Parnassus has lost a member: Dr Goldsmith is dead of a purple fever, and I think might have been saved if he had continued James's powder, which had had much effect, but his physician interposed.'[81]

If Goldsmith's name was linked with James, Henry Fielding became known in a similar way as a staunch defender of Joshua Ward. Ward gained custom, wealth and notoriety with his 'pill and drop', a quack panacea widely used for stomach complaints.[82] Edward Gibbon's father, seeking to reconcile his son to his second wife, claimed that she had saved Edward's life 'by recommending Dr Ward when you was given over by the regular Physicians'.[83] The general public continued loyal to Ward's medicine, and, as with James's Powders, regular doctors also sometimes prescribed it. Farington records how Dr Reynolds called to treat Eliza, his sister-in-law; and the eminent doctor 'reccomended Dr. Wards drop to be taken by Mrs. Miers, as an antiscorbutic, for the humour in her face. He reccomended one drop to be taken at night and one in the morning in half a pint of Sarsaparilla tea for a month.'[84] Farington wanted to know what Reynolds made of the use of such a nostrum:

> Dr. Reynolds told Eliza that Dr. Ward was a very able man whose medicines were in great repute [at] the beginning of the present Kings reign: That the use of them having become very general they were now considered as Quack medicines but He had known instances of extraordinary cures having been wrought by them. Two instances of Leprosy having been cured. He had taken Wards medicines in the early part of his life for an erruption in his face: it was while He was studying Physick, at which time He fancied himself afflicted by half the disorders He read of.[85]

Henry Fielding, whose health gave way in the 1740s, was a vocal advocate of Ward's medicines. Failing with dropsy and a multiplicity of complaints, he found no relief from 'The Duke of Portland's Medicine', as recommended to him by Ranby, the King's surgeon. Being judged a 'Bath case', he tried the waters, but equally to no avail. Berkeley's tar-water did not help, either. In desperation, he 'became the patient of Dr. Ward, who wished I had taken his advice earlier': 'By his advice I was tapped, and fourteen quarts of water drawn from my belly. The sudden relaxation which this caused, added to my enervated, emaciated habit of body, so weakened me that within two days I was thought to be falling into the agonies of death.'[86] But, in fact, he began to pull through: 'From that day I began slowly, as it were, to draw my feet out of the grave; till in two months' time I had again acquired some little degree of strength.'[87] Fielding was happy to broadcast his gratitude to Ward: 'The powers of Mr. Ward's remedies want indeed no unfair puffs of mine to give them credit.' Hence, he continued, 'Obligations to Mr. Ward I shall always confess; for I am convinced that he omitted no care in endeavouring to serve me, without any expectation or desire of fee or reward.'[88]

Yet Fielding denied that Ward's pills were a panacea: indeed, the very idea of a cure-all had to be taken with a pinch of salt – Fielding made fun of those who had thus praised Bishop Berkeley's tar-water:

But even such a panacea one of the greatest scholars and best of men did lately apprehend he had discovered. It is true, indeed, he was no physician; that is, he had not by the forms of his education acquired a right of applying his skill in the art of physic to his own private advantage; and yet, perhaps, it may be truly asserted that no other modern hath contributed so much to make his physical skill useful to the public; at least, that none hath undergone the pains of communicating this discovery in writing to the world. The reader, I think, will scarce need to be informed that the writer I mean is the late Bishop of Cloyne, in Ireland, the discovery that of the virtues of tar-water.[89]

Rather than relying on a single nostrum, Fielding attempted to integrate his recourse to Ward's medicines within a unified curative strategy. He was 'tapped a second time': 'I had one quart of water less taken from me now than before; but I bore the consequences of the operation much better. This I attributed greatly to a dose of laudanum prescribed by my surgeon. It first gave me the most delicious flow of spirits, and afterwards as comfortable a nap.'[90] He also, in the time-honoured way, moved home for the sake of his health, visiting 'a little house of mine in the country, which stands at Ealing, in the county of Middlesex, in the best air, I believe, in the whole kingdom, and far superior to that of Kensington Gravel Pits.' What made the air so good? 'The gravel is here much wider and deeper, the place higher and more open towards the south, whilst it is guarded from the north wind by a ridge of hills, and from the smells and smoke of London by its distance; which last is not the fate of Kensington, when the wind blows from any corner of the east.'[91]

Racked with gout, Fielding also patronized Dr Thomas Thompson, giving him favourable puffs in *Amelia*, in the *General Advertiser* and in the *Covent Garden Journal*.[92] Fielding's introduction of Thompson into the story of *Amelia* has been summarized thus: 'When one of Booth's children . . . was brought to the point of death by the erroneous treatment of an unnamed physician, the distracted parents summoned Dr. Thompson, who threw all the physic of his predecessors to the dogs, and by simple remedies cured the little patient in three days. Dr. Thompson's remedies also had the same marvellous effect on Sergeant Atkinson after he had been given over by several very good doctors.'[93]

Thompson was more famously patronized, however, by Alexander Pope. An ambiguous figure, and a coffee-house wit, Thompson does not seem to have sold nostrums; but apparently won himself a large practice amongst the fashionable by contradicting other practitioners and ingratiating himself with the sick through his sociable presence. He was protected by Lord Melcombe, and apparently attended Frederick, the Prince of Wales. His vocal differences of opinion with the other physicians at the prince's deathbed won him some éclat.[94]

Thompson appears to have been a dangerous practitioner, being recklessly heavy in his dosing. He gave Pope heroic medicines for what was diagnosed as dropsy; and he was widely thought to be responsible for the death of Thomas Winnington, paymaster to the forces, by excessive venesection. Horace Walpole noted Winnington's foible, as a man with 'a strong aversion to all physicians' who nevertheless put himself in Thompson's hands when 'seized with an inflammatory rheumatism, a common and known case, dangerous, but scarce ever remembered to be fatal'.

> This man [Thompson] was the oracle of Mrs Masham's sister, and what one ought to hope she did not think of, co-heiress to Mr. Winnington: his other sister as mad in Methodism as this in physic, and never saw him. This ignorant wretch [that is, the doctor], supported by the influence of the late sister, soon made such progress in fatal absurdities, as purging, bleeding, and starving him, and checking all perspiration, that his friends Mr. Fox and Sir Charles Williams absolutely insisted on calling in a physician.[95]

Instead of this leading to a confrontation between the quack and a newly-summoned regular, the reverse happened:

> Whom could they call, but Dr. Bloxhome, an intimate old friend of Mr. Winnington, and to whose house he always went once a year? This doctor, grown paralytic and indolent, gave in to everything the quack advised; Mrs. Masham all the while ranting and raving. At last, which *at last* came very speedily, they had reduced him to a total dissolution, but a diabetes and a thrush; his friends all the time distracted for him, but hindered from assisting him; so far, that the night before he died, Thompson gave him another purge, though he could not get it all down.[96]

Something little short of pandemonium then set in, when the eminent Dr Hulse was brought in 'by force':

> it was too late; and even then, when Thompson owned him lost, Mrs Masham was against trying Hulse's assistance. In short, madly or wickedly, they have murdered a man to whom nature would have allotted a far longer period, and had given a degree of abilities that were carrying that period to so great a height of lustre, as perhaps would have excelled most ministers, who in this country have owned their greatness to the greatness of their merit.[97]

In the complex dealings between regular and unusual doctors, and their mutual lay champions we see an epitome of the world of patient choice which was Georgian medicine.

Patient power – in the last resort the power of the purse – thus flourished in a symbiosis with medical pluralism in Georgian England.

During the course of the nineteenth century, it is arguable that 'medical orthodoxy' and 'medical fringe' were slowly but surely differentiated from each other more rigidly, more visibly.[98] Regulars were able to define and defend themselves behind a new stockade of legal privileges; the fringe, for its part, developed its own populist ideologies of plebeian radicalism. Such a pattern can hardly be said to apply to the eighteenth century. Both regulars and irregulars practised as individual operators, and patients habitually shopped around, drawing upon whatever forms of medical services were available and eligible. It would be historically silly to attempt to obliterate all distinction between *bona fide* healers and knavish quacks. But it would be equally misguided to be blind to the common ground shared by regulars and irregulars alike in Georgian medicine, or to deny that, in many circumstances, the sick would choose, or would feel obliged, to treat all available healers with comparable caution.[99]

PART III

Doctors

7

The Economy of Medicine

On 19 August 1737, Richard Kay of Bury in Lancashire, just embarking upon medical practice, had a nightmare: 'This last Night I dream'd that my dear Father (who under God is the chief Support and Comfort of my Life) was dead.'[1] Freudians would, of course, see disguised here the wish to murder his father, the senior partner, and run the business himself. In his dream, Kay had to soldier on: 'Patients came as usual, yea I imagin'd we had a Throng of Patients, and fanc'd myself often at Loss to know what Remedies to apply to Persons with Different Disorders; I thought after my dear Father's Death that Persons soon began to impose upon us.'[2] Perhaps a saner interpretation of the dream is that Kay was experiencing profound anxiety about the burdens of medical practice. How was he to combat disease, to know the right remedies? How was he to deal with difficult patients?

So far in this book we have examined the relations between patients and medical practitioners chiefly from the patients' point of view. Now we will switch perspective and examine the problems and opportunities facing pre-modern practitioners, assessing what Samuel Johnson called 'the fortune of physicians', in terms of practice, remuneration and social status.[3]

Patient power and disease power between them rendered the physician's lot quite precarious. His capacity to cure was often slight; and he could not count on the state and professional protection that nowadays safeguards the incorporated profession of medicine. Relations between individual practitioners were commonly acrimonious,[4] and intra-professional conflicts flared between the physicians and the apothecaries, between general practitioners, druggists and chemists, and between the regulars and quacks.[5] At all stages of a career, as William Hunter emphasized, the practitioner had to be alert to the perils of practice.

Yet, as he affirmed to his students, the astute and successful doctor had the opportunity to rise:

> I firmly believe, that it is in your power not only to *chuse*, but to *have*, which rank you please in the world. An opinion the child of spleen and idleness, has been propagated, which has done infinite prejudice to science as well as to virtue. They would have us believe that merit is neglected, and that ignorance and knavery triumph in this world. Now, in our profession it seems incontestable, that the man of abilities and diligence always succeeds. Ability, indeed, is not the only requisite; and a man may fail, who has nothing besides to recommend him; or has some great disqualifications either of head or heart. But sick people are so desirous of life and health, that they always look out for ability; and surely the man who is really able in his profession, will have the best chance of being thought so. In my opinion, a young man cannot cultivate a more important truth than this, that merit is sure of its reward in this world.[6]

BUILDING A CAREER

Beginners had to start somewhere. Some, like Kay, advanced by joining their fathers in practice, or being taken into partnership with the apothecary or surgeon to whom they had been apprenticed. Some married the daughters of their masters. At one point, it seemed as though the young William Hunter, new to London, would wed the daughter of his patron and landlord, the surgeon, James Douglas.[7] In more ways than this, Hunter's early London career offers a splendid instance of how being a leading practitioner's protégé could provide an enviable sequence of openings. Hunter moved into Douglas's home, tutored his son, took over some of his practice and ended up appropriating his specimens and research.[8]

Becoming the favourite of an eminent practitioner and stepping into his shoes was a short-cut a fortunate few were able to exploit. Young Richard Mead succeeded in buttering up the ageing John Radcliffe. He was able to inherit Radcliffe's lucrative practice, indeed his house.[9] Later in the century, young Matthew Baillie had the similar good fortune to be the nephew and surrogate son of William Hunter.[10] Such transitions were not always so smoothly effected. John Fothergill had a vast London practice. On his death in 1780, his sister brought in one Dr Hird, her nephew, from Leeds, to take it over. He soon died, to be succeeded by Dr Gilbert Thompson, who was a failure, as, successively, was a distant relation, Anthony Fothergill. At last, John Coakley Lettsom was found to fill the breach.[11]

Such patterns of advancement through personal contacts were repeated endlessly at lower levels of the profession, as the young doctor, Robert

Simpson, discovered to his delight in early nineteenth century-Bradford. Blood was obviously thicker than water: 'A poor woman of the name of Ann Dale came today to consult me', he wrote, 'all the way from Snowden in the Forest of Knaresbrough, a distance of seventeen miles, coming and returning on horseback the same day. She has been ill eight years: her complaint is dropsy dependent on diseased liver. She may become relieved but I am afraid not cured.'[12] Why had she sought out this unknown young practitioner? 'The people about Knaresbrough and in the Forest have great faith and confidence in my family as medical men. Indeed the profession of medicine seems to be hereditary in the family for we have had several generations of medical men.'[13]

Despite such breaks, Simpson found the going tough. Business was slack for a junior like himself, he groused, in a profession which already seemed to him 'quite overstocked'.[14] Setting up in independent practice was rarely easy for a young man, because established practitioners were fiercely territorial. Matthew Flinders, operating from Horncastle in Lincolnshire in the 1790s, managed to head off such 'opponents in business'.[15] And even if the young doctor attracted custom, collecting his fees might prove another matter. It was ungentlemanly, and simply self-defeating, to press genteel clients to pay (they, in turn, would have thought it vulgar to pay with alacrity). As Judith Lewis has documented, early in their careers practitioners such as Thomas Denman or Richard Croft might find themselves in straitened circumstances, because fashionable clients might be eighteen months in arrears with their bills.[16]

Yet success and reward are relative, and Simpson, despite his fears and grumbles, did not do too badly. He recorded, for example, attending a consumptive teenage girl over the course of several months and taking thirty guineas in fees.[17] The prospects of the typical young practitioner probably deteriorated somewhat during the nineteenth century. In the 1880s Conan Doyle wrote his early stories while kicking his heels as a patientless young practitioner in Southsea.[18]

To become established, contacts were needed. Some had a lucky break: the myths adorning the careers of successful physicians commonly included a fortuitous encounter with a socially distinguished patient, who, relieved or cured, then broadcast the darling young practitioner's name, thus launching his reputation. But not least, in a world where fashion increasingly ruled, it was widely believed the young doctor could succeed only if he were an astute self-publicist.

The prosperous Erasmus Darwin gave copious advice, via his son, Robert Waring Darwin, to a young man about to set up in practice in Lichfield. Of crucial importance, thought the worldly-wise physician, were visibility and sociability – one had to make one's face known:

I should advise your friend to use at first all means to get acquainted with the people of all ranks. At first a parcel of blue and red glasses at the windows might gain part of the retail business on market days, and thus get acquaintance with that class of people. I remember Mr Green, of Lichfield, who is now growing very old, once told me his retail business, by means of his show-shop and many-coloured window, produced him £100 a year. Secondly, I remember a very foolish, garrulous apothecary at Cannock, who had great business without any knowledge or even art, except that he persuaded people he kept good drugs; and this he accomplished by only one stratagem, and that was by *boring* every person who was so unfortunate as to step into his shop with the goodness of his drugs. 'Here's a fine piece of assafoetida, smell of this valarian, taste this album graecum. Dr Fungus says he never saw such a fine piece in his life'.[19]

There were other ploys, too, whereby a young practitioner could bring himself into the public eye: 'Thirdly, dining every market day at a farmers' ordinary would bring him some acquaintance, and I don't think a little impediment in his speech would at all injure him, but rather the contrary by attracting notice. Fourthly, card assemblies – I think at Lichfield surgeons are not admitted as they are here; – but they are to dancing assemblies; these therefore should be attended.'[20] Of course, self-publicizing could be carried too far, with the risk that the doctor would lose face: 'Dr K---d, I think, supported his business by perpetual boasting, like a Charlatan; this does for a blackguard character, but ill suits a more polished or modest man.'[21]

The doctor had to keep in the public eye. How best to do so, required judgement. It would not do, Erasmus Darwin thought, to get too much of a reputation as a scholar or a scientist, for thereby the young physician was in danger of being thought singular and eccentric. Darwin himself was always careful to publish his poetry anonymously – his authorship was an open secret – lest it be held against him as a physician. But he was eager for his physician son to become a Fellow of the Royal Society and to publish in the *Philosophical Transactions*.[22]

Darwin's junior contemporary, the American, Benjamin Rush, held comparable views on the art of succeeding in medicine. Departing on his travels, the medical student, John Foulke, was sent 'a few hints' by Rush to help him to win friends, influence people and learn the ways of the world. 'In your visits to great men, attend to all their peculiarities', Rush told him, 'and record them.' Then, for example, especially with an eye to the *ton*:

Attend the most celebrated hospitals. Record the recipes and modes of practice that are new or even common of each physician and surgeon, together with the most *fashionable*, I do not say powerful medicines . . .

Gain access to and cultivate an intimacy with a few eminent physicians and surgeons. You will profit more by asking them questions in a few hours than by attending hospital practice for years.[23]

Rush was nothing if not worldly wise. He recognized that the practitioners really *au fait* with the secrets of seducing the public were charlatans. If you could not beat them, you could at least take a leaf out of their book: 'Converse freely with quacks of every class and sex, such as oculists, aurists, dentists, corn cutters, cancer doctors, etc. etc. You cannot conceive how much a physician with a liberal mind may profit from a few casual and secret visits to these people.'[24]

If by such means the student grew wise in the ways of the medical world, how was he best to set up in business? Once again, Rush was ready with tips as to how the young physician should emplace himself as a respectable and respected member of the community: 'Take care of the poor', he advised

1 By becoming faithful over a few, you will become a ruler over many. When you are called to visit a poor patient, imagine you hear a voice sounding in your ears, 'Take care of him, and I will repay thee.'
2 Go regularly to some place of worship. A physician cannot be a bigot, Worship with Mohamitans rather than stay at home on Sundays.
3 Never resent an affront offered to you by a *sick* man.
4 Avoid intimacies with your patients if possible, and visit them only in sickness.[25]

Questions of financial reward were of some moment. The physician should ensure liberal reward for his labours, but be sure to avoid a reputation for being grasping:

5 Never *sue* a patient, but after a year's services get a bond from him if possible.
6 Receive as much pay as possible in goods or the produce of the country. Men have not half the attachment to these things that they have to money . . .
8 Never dispute about a bill. Always make reductions rather than quarrel with an old and profitable patient.
9 Don't insert trifling advice or services in a bill. You can incorporate them with important matters such as a pleurisy or the reduction of a bone.[26]

It was of paramount importance to wear the appearance of humanity, sobriety and concern:

10 Never make light (to a patient) of *any* case.
11 Never appear in a hurry in a sickroom, nor talk of indifferent matters till you have examined and prescribed for your patient.[27]

MOVING UP-MARKET

The profession of medicine as a whole won real advances in prestige during the course of the eighteenth century. As hinted above, the old sawbones surgeon – if such a breed ever existed in large numbers – became much rarer, and was replaced by more highly skilled operators.[28] The shop-counter apothecary turned himself into a general practitioner,[29] paying house calls, occasionally equipped with a carriage of his own and an air of gentility. In part, this rise in status reflected better training and education. Trainee practitioners exercised themselves to obtain the best possible education and credentials. Richard Kay spent a year at the London hospitals in the 1730s improving his skills, not least his operating techniques. Guy's, he thought, was the 'Fountain Head for Improvement'.[30]

The same spirit of self-improvement is conspicuous in Hampton Weekes, a medical student at St Thomas's at the turn of the nineteenth century. His account of his examinations at St Thomas's reveal testing standards of practical anatomy and therapeutics.[31] Weekes was being groomed to take over his father's practice in rural Sussex. His letters home from the hospital show he was well aware that advanced London-acquired skills would make him a highly marketable commodity on his return. He knew equally well that those were days in which a successful country practitioner could make an income running into thousands – old Henry Cline, for instance (father of a more famous son), was earning '3000 pound a year of his business, the first business in the County of Kent. Keeps a Chariot. Chaise. 5 horses 2 assistants & Apprentice'.[32] Yet to make a successful appeal to the rural gentry, or even the snobbish farmers, the practitioner needed a genteel mien. '*Suaviter in modo*' had become the passport to success for a young practitioner in a polite society.[33]

This truth applies most spectacularly to the cream of the profession, the top dozen or score of physicians and surgeons in London, a smaller number in Bath and a sprinkling of other luminaries dotted about the nation.[34] From the heyday of Radcliffe, Sloane and Mead near the beginning of the eighteenth century, fashionable physicians achieved an astonishing and hitherto unsurpassed social éclat. Those commanding clienteles amongst royalty and the aristocracy, in Parliament, in the newly fashionable West End and, not least, amongst literary London circles, became famous and rich, earning incomes of £5000 a year or more, equivalent to the rent-roll of a really substantial member of the gentry. Their names were listed in publications such as the *Royal Kalendar* just as, later, provincial physicians were listed in numerous trade directories. Some became household names. At the end of the Georgian era, Sydney Smith was staying with Sir Henry Holland, perhaps the leading society physician of his time: 'In coming home last week from a dinner party our Carriage was stopped and as I was preparing my Watch and Money a man put his head in the Window and said, We want Dr Holland. They took him out and we have heard nothing of him since; we think of advertising.'[35]

THE ELITE

How did the cream of the Georgian doctors achieve fame and glory hitherto beyond the grasp of medical men? Their success did not stem from advances in medical science or from spectacular breakthroughs in therapeutics. They were rather valued, above all, as clinicians. Physicians such as John Fothergill, John Coakley Lettsom, William Heberden and Matthew Baillie built glowing reputations as expert diagnosticians and sympathetic case managers; they were trusted judges of both syndromes and clients.[36] Joseph Farington thus recorded Dr Lawrence's favourable comments upon Baillie: 'Lawrence came . . . He was at Mr. John Angerstein's yesterday when Dr. Baillie came to see Mr. Lock who, with His family, is there. He observed that at once you see that Dr. Baillie is a man of a strong & clear understanding.'[37] How did one discern this from his clinical approach?

> Mr. Lock's illness commenced with a cold & cough, which has been attended with a fever & loss of appetite. – Dr. Baillie said That considering His time of life, 76 – or 7, – there was danger. Dr. Baillie spoke concisely but in a few words conveyed a clear meaning. He sd. that the fever must *have its way*; that medicine could do nothing against it, but that medicine might do good by counteracting some of the effects of fever. If the Bowels shd. be disordered, medicine might give relief.[38]

London doctors thus formed an elite, exercising sway not because of statutory authority but because of celebrity. This corps consolidated its prestige and enhanced its fortunes as the century wore on. Farington was informed that near the beginning of the century 'Dr Mead only recd. half-guinea fees', and that in Mead's day the physicians used to sit around in coffee-houses and taverns listening to apothecaries' accounts of cases, whereupon they would prescribe, sometimes hardly sober.[39] Thus the demeanour of the fashionable physicians of the early Georgian age was retrospectively perceived to have been rather indecorous, over-familiar and mercenary. Things had changed. For the sub-text of Farington's tale was that such practices would have been regarded as utterly undignified – indeed, inimical to good medical practice – by the age of William Hunter or Baillie. Imagine the sober Quaker, Lettsom, making snap diagnoses amid the hubbub of a coffee-house. By the close of the century, good practice and good form required that physicians would always visit patients personally – and, incidentally, thereby obtain fatter fees.

The elite amongst the physicians certainly cultivated social visibility. Sloane became President, first of the College of Physicians and later of the Royal Society, and the greatest dilettante of the age. He bequeathed his collections to form the core of the British Museum.[40] Richard Mead gathered one of the largest private libraries in London.[41] Both were noted for their soirées, encompassing the fashionable, literary and intellectual worlds. Political allegiance and patronage were probably important too in the building of careers. The courtly Mead did far better than John Freind in early Hanoverian times, partly because he was a staunch Whig, whereas Freind was Jacobitical. Mead quickly rose to become court physician. Half a century later, physicians were independently doing so well with their private practices that they might even turn their noses up at that honour. Thus, William Heberden had the temerity to decline such an appointment under George III; attendance at Kew, he feared, would detain him too much from his fashionable Town practice.[42]

Physicians made their mark upon the metropolitan social scene. Early in the century in particular, some – notably John Arbuthnot – shone amongst the wits;[43] others won reputations as poets, such as Samuel Garth and Mark Akenside, or were active in the coffee-house and clubbish sets of the world of letters.[44] Still others cultivated science, or like Fothergill and Lettsom, championed the cause of social betterment, humanitarianism and reform.[45]

And some index of the growing public prominence of top doctors is afforded by the barrage of satire being fired against their fame, wealth, pomp and pretensions.[46] Physicians were lampooned for allegedly deploying devious devices for keeping themselves in the public eye – for example, being noisily called out of church on a Sunday for purely fictitious emergency cases, and then hurtling around London in their ostentatious chariots. When the top physician, Sir Samuel Garth, published his *Dispensary*, a mock heroic epic, satirizing the titanic struggles fought between the College of Physicians and the Society of Apothecaries over the establishment of a free public dispensary for the poor, it immediately went through multiple editions: medical politics became the talk of the town.[47]

Later in the century, a burlesque against the Quaker, John Coakley Lettsom, captured that hypocritical mélange of professional high-mindedness and mercenary ambition that critics found offensive amongst late-Georgian physicians. This exposé of 'Dr Wriggle', subtitled 'The Art of Rising in Physic', dissected the ploys to which top doctors allegedly resorted to ensure the limelight upon the medical stage:

> Dr. Wriggle has the skill to cover an artful and designing disposition, with the utmost semblance of gravity and simplicity. He passes with the public for a man of humanity and deep learning; and has had the address to work himself into considerable practice by his subtle conduct . . .
>
> I shall not trouble you with a recital of his intriguing with Apothecaries and nurses, of being called out from company; and a long catalogue of other artifices (all of which he has adopted with success), but proceed directly to what may properly be called *his own*.
>
> His first great maxim is: '*Bring your name before the public; it will, by degrees, become familiar to them and they will at length think you a man of consequence.*' For this purpose, the doctor contrives to have his name appear every now and then in paragraphs in the newspapers which everybody reads.[48]

The author went on to offer instances of such gratuitous, self-interested, self-promoting newspaper puffery:

> 'Yesterday as Dr. Wriggle was returning *in his chariot* from such a place, he was attacked by two highwaymen, who demanded his money etc', – Or,
>
> 'On Wednesday last, as Dr. Wriggle and his lady, etc'. But Dr. Wriggle was never robbed.
>
> No. It was a mere invention; a pretext *for bringing his name before the public*. There are a variety of other methods by which a man may *bring his name before the public* in the newspapers, all which Dr. Wriggle has successfully employed.
>
> His second great maxim is : 'Let everything about you speak learning and gravity'.
>
> The hall of the Doctor's house, for example, is a perfect *museum*. A patient no sooner has the street door opened to him than he is struck with the appearance of mosses, shells, dried foreign animals and the like. He is led immediately to conclude that the Doctor, like Solomon, is a very *deep* man, as indeed he is in *one* sense of the word.[49]

Such satires were, evidently, indirect tributes to the success of the medical elite in securing their place in the sun during the Georgian age. Great physicians became associated in the public mind with great men: Sir Walter Farquhar, for example, was Pitt the Younger's physician, while Sir Richard Warren was the darling of the Whig grandees. And the public gossiped about physicians and their bank-balances much as people might discuss movie stars today. 'R. Price's I dined at. Much conversation abt. the Physicians of London', recorded Farington:

Dr. Baillie allowed to be first in practise, & makes probably £10,000 a
yr. – Sir Walter Farquhar had a run for sometime, being supported by
the Duchess of Gordon, – Mr. Pitt etc. – but He is now only in the 3rd.
or 4th. line. – He never had the opinion of the other Physicians with
Him, & it has been observed that unless a Physician is supported in His
reputation by the acknowledgement of his claim by the Corps of Physician
His reputation will only be temporary. – Dr. Reynolds was sd. to have
[a] good practise, – to be abt. the 3rd. or 4th.[50]

THE RANK AND FILE

It was not only the medical elite that lived in the broad sunshine of life
during the long eighteenth century. Times were good, as contemporaries
recognized, for smaller fry as well. In his *London Tradesman*, Robert
Campbell paraded the opportunities: 'An ingenious surgeon, let him be
cast on any corner of earth, with but his case of instruments in his
pocket, he may live where most other professions may starve.'[51]
   Apothecaries, too, seemed to be enjoying the Georgian pudding time.
Parson Woodforde recorded, perhaps with a trace of disdain, that widow
Davy was in the thick of a 'love affair' with a Mr Rand, 'who is
distracted after her'. 'Mr Rand is a man of very good fortune, keeps a
carriage and' – the crunch – 'is an Apothecary and has great Business.'[52]
What times! For an apothecary to keep a carriage and attract a rich
widow would have been scarcely thinkable in 1660, but had become
commonplace by the late eighteenth century. In fact, apothecaries seem
to have been lucky in love. Lady Sarah Lennox reported the bizarre
match between Lady Camilla Fleming and 'a Bath apothecary [who
wore] a true apothecary's wig'.[53]
   The growing affluence and airs of the rank-and-file of the profession
excited astonishment and envy. Adam Smith remarked that 'apothecaries'
profit is become a by-word, denoting something uncommonly extravagant'. Yet, as a social observer and economist, he saw fit to defend
them: 'This great profit, however, is frequently no more than the
reasonable wages of labour. The skill of an apothecary is a much nicer
and more delicate matter than that of any artificer whatever; and the
trust which is reposed in him is of much greater importance.'[54] In any
case, the apothecary, having now become a general practitioner to many
classes, had become utterly socially indispensable: 'He is the physician
to the poor in all cases, and of the rich when the distress is not very
great. His reward, therefore, ought to be suitable to his skill and trust,
and it arises generally from the price at which he sells his drugs.'[55]
Assuredly, these drugs might cost the apothecary rather little wholesale

(perhaps 'thirty or forty pounds'), whereas he might be able to sell them 'for three or four hundred, or at a thousand per cent profit'. This seemed extravagant but: 'This may frequently be no more than the reasonable wages of his labour charged, in the only way he can charge them, upon the price of his drugs. The greater part of the apparent profit is wages disguised in the garb of profit.'[56] Though a physician, Thomas Percival endorsed the wisdom of Smith's account: the public could not expect skilful general practitioners without paying the price.[57]

The humble surgeon-apothecary thrived by making himself indispensable in providing the entire range of services demanded by the medical consumer.[58] In an analysis both descriptive and prescriptive, James Nelson emphasized that physicians, being expensive, were bound to be called in only after careful consideration. In such circumstances, people summoned the apothecary to do the physician's job, and perhaps, in his down-to-earth way, he did it better:

> While the Physician is labouring at Theories, the Apothecary is perhaps deeply immers'd in Practice: and as all allow that nice Observation is of vast Use in Physic, while the one is searching into Causes, the other, if he improves as he ought the Opportunities he is furnished with, gains a Knowledge of Effects. Hence it appears, that an Apothecary is capable of being, not merely an useful, but a valuable Man to Society.[59]

The great virtue of apothecaries lay in being ready, willing and able to perform all manner of medical-social functions which physicians would not, or could not:

> Who is it that gives the Patient that close Attendance he frequently wants, but the Apothecary? Who is it that has the Trouble of applying Leeches, of applying dressing Blisters, of administering Vomits, etc. of watching the various Changes that arise, and of running in Pursuit of the Doctor to check some threatening Symptom, but the Apothecary? And who is it, in fine, that on every Emergency, in every real or fancied Danger, is called out of his Bed to administer some speedy Relief, or appease some groundless Fears of the Patient, or their Friends, but the Apothecary?[60]

Thus presented, the new-style surgeon-apothecary seemed perfectly tailored to meet the wide-ranging needs of a public who could afford a single, reasonably cheap, multi-purpose practitioner. Nelson tendered clear advice as to the medical pecking-order: 'Those who are rich, let them at once send for the Physician, especially if it be a Matter of Moment; . . . those who cannot reach the best, let them take the next best . . . employ a good Apothecary.'[61]

Nevertheless, these developments were greeted with mixed feelings, as Smith's parrying of the outrage against apothecaries' profits shows. Medicines were being prescribed in ever greater quantities. As Loudon has shown, it was not unknown for a family's apothecaries' bills to exceed a hundred pounds a year.[62] In his *Medical Ethics*, Percival stressed that it would be wrong for physicians and surgeons to be niggardly with drugs, and it seems they heeded his advice.[63] One consequence of the rising status of the medical profession was a growing public concern against physician-inaugurated, apothecary-engineered overdosing.[64]

MEDICAL ENTREPRENEURS

Eighteenth-century doctors were not ashamed to display an entrepreneurial bent. The Prussian traveller, Von Archenholz, was staggered at the commercial aggressiveness evident in the advertisements of English practitioners: 'One person informs you that his Mad-House is at your service; a second keeps a boarding-house for idiots; a good natured man-midwife pays the utmost attention to his ladies in certain situations, and promises to use the most scrupulous secrecy. Physicians offer to cure you of all manner of disorders, for a mere trifle.'[65]

The development of smallpox inoculation offered another medical opportunity for easy profits. 'Inoculation has arrived at its "ne plus ultra" in England', proclaimed young Benjamin Rush, noting that the Sutton family had done much to make it safe, successful and profitable.[66] They had set up private hospitals for wealthy inoculees.[67] Inoculation became a flourishing trade, because there were plenty of customers to treat and doctors tailored fees to suit individual pockets. Parson Woodforde paid for his whole household to be inoculated *en masse*, and was pleased to find he could have four done for a guinea. The Revd John Penrose, recuperating in Bath, noted, by contrast, that the Hertfordshire practitioner, Thomas Dimsdale, charged no less than five guineas to inoculate a gentleman.[68]

The Sutton family – originally humble Suffolk surgeons – offers a good illustration of Georgian medical entrepreneurship. Lady Mary Coke saw one of Robert Sutton's sons at close quarters, operating in Paris just when Louis XV was apparently dying of smallpox at Versailles: 'When the physicians began to despair they advised sending for Sutton . . . He arrived & offer'd to give a remedy, which he said had hitherto been successful in very desperate cases.'[69] Sutton obviously had a secret nostrum. Mention of it immediately precipitated a crisis of authority. Would the provincial surgeon be allowed to barge into the French Court with its complex hierarchy of medical power? 'The King's physicians told him he must not give it unless he wou'd acquaint them with the ingredients: this Sutton refused, saying the secret was his fortune, &

return'd immediately to Paris.'[70] Thereafter, a game of bluff and counter-bluff was played with the nostrum-monger.

> *Monday.* – Sutton was again sent for this morning, & they ofer'd him any sum of money if he wd communicate the composition of the medicine he proposed giving to the King; he nobly answer'd [is Lady Mary being ironical?] he wou'd not sell the secret for a million, but that as the King's life was in question he wou'd tell the first physician the ingredients, provided he wou'd take a solemn oath not to reveal it. This was immediately consented to; the secret communicated . . .[71]

So far so good, but 'the physician then desired to know the quantities of each ingredient, which Sutton told him was not in his power to tell him, as the medicine was prepared by his Brother. This again was the objection to their permitting the King to take it, tho' they all thought he had but a few hours to live . . .'[72]

Did people deprecate Sutton's sharp practice, or rather admire his effrontery in trying to preserve the secret of his nostrum? Maintaining 'industrial secrets' in drugs was commonly practised. There were no overwhelming ethical grounds against reputable doctors selling nostrums or patenting medicines. 'In Dr James's time', Francis Newbury claimed, 'it was not considered derogatory in the profession to sell a nostrum. Sir Hans Sloane, the President of the Royal Society, vended an eye salve, and Dr Mead, the Court Physician, sold a nostrum which it was pretended would cure the bite of a mad dog.'[73] Robert James, as mentioned above, was the originator of the most widely used patent medicine of the age – some two million doses were sold in twenty years.[74] In the early nineteenth century, Thomas Bakewell, the respected proprietor of a lunatic asylum in Staffordshire, boasted a specific against insanity, which, he claimed, he was duty-bound not to reveal to the public, since he had overriding duties to preserve his family income.[75]

Doctors proved adroit self-publicizers, learning from the tricks of the quacks. William Rowley, an Oxford MD and author of numerous popular medical works, was notorious for parading his name before the public. 'A few days since', began a newspaper story,

> Mr. Hankey, a gentleman of considerable fortune in Harley-street, Cavendish Square, swallowed, by an unfortunate mistake, a tea-cup full of Goulard's extract of lead, one of the most destructive and certain poisons in nature. Mr. Hankey, it seems, sustained himself with an uncommon firmness under this alarming situation, expecting immediate death, from which, however, he has been preserved by the skilful assistance of Dr. Rowley, an eminent physician of the same street; and we have the pleasure to inform the public, Mr. Hankey is now perfectly recovered.[76]

Doubtless such an item was inserted by Rowley or his friends.

FEES AND INCOMES

The rising status of medicos found expression in the growing capacity of the profession to command substantial fees. There is no 'country in the world', thought Lady Mary Wortley Montagu, 'where the doctors raise such immense fortunes'.[77] 'Sir Andrew Fountain lies still extremely ill', Swift told Stella in 1711, 'it costs him ten guineas a day to doctors, surgeons and apothecaries, and has done so these three weeks.'[78] Certain cases became notorious. Around 1730, William Pulteney, later the Earl of Bath, was ill of a pleuretic fever. According to Timbs:

> This illness cost him an expense of 750 guineas for physicians; . . . Dr. Hope, Dr. Swynsen, and other physicians from Stafford, Lichfield, and Derby, were called in, and carried off about 250 guineas of the patient's money, leaving the malady just where they found it. Dr. Friend went down post from London, with Mrs. Pulteney, and received 300 guineas for the journey. Dr. Boxholm went from Oxford, and received 200 guineas. When these two physicians, who were Pulteney's particular friends, arrived, they found his case to be quite desperate, and gave him over, saying that everything had been done that could be done.[79]

Pulteney was said finally to have recovered by 'drinking small beer'.

Doctors' greed riled patients. Writing from the Newfoundland fishing grounds near the close of the eighteenth century, Aaron Thomas remarked on what seemed to him a grasping practice 'which destroys that little dignity we sometimes find attached to the Sons of Galen':

> It is a rule with the doctors for to give you Medicines for the Fishing or Summer Season. Ill or well the money must be paid at the Fall of the year. You enter your name on the Doctor's book on arrival and, if he doth not see you untill the close of the year, you pay all the same. If you propose to stop all the year round you must pay 10/- under the same regulation as the first. Having made these premizes, I have to mention that part of the business which reflects disgrace on these disciples of Warwick Lane.[80]

It was, of course, a money-conscious age, but the fees of physicians seem to have excited a peculiar fascination throughout the Georgian century: the wealth of Radcliffe or of Astley Cooper remained perennial talking points.[81] Certain practitioners won reputations for being notably mercenary. Gossip had it that when Richard Warren looked at his tongue in the mirror in the morning, he transferred a guinea from one pocket to another. Likewise, it was said that one could always recognize Dr Caleb Parry walking along the street in Bath from the sound of the guineas jingling in his pocket.[82] The wealth of physicians was exciting public concern and even jealousy.

Incomes were certainly on the rise. A graduate physician, Claver Morris, operating in Wells at the turn of the eighteenth century, seems to have been able to charge his better-class clients a standard guinea per consultation: others paid half a guinea, as his account book shows:[83]

June 16	Of Captain Piers of Wells a Guinea . . . 01–01–06.
1690	
Oct: 16	Of Mr Grove of Zeales . . . 01–01–06.
17	Of ye Right Honourable ye Lady Viscountess Weymouth . . . 01–01–06.
1691	
May 12	Of Colonel St Loe of Little Fontmell in Dorst . . . 03–04–06.
June 6	Of a Woman yt would not be known . . . 00–10–06.
1692	
May 23	Of My Lord Bp Kidder . . . 01–01–06.
May 24	Of Mr Gravener of Vbley . . . 00–10–06.
Sept: 12	Of Mine Heere Copeman . . . 01–01–06.

Morris's income remained modest, however, never rising above a couple of hundred pounds a year, because he seems to have had few patients. But, as Loudon has shown, ordinary surgeons were earning considerably more than Morris by the close of the eighteenth century.[84] This was not because individual fees increased but because doctors were being called in more commonly for a wider range of conditions and a greater number of times per illness. When Thomas Turner's wife was gravely ill, she was treated by a physician, Dr Poole, and also by the local surgeon-apothecary, Mr Stone. On occasions, Poole would drop by on his own initiative, to see how his patient was doing, and charge half a guinea for his services. Turner's blood boiled: 'Really a fine thing it is to be a physician who can charge just as they please and not be culpable according to any human law.'[85] Some practitioners generated a great deal of business (though doctors always claimed to be busy: Dr Denton wrote to Ralph Verney in 1648, 'I have since thursday last . . . beene almost confounded with business').[86] It was said that, during an influenza empidemic in Bath, Caleb Parry treated 120 people in two days.[87]

Being busy, as Erasmus Darwin would have said, was good for business. Doctors grew more socially visible, assuming larger parts in the community. Many Georgian doctors were prominent in the voluntary hospital movement,[88] others were conspicuous in local charities. Leaders of public conscience, they often promoted improvements and reform in fields such as education and the care of unfortunates.[89] In the latter half of the century, they contributed actively to cultural movements such as the Literary and Philosophical Societies.[90] At a humbler level, surgeons and apothecaries became increasingly involved in the community, through working as Poor Law surgeons.[91]

As Geoffrey Holmes rightly perceived, during the eighteenth century the common doctor began to claim his place in modern society. This was not, *pace* the assertions of much medical sociology, through the claims of professional collective muscle power, but through a capacity to appeal to the individual and the community.[92] There may be much to be said for Holmes's implied view that medicine became a successful profession (in the rather broad traditional sense of occupation) before it invested vast efforts in the nineteenth century in more formal 'professionalizing' strategies. There certainly appears a marked contrast between Georgian England, where practitioners undoubtedly throve by grasping market opportunities with both hands, and the far more limited inroads made by orthodox practitioners in *ancien régime* France where stricter corporate control kept practitioners scarcer, more aloof and pricier, and thereby guaranteed irregulars a place in the sun.[93]

8

The Doctors' Point of View

In earlier chapters we have examined, chiefly from the patient's point of view, the dynamics of clinical interaction during the long eighteenth century. We argued that questions of choice, confidence, trust and power often weighed more heavily in forging and modifying such ties than supposedly 'objective' considerations of 'correct' therapy as adjudged by medico-scientific criteria. The sick – those footing the bills – rarely resigned their health and lives unequivocally into doctors' hands, and commonly skirmished with them over diagnosis and treatment.

The previous chapter surveyed the socio-economics of medical practice in Georgian England. Here, we proceed to examine how doctors themselves negotiated the personal, face-to-face aspects of this unstable and potentially explosive world of patient power, patient protest and perhaps patient control – how they tried to achieve an ascendancy over their patients.

DOCTORS' DISTASTE

Doctors were sick of the scurvy treatment their patients accorded them. 'The ten leapers praid aloud in trouble', complained the Stratford practitioner, John Ward, 'but they being once cured, nine in ten are as mute as fishes; so itt is with physitians' patients, they promise fair till they are cured, but then never so much as come back and thank you.'[1] No sooner was a sick man healed, doctors complained, than the physician was forgotten: 'God and the Doctor we do both adore – Just on the brink of danger, — not before – The danger o'er, both are alike requited, – God is forgotten, and the Doctor slighted.'[2] In the no-nonsense idiom of the eighteenth century, George Cheyne rang the changes on the same indictment. 'Fine folks', he remarked, 'use their physician as they do their laundresses, send their linen to them for it only to be dirtied again.' It was hardly flattering for a physician to be regarded as such a menial.[3]

The medical profession felt continual irritation at the residual power lodged with the laity and the degree to which they had to humour lay foibles. The public at large were medically ignorant, many doctors stated or implied, yet they puffed themselves up with a simulacrum of medical knowledge, pretending to be what James Makittrick Adair called 'lady and gentlemen doctors'.[4] In his *Domestic Medicine* (1769), a work aimed to dispel some of that ignorance, William Buchan painted a picture of the children's nurse, perpetually with her 'Godfrey's cordials, Daffy's elixirs &c. at hand' to pacify her infant charges, sending them at best into a narcotic haze, at worst into oblivion.[5] But ignorant self-dosing was not restricted, it was alleged, to the uneducated. Consider 'persons of the nervous temperament' with sedentary occupations. Such people, argued the Newcastle practitioner, Thomas Trotter, typically developed 'a constipated state of body', which they then hoped to relieve by foolish self-dosing with laxatives. The consequences of such 'frequent recourse to medicine for opening the bowels' were dire: 'Some of the most drastic purgatives, such as aloes and scammony, come at last to be in common use with them. This custom soon begets a habit; when the bowels are brought to that torpor and inactivity as never to be moved without the aid of a drug.'[6] Self-dosing thereby led to habituation and addiction.

The laity, so doctors such as Thomas Beddoes alleged, just as easily addicted themselves also to medical pretensions, becoming infatuated with quack remedies, old wives' tales and a bogus lay wisdom:[7] 'The hasty cure', judged Buchan, 'turns out to be no cure at all.'[8] Adair believed, with Pope, that a little learning was a dangerous thing. 'The credulity of mankind in regard to medicine, is truly astonishing', he noted in a phrase perhaps more ambiguous than he intended: 'Even those who affect to be sceptical in other matters are the easy dupes of every pretender to a secret medicine: they will neglect the advice of the most skilful physician.'[9] The answer as Buchan saw it, was not still further to restrict lay medical knowledge – a self-defeating strategy – but to broadcast proper understanding more effectively.[10]

Physicians did not merely complain about lay medical know-alls; they feared improper relations between their clients and other branches of the profession. One of Bernard Mandeville's *bêtes noires* was the duplicity of apothecaries in exploiting patient gullibility and foisting unnecessary and harmful medication upon them. For example, an apothecary would make house-calls on spec:

There happened to be nobody at home but children and servants who from the highest to the lowest were all in perfect health; if here he came for business (you'll say) he was disappointed; but you are mistaken; the courteous gentleman with an engaging familiarity accosts every servant in the house and puts off a purge to the cook, a vomit to the butcher, a box of pills to one of the footmen, and a pot of lucatellus balm to old Nurse.[11]

Not even the children were spared the attentions of such a leech:

The children absolutely refused to take any physic . . . [but] at last he coaxes the little master into the use of a charming dentifrice and a sweet scented collyrium to rinse his mouth with after it . . . to pretty miss he'll send a lotion for her hair and a paste for her hands . . . with a beauty wash for their maid that assisted in the pursuit of them . . . The children are pleased, the servants commend him, my lady is obliged to him . . . and probably drives to thank him for the care he took of her family in her absence.[12]

It was also implied that the sick themselves were just as eager, rather improperly, to consult with apothecaries rather than physicians in the first instance, in order to save money. And if apothecaries could thus be a menace, no less dangerous (doctors moaned) were those practitioners who churned out irresponsible hack-works of medical popularization, deadlier than a lancet in the wrong hands. 'The Lady and Gentlemen Doctors' (that is, well-meaning amateur healers, who killed by kindness), complained James Makittrick Adair, 'since the publication of some popular medical books, proceed with more confidence in their private practice than their predecessors; as deeming those books sufficient guides in every case that can occur; and when they deign to consult a physician or apothecary, it is rather with an expectation of having their medical sagacity applauded, than their errors corrected.'[13] Such Ladies Bountiful, it was alleged, regarded practising their own medical skills on their servants as an act of charity. As a result, there were many who 'seldom ask my advice', complained Edward Jenner (rural general practitioner as well as pioneer of vaccination), 'until things come to extremes', because first they 'go to so-and-so, who has "a desperate good receipt"'.[14]

'I knew a Gentlewoman', claimed the anonymous author of *Letters to a Sick Friend* (1682), 'who coming to visit a sick Friend, much blamed the Doctors Prescriptions, and perswaded the Patient to the use of a Pill, which she found commended in a printed Bill.' It proved a disaster: 'he took it, and dyed that night: which so troubled the Gentlewomans mind, for medling without just call, that it cost her Husband ten pounds to prevent her real distraction; she is not as yet fit to be left alone.'[15] How could this be charity? A truly philanthropic gesture towards the poorer classes, the *Letters* went on to argue, would be to 'gratifie Physitians for their advice, and to be at the charge of their Medicines when prescribed by the Learned'.[16] Worse still, however, was the ready recourse the sick made to quacks. Secret medicines were an unmitigated evil 'Sir, let me tell you, I have often found those kind of Medicines but meer Cheats, and Springes to catch Woodcocks; and yet men will not learn Wisdom, until the dust of the Grave, that Powder of Experience, be cast in their Eyes. He that will venture his life with the use of such a Medicine, will give the world cause to suspect, he stands in need of a large dose of Hellebore.'[17]

Only when charlatans had thoroughly destroyed their health did the sick finally and sheepishly apply to the regular physician – but, all too often, too late. In 1684 Mr. Duke's daughter, of St Mary Axe in the City of London, went into a decline. Foolishly (reported the physician, Richard Morton), 'the Spring following, by the Prescription of some Empirick, she took a *Vomit*, and after that I know not what *Steel* Medicines, but without any Advantage' (steel was meant to strengthen). The failure of all such nauseous quack remedies caused her to reject regular medicines for two years, by which time she had sunk into an utter consumption. Morton was then called in, and, heroically, by the use of proper medicines, *almost* saved her life.[18]

Apart from the fact that such empirical healers were typically hucksters, physicians claimed the very basis of treatment via instant nostrums was unsound, for no medicine could radically cure unless it was carefully tailored to the precise needs of the particular patient, calculated through an intimate knowledge of his constitution. Thus fly-by-night itinerants, with their ready-mix panaceas, at best wrought a superficial amelioration, but all too often in the process masked the deterioration of a mild disease into a severe one. 'The retained Physician hath been long acquainted with the Patients constitution and distempers', argued *Letters to a Sick Friend*, 'and hath often relieved him'. The itinerant, by contrast, 'hath no acquaintance with the Patient but . . . shall pretend to great skill in such or such a disease, and yet knows nothing but only how to kill people dexterously.'[19] What appalling harm the irresponsible quack could do, especially through transforming minor disorders into grave and chronic ones! 'If violent distempers surprize the brain and cause want of sleep, in comes a loving Friend and recommends Syrup of *Poppies* or else some other sleeping medicine, which Translates the Morbifick humour to the Brain, causing a Phrensie or such a sleep which only the last Trumpet can awake.'[20]

If quacks and well-meaning meddlers were widely condemned, the other pet hate was the disobedient patient: 'Many sick Patients are like the *Babel* Builders, . . . if the repetition of a Medicine be requisite, the

Patient is presently weary: as if a wound could be cured immediately upon the Application of a Plaister, before it hath lain a quarter of an hour[21] – and then, when an instant cure is not obtained, the patient leaps to blame the doctor,' 'as if the Cook were to be blamed because a Morsel of Meat doth not allay hunger, when it may be a pound is requisite.'[22] The sick had only themselves to blame for their fate: 'The Failing is in the *Patient* himself', George Cheyne accused, 'who will not, or cannot *deny himself* for a Time sufficient to bring about the Cure.'[23]

At the root of all these evils, it was argued, lay the vulgar, demotic spirit of the age, encouraging the silly idea that everyman could be an expert. 'Every individual of the least penetration', grumbled Willich, 'now claims the privilege of being his own physician.'[24] Health was too important, too delicate, to be left entirely to the laity. Hence, doctors standardly argued that the duty of the sick – under many circumstances at least – was to consult a regular doctor for sound advice.[25]

DOCTORS ACQUIESCE

Doctors wrote millions of words along these lines, berating the ignorant folly of headstrong self-medicators and the intrigues of quacks and others. Such self-righteous indignation helped them let off steam, at least. Nevertheless, the medical profession lived in the real world. In practice, therefore, doctors acquiesced in patient power, for the very pragmatic reason that George Bernard Shaw formulated over a century later: 'the doctor learns that if he gets ahead of the superstitions of his patients he is a ruined man; and the result is that he instinctively takes care not to get ahead of them. That is why all the changes come from the laity.'[26] The practitioner who would not placate his patients would end up with none. As Lydgate, over-zealous for modern medical science, was told, 'a young doctor . . . has to please his patients in Middlemarch.'[27] The foibles of the sick had to be taken into account, argued Thomas Percival: humanity and prudence advised it, but it also made good therapeutic sense. Not least, he averred, 'the *feelings* and *emotions* of the patients, under critical circumstances, require to be known and to be attended to no less than the symptoms of their diseases.' 'Thus, extreme *timidity*, with respect to venaesection, contraindicates its use, in certain cases and constitutions. Even the prejudices of the sick are not to be condemned or opposed with harshness. For though silenced by authority, they will operate secretly and forcibly on the mind, creating fear, anxiety and watchfulness.'[28]

Thus there was a further reason why the astute physician indulged the ways and whims of his more prestigious patients. In an age of patronage, the doctor owed his standing not, as perhaps today, to his reputation amongst his peers, but to his public fame. It was therefore paramount to the practitioner that he should ingratiate himself with polite society.

Hence, career manuals and works of medical ethics constantly reminded young doctors of the influence wielded by paying patients. It was within their power to initiate multiple consultations or change their physician as they would change their milliner – so long as they did so genteelly. Such rights did not extend all down the social scale. Thomas Percival emphasized that charity patients in hospitals could not expect to choose or change their physician, and would have to accept whatever medication was given them, without cavill.[29] Indeed, doctors seem to have felt entitled to decline attendance upon undesirable patients. Claver Morris 'refus'd to have anything to do with' a certain Mrs Franklin, 'dangerously ill of the Small-pox', she being a 'vicious woman' (was it her tongue or her morals, or did she not pay her bills?).[30] One of Harriet Martineau's indictments against regular doctors stemmed from an occasion when physicians refused to visit a sick baby after a friend of hers had given it mesmeric treatment.[31]

There is a larger sense in which the medical profession necessarily acquiesced in an active lay sickness culture: for they were themselves partly responsible for creating and sustaining it in the first place. Not only did scores of medical men write books and pamphlets targeted at the public, laying medicine open (to some degree at least) to popular understanding. But they sometimes specifically whipped up public resentment against the apparently restrictive practices of the profession. 'The period is not yet arrived when medical publications may be addressed to the people with impunity', contended the impassioned William Buchan, alleging that he had been the target of a 'spirit of persecution' from some official quarters for his temerity in writing *Domestic Medicine*: 'In all probability some ages will elapse before physicians can be convinced that their art will never be truly honourable, nor extensively useful, till its doctrines are laid open, and candidly submitted to the examination of all men.'[32] Buchan was convinced that the genuine interests of the medical profession lay in keeping the laity well informed. Only thus would the competition of quackery be defeated and the true cause of health advanced: 'While disguise of any kind is practised, quackery will prevail, and medicine will be little better than a piece of mummery.'[33]

Of course, it was a Herculean task, even a forlorn hope, for doctors to try to educate the laity in matters of health without risking usurpation of their own functions and dignity. Buchan argued how extensively the laity should take health care into their own hands, yet he also tried to draw the line:

> Surely the man who writes a catechism does not intend to qualify his readers for becoming doctors in divinity; yet such is the folly of men, or rather the prejudice of the faculty, that whoever attempts to throw a little light on the public mind, with regard to diseases, is immediately branded with the intention of making every man a physician. Would to God that physicians were so easily made! To be a physician is the business of a man's life, and the candid will confess that, to the last, he has still much to learn.[34]

In a Protestant nation, which had long since proclaimed the priesthood of all believers, this rang somewhat hollow.

MEDICAL MANIPULATION

In Britain, the medical profession enjoyed scant statutory powers protected by legislation. Doctors were typically dependent upon paying patients, many of whom would be fickle, few of whom would prove prompt payers. In such circumstances, medical authority had to be asserted indirectly, largely through custom, convention and civility, through forces of personality and a skilful and even theatrical capacity to exploit the emotional possibilities of sickness. The prime way practitioners coped with their somewhat ambiguous situation in face-to-face clinical encounters was through personal management. They had to cultivate arts of probing below the surface of difficult and demanding patients, but in such a way as not to erode confidence. In taking a history, for example, the doctor had to listen to the explicit account the patient offered. But it was equally important to read between the lines, gathering vital information from the apparently chance remark. Anna Seward was generally critical of Erasmus Darwin as a browbeating bully of a man; nevertheless, she admired him for his penetrating clinical acumen. 'Extreme was his scepticism to human truth', she reported: 'From that cause he often disregarded the accounts his patients gave of themselves, and rather chose to collect his information by indirect inquiry and by cross-examining them, than from their voluntary testimony. That distrust and that habit were probably favourable to his skill in discovering the origin of diseases, and thence to his preeminent success in effecting their cure.'[35] Even so, Miss Seward thought Darwin only half successful because he was needlessly blunt with his patients: 'apt to wound the ingenuous and confiding spirit, whether seeking his medical assistance, or his counsel as a friend. Perhaps this proneness to suspicion mingled too much of art in his wisdom.'[36] Mary Anne

Schimmelpenninck, by contrast, believed that Darwin's bold and frank manner was spot on, inspiring confidence in his patients: 'The doctor's eye was deeply sagacious, the most so I think of any eye I remember ever to have seen; and I can conceive that no patient consulted Dr. Darwin who, so far as intelligence was concerned, was not inspired with confidence in beholding him: his observation was most keen; he constantly detected disease, from his sagacious observation of symptoms apparently so slight as to be unobserved by other doctors.'[37]

There were many ways to angle for ascendency over a patient. A doctor could sometimes impress through declining to prescribe and refusing to take a fee – proving his high-minded superiority to mere mercenary matters. 'Fothergill came, would not write, said go on as usual, etc; he would take no fee', recorded John Baker. Joseph Gutteridge similarly recalled how, in his childhood, 'one old physician, a Quaker, named Dr Southam, refusing to prescribe for me', rather ambiguously 'remarking that the money on my case would be wasted'.[38]

Medical authority had many mysteries. Percival cautioned doctors against unnecessarily multiplying 'visits to the sick', partly because 'they tend to diminish the authority of the physician', while at the same time exciting suspicions of excessive love of lucre.[39] But if doctors should not be over-familiar, it was important to get the patient to be completely frank. He had to tell all. 'Some patients think it is the business of the doctor to find out their disorders, without being told any thing about them', grumbled Buchan. Such want of candour was hopeless:[40] 'They treat physicians as conjurors, and think they need no information. A patient, who wishes for a cure, cannot be too open and explicit with his doctor. He should not only impart every circumstance he knows concerning his disease, but follow the doctor's directions, as far as it lies in his power.'[40]

In some cases, above all with charity patients, true medical authority came from commanding. As Percival put it, 'greater *authority* and greater *condescension* will be found requisite in domestic attendance on the poor.'[41] How should one deal with a habitual drunkard? asked Thomas Trotter. It was useless to attempt to negotiate through sweet reason with those of diseased will. Only decisive action would work. It was vital to forbid them drink at a stroke; only such a move would impress the gravity of the situation upon their diseased minds. Trotter told an exemplary tale of how he had informed a habitual drunkard's husband, within her earshot, of the complete hopelessness of her case. Hearing such words had stirred the patient into deep remorse, and the ending was happy.[42]

But there were times and places where the astute physician believed it prudent to pander to patients' whims. Occasionally, Trotter suggested, it was best to be easy with hypochondriacal cases (this 'class of diseases, so variable in appearance, and equivocal in their symptoms, requires a full share of experience and discernment, and not a little patience in actual attendance'): 'The physician must often take a very circuitous route to put questions to his patients, that he may learn the real genius of the distemper. He must in many cases be guarded in his inquiries, lest he excite fears and suspicions in the irritable mind, which is observant of every trifle, jealous of a whisper, and when once alarmed, however falsely, not easily quieted again.'[43]

Thus it was a dictum of eighteenth-century medicine that the clinical encounter depended for its success very largely on the personality, foresight and sagacity of the doctor himself. Thomas Withers, physician to the York Hospital, waxed lyrical over the healing power of such physicians, who were blessed with 'an humane and generous disposition'.

> They feel for their fellow-creatures in distress. Humanity forbids them to increase the uneasiness of their minds, and generosity teaches them to disdain every little consideration of interest, which is not perfectly consistent with the patient's condition in life. Their conversation, which is manly, rational, and untainted with the low deceits of craft, both soothes and animates the mind. It affords at once entertainment and instruction, social pleasure and rules of health. The physician should study and humor the different dispositions of his patients. The careless should be brought to a sense of their situation by a cautious admonition of their danger.[44]

Thus, Withers argued, the physician had to be more than a mere clinician: he needed to be a sage, a hero, a 'man of the world', as well:

> He should be able to read internal characters from external signs. He should not study men and manners in the common superficial way [but] . . . he should endeavour to penetrate at once into the mind, and to ascertain with a cautious exactness the ruling passion. He should observe countenances, gestures, words and actions, and yet seem as perfectly regardless of these things as if he made no observations upon them. He should with all possible care gain the confidence of his patient; and if he should happen to be intrusted with any family secrets or to be informed of any family distresses, he should act with the utmost regard to honour and humanity.[45]

Not least, it was crucial that the doctor should be the master of the use of speech. Many doctors believed, with Giorgio Baglivi, that words themselves could act as drugs: 'I can scarce express what Influence the Physician's Words have upon the Patient's Life, and how much they sway the Fancy.'[46] Thus Baglivi stressed, in tune with his times, the sheer captivating importance of imagination: 'for a Physician that has his Tongue well hung, and is Master of the Art of persuading, fastens, by the mere Force of Words, such a Vertue upon his Remedies, and raises the Faith and Hopes of the Patient to that Pitch, that sometimes he masters difficult Diseases with the silliest Remedies; which Physicians of greater Learning could not do with nobler Remedies, merely because they talk'd faintly, and with a soft dead Air.'[47]

As this view suggests, most Georgian doctors believed that civility smoothed the path to success. Yet certain famous doctors were renowned for their rudeness. At the turn of the eighteenth century, John Radcliffe notoriously spoke his mind. On one occasion, he allegedly informed William III that he would not want the King's two legs for all his three kingdoms. Rudeness of that order meant exclusion from Court. Yet Radcliffe continued to boast many eminent patients, who evidently approved of his plain-speaking.[48] When Richard Mead was about to take over his practice, Radcliffe told him: 'There are two ways, my boy, for a physician to treat his patients; either to bully or to cajole them. I have taken the first course and done very well, as you see. You may take the latter and perhaps do as well.'[49]

Later in the century, Sir Richard Jebb was noted for being at best laconic and at worst surly. 'That is my way', he is reported as saying to a noble patient, astonished at his peremptoriness. Stories abounded about his rough ways with patients:

> To questions about diet Jebb would reply testily. 'Pray, Sir Richard, May I eat a muffin?' asked a lady. 'Yes, madam, the best thing you can take'. 'Oh dear, Sir Richard, I am glad of that. The other day you said it was the worst thing in the world for me'. 'Good madam, I said so last Tuesday. This isn't a Tuesday – is it?' To another lady, who asked what she might eat, he said contemptuously, 'Boiled turnips'. 'Boiled turnips?' was the answer; 'You forgot, Sir Richard, I told you I could not bear boiled turnips'. 'Then, madam, answered Sir Richard, sternly, 'you have a d---d vitiated appetite'.[50]

Even aggression was tried. John Ward told stories of quite brutal cures by doctors: 'Dr. Trig cured a woman that was troubled with hysterical fitts this way: he laid her uppon the ground with her face downwards, then took up her coats and gave her three or four slaps on the arse; he did this before much companie, which I scarcely believe.'[51] The profession presumably enjoyed retailing such tales precisely because doctors normally felt constrained to wear a mask of civility, which they found irksome. Indeed, *suaviter in modo* was their general watchword. At the beginning of the nineteenth century, the country practitioner, Richard Weekes, told his son, Hampton, a student at St Thomas's:[52] 'Your situation at a public Hospital must have enabled you to see how necessary it is for a medical [man] to have thorough knowledge of his profession but it is in private practice only that you can see the necessity of Address, attention, & assiduity without which few men get on in life, & still fewer get fortunes.'[52]

Behind the civil expression, the doctor had room for manoeuvre and vast manipulative powers at his disposal. If sickness itself could readily dupe the doctor, so could the physician manipulate the patient in the interests of higher therapeutic ends. Folklore about doctors abounds with the conceit that great practitioners sometimes had to outwit patients for their own good. Thomas Sydenham is said to have cured a hypochondriac by sending him off to Scotland to consult with what turned out to be a non-existent physician. The expectancy, the exercise and the resultant rage at being sent on a fool's errand, cured the patient despite himself.[53]

Doctors liked to think patients gullible. Quacks (they said) duped the sick for selfish purposes; the true physician would play psychological games for entirely laudible therapeutic goals. Thus, under certain circumstances, the physician might 'give them any disguised nostrum, and they will use it; but they have no faith in the virtues of plain water.' The wise and humane clinician had to exploit such prejudices.[54]

THE MARCH OF MEDICINE

The medical art, William Heberden remarked, echoing Hippocrates, was dark, difficult and obscure.[55] No great breakthroughs in medical science or in professional organization during the eighteenth century dramatically bolstered the doctor's authority. Nevertheless, during this period medical men came to exercise greater control in many sectors, through informal modes of 'medicalization'.

Practitioners extended the range of their competence into new fields. One instance is the understanding and treatment of alcohol-related problems. Before the eighteenth century, few doctors paid special attention to drunkenness; it was classically handled as a vice or a sin, a problem of public order and moral discipline. But in the Georgian era, numerous practitioners – from Mandeville and Cheyne near the opening of the century to Thomas Trotter at its close – approached habitual drunkenness with assiduity, both diagnostically and therapeutically.[56] Alcohol addiction was increasingly cast as a medical problem; indeed, Trotter explicitly argued that it was not just a disease, but a disease of the mind. Certain practitioners, notably Erasmus Darwin, made campaigning against the dangers of drink central to their dreams of a healthy future. Doctors came to recognize the special problems of co-operation posed by the habitual drunkard.[57]

As already hinted, the treatment of the hypochondriac offers a comparable instance of the enlargement of the medical domain and of medical expertise during the Georgian age, another field in which the doctor could display subtlety – virtuosity even – in handling particularly refractory patients.[58] The following chapter will pay attention to ways in which women's and children's disorders became areas of medical specialization.

One further, and rather spectacular, extension of the field of doctoring during the eighteenth century deserves a brief mention: the rise of the mad-doctor. A small number of doctors were already making a speciality out of treating the mad before the eighteenth century: Richard Napier is a classic instance.[59] But it was principally during the Georgian era that practitioners first devoted themselves in sizeable numbers to mental disorder, and the 'trade in lunacy' began to shed its stigma and grow in prestige. Above all, treating the mad became utterly bound up with running a madhouse, as part of the very English development of a free market in institutionalized psychiatry. Asylum proprietorship was both a tangible and a highly profitable expression of power and control.[60]

We have so far been suggesting in this chapter that doctors responded to a patient/doctor contract that potentially granted great latitude to the sick by developing their own counter-strategies for managing the relationship. Authority was exercised, sometimes through charisma, often by the deft use of therapeutic discretion and clinical judgement, and, not least, by extending medical control over areas – such as obstetrics, children's diseases and madness – never hitherto medicalized to any great degree.[61] This chapter concludes with an extended discussion of one final such area: the medicalization of dying.

DYING AND THE DOCTORS

In traditional notions of the good death, medical procedures for treating fatal illness remained in the shadows: secondary, almost irrelevant. Both medical theory and practice respected the fact that living and dying lay in Nature's hands, as the best Classical medicine stipulated, or were directed by Providence. The art of physic as handed down from the Hippocratics was the business more of diagnosis and prognosis than of cure, and certainly not of 'miracle cure' (snatching people back from the dead).[62] Doctors and laymen equally accepted that death was inexorable, implacable. A late seventeenth-century children's rhyme, 'Tom Thumb, his Life and Death', put Death's sovereignty thus,[63]

> Where lying on his bed sore sicke
> King Arthur's doctor came
> With cunning skill by physick's art,

To ease and care the same.
His body being so slender small,
This cunning doctor tooke
A fine perspective glasse with which
He did in secret look
Into his sickened body downe
And therein saw that Death
Stood ready in his wasted guts
To sease his vitall breath.[63]

Hence, except in special cases such as the lives of sovereigns, doctors did not attempt heroic intervention to delay or defy death. Indeed, the excruciatingly painful death of Charles II, surrounded by a swarm of meddling doctors (the King civilly apologized to them for being an unconscionable time a-dying), perhaps indicates that the faculty was wise to shun futile heroics.[64]

What then did doctors do? Pre-modern physicians seem to have believed their role was to make a prognosis, informing the dying of their imminent fate so that they could good put their affairs in order.[65] Physicians practised upon themselves what they preached. At the turn of the eighteenth century, Dr Samuel Garth, suspecting his own end to be nigh, summoned fellow physicians to give a frank prognosis.[66]

Impending death was often announced (it was said that people were 'given over'). Thus, reported Woodforde, 'Poor Henry Nobbes continues near in the same terrible Situation, if any thing, worse. His Death has been daily expected for near two months, as the Faculty then declared that his case was incurable, that nothing could be done for him to any effect whatever. Pray God! release him out of his misery.'[67]

Once a patient was 'given over', the physician was released: doctors did not necessarily attend the dying. Radcliffe would not come to the bed of the dying Queen Anne, arguing that attendance was futile.[68] Similarly, the Verneys' physician, Dr Denton, was informed in 1656 by his kinsman, Alexander, that he was 'much troubled for my Brother [George]. I can hardly persuade the Doctors to come to him, for they say they cannot helpe him. Neither can I procure a Minister to come to him, which troubles me very much hee being so insensible of Dying.'[69] Samuel Garth was said to be notoriously indifferent to those whose ends were near. When drunk, and failing to attend his patients he is reported to have exclaimed: 'It's no great matter . . . whether I see them to-night or not, for nine of them have such bad constitutions, that all the physicians in the world can't save them; and the other six have such good constitutions, that all the physicians in the world can't kill them.'[70] Thus, only in rather special circumstances would the traditional doctor continue to visit the dying patient right up to death.

'My Brother continues much as he was', William Cowper reported:

> His Case is a very dangerous one. An Imposthume of the Liver, attended
> by an Asthma & Dropsy. The Physician has little Hope of his Recovery.
> I believe I might say none at all, only, being a Friend, he does not
> formally give him over by ceasing to Visit him, lest it should sink his
> Spirits. For my own part I have no Expectation of his Recovery except
> by a signal Interposition of Providence in Answer to Prayer. His Case is
> clearly out of the Reach of Medicine.[71]

In other words, traditional medical etiquette required that the dying
patient be informed of his likely fate. Then, their part in the proceedings
complete, physicians would withdraw, leaving the dying man to compose
his mind and his will, and make peace with God and his family. Case-
notes show that Stuart practitioners followed these protocols, quitting
their patients after 'giving them over'. 'He groaned horribly like a dying
man . . . then judging the issue to be settled I bade farewell to him and
his friends. At evening he died', concluded Thomas Willis's notes on
one of his patients in the middle of the seventeenth century.[72] We
should not attribute the doctor's departure to callous indifference, but
rather to a sense of place, proper resignation, humility and dignity.
Physic was for the living. Death was hardly on the medical agenda at
all. Robert James's huge *Medicinal Dictionary* did not even have an
entry for it.[73]

There was no sudden change of mind or practice with the coming of
the eighteenth century. But a new ideal of dying gradually came into
vogue, dying seen not as a Christian heroic struggle against Death but
as a peaceful falling asleep; and this had major implications for the
doctor's role.[74]

So what part did the physician play in this new paradigm of dying?
Did the profession help to establish it in the first place? And did they
play a leading part in it? The answer, in particular to the second
question, is 'yes', but that role is not quite the one depicted by
recent historians. Illich, in particular, has argued that, swollen with
Enlightenment hubris, doctors began to nurse the illusion that they
could actually conquer ageing and even death. Medicine became fired
with the Baconian ambition of the prolongation of life. Indeed, perhaps
wilfully blind to the irony of Swift's prescient presentation of the
wretchedly immortal Struldbruggs in *Gulliver's Travels*, Godwin,
Condorcet and other *philosophes* began to entertain conjecture of a this-
worldly immortality, grounded upon new laws of health.[75] There is
some truth in Illich's interpretation of a new prometheanism amongst
doctors, for in hospital foundations, smallpox inoculation and the rise
of public health, medicine undeniably took the offensive against disease.

Certain developments – above all the Humane Movement – clearly mark a medical campaign to snatch people back from the jaws of death itself.[76]

But it would be wrong to infer from this, with Illich, that the deathbed became a new battleground, witnessing a fight – to the death! – to keep patients alive at all costs, with the physician as the generalissimo. Evidence suggests the contrary. Dr John Ferriar insisted, at the dawn of the nineteenth century, 'the physician will not torment his patient with unavailing attempts to stimulate the dissolving system, from the idle vanity of prolonging the flutter of the pulse for a few more vibrations'.[77] And, taking a broader perspective, the public involvement of doctors with the whole phenomenon of death remained fairly marginal: for example, well into the nineteenth century, no medical competence was required of coroners. In England, though less so in Scotland, morbid anatomy and legal medicine, with their key roles in establishing the causes of death, remained backward.[78]

Yet in one respect, death was undoubtedly becoming medicalized: the development of the management of death at the bedside. Looking back from the late eighteenth century, physicians often remarked with surprise upon the absence of their predecessors from the deathbed. Sir William Temple had explained it thus: 'an honest physician is excused for leaving his patient, when he finds the disease growing desperate, and can, by his attendance, expect only to receive his fees, without any hopes or appearance of deserving them.' Countering this view, Thomas Percival argued that there was much the conscientious physician ought to be doing around the deathbed, 'by obviating despair, by alleviating pain, and by soothing mental anguish'. The old 'fanciful delicacy' over accepting fees ought to yield to this higher 'moral duty'.[79] John Ferriar agreed: 'When all hopes of revival are lost, it is still the duty of the physician to sooth the last moments of existence.' The doctor should decide: 'it belongs to his province, to determine when officiousness becomes torture'.[80] For Ferriar, the physician's continued presence in a position of authority was vital, not least to curb the excesses of nurses and servants eager to employ what he saw as their cruel folkloric techniques for trying to revitalize the dying.[81]

Possibly paralleling the role professional undertakers were newly assuming in stage-managing funerals,[82] physicians increasingly argued they should attend deathbeds not as doctors but as friends; as Richard Kay put it, faced with his dying brother, 'as a Physician I cannot help you: As a Christian and as an affectionate Friend and a loving Brother I must pity and pray for you'.[83] Moreover, they claimed they possessed unique experience in piloting the optimum course – therapeutically and emotionally – for managing the last weeks, days, hours, of the dying. Thus, to some degree, the dying person ceased to be in charge of his own death, which instead became orchestrated by the physician, with the agreement of the family.

This argument might *prima facie* sound wildly anachronistic; for it so closely resembles the accusations made against today's medicine of the terminal ward, the life-support system and of pious lies and evasive euphemisms. But not so, for it was explicitly levelled by contemporaries. People were no longer allowed their own deaths, Thomas Sheridan contended in the 1760s; for, in the name of sympathy and minimizing distress, their families and doctors were arranging for them to slip away oblivious to their fate: 'very few now die [he told Boswell]. Physicians take care to conceal people's danger from them. So that they are carried off, properly speaking, without dying; that is to say, without being sensible of it.'[84]

Evasion on that scale may have been unusual. But as the eighteenth century wore on, and as fashionable physicians raised their aspirations to become trusted family advisers and intimates, they adopted a more managerial approach to the deathbed. The most spectacularly successful practice of this medicalization of dying appears in the career of Sir Henry Halford in the early nineteenth century. Halford became physician on an unparalleled scale to royalty and the aristocracy, not least because of his diplomacy in helping to implement what had become the widespread desire for easy death.[85] With patients he recognized to be dying, it was Halford's policy long to mask the truth, and instead to prevaricate or give cheerful prognostications. Optimism was therapeutically valuable. The second stage lay in preparing sufferers and divulging the truth, at the appropriate moment, in time for the dying person to set his house in order.

By no means, however, did that signal the end of the physician's role. Indeed, the most difficult, but valuable, part was just beginning. For, lastly, the doctor must manage the actual process of ceasing to be. Here, Halford – who had, we are told, an 'innate shrinking from bodily pain' – stressed that the true priority must be to 'smooth the bed of death',[86] or in other words, to undertake the management of pain, thereby overcoming fear and restoring tranquillity, orchestrating an end serene and blissful. In this, Halford made it his 'rule in all cases of ministering to them such aid as medicines could supply', often using his own individual preparations.[87] He became the premier physician of his age precisely because his patients had confidence that, through generous medication, he would not let them die in agony. Rumour had it that: 'A lady of the highest rank . . . declared she would rather die under Sir Henry Halford's care than recover under any other physician.'[88] Halford's own dying was 'only partially relieved by full doses of opium',[89] lamented his biographer, Dr William Munk. Munk went on to write *Euthanasia, or Medical Treatment in Aid of an Easy Death* (1887).[90]

What Halford turned into an art was, however, already becoming common practice long before. During the eighteenth century, physicians seem increasingly to have shrunk from telling patients outright of their impending quietus. Dr William Buchan, for example, repudiated the ancient practice of 'prognosticating . . . the patient's fate, or foretelling the issue of the disease', on the grounds that 'we do not see what right any man has to announce the death of another, especially if such a declaration has a chance to kill him.' Instead of this 'vanity', Buchan recommended something altogether more tactful: 'a doubtful answer . . . or one that may tend rather to encourage the hopes of the sick, is surely the most safe.'[91] Therapeutic management came to the fore. In this, Matthew Baillie's approach was exemplary. He was called in to treat the failing Mrs Wynne. 'Dr Baillie saw Mama', recorded her daughter, 'he says he cannot cure her, but hopes to relieve her and to prevent her illness from getting worse with a prospect of getting better.'[92]

Above all, in the management of desperate cases, it became medical policy to prescribe optimism as the most effective psychotherapy. Parson William Jones mentioned the doctors around the deathbed of his friend, Mills: 'Mr Worthington, who attended poor Mills at first, and Mr Harold who succeeded him, . . . endeavoured to buoy him & Mrs Mills up with hopes of his recovery, whereas I pronounced him, from the first, to all but himself, a condemned man & his case a lost one.'[93] Symptomatically here, in this new age of supercharged sensibility, even the parson declined to inform the dying man of his impending fate.

Above all, doctors devised strategies in which divulgence of truth to their patients became gauged by their own yardsticks of therapeutic appropriateness. 'Physicians are sometimes called upon to mention the deaths of relations to their patients', noted Benjamin Rush: 'This should never be done at once. They should be first told that they were sick, and in great danger, and the news of their death should not be communicated until after a second or third visit.'[94]

Death without fear, thought Dr John Ferriar, should resemble 'falling asleep'.[95] Effective sedatives were indispensable to that strategy. It was widely accepted that Halford drew liberally upon a range of soporific draughts, doubtless mainly opium-based, to help his patients glide towards oblivion. We sometimes assume that our own generation is the first in which dying typically involves heavy sedation. That would be a great mistake. For the first golden age of the stupefying drugs was the eighteenth century. If medicine could not delay death, it could make it much less agonizing. Of course, the Georgian age remained the 'Age of Agony'.[96] But relative to earlier times, it was an anaesthetized age, precisely because of the startling surge in the use of powerful narcotics, particularly alcohol and opium and its derivatives, laudanum and paregoric. It was a habit sanctioned by regular doctors, and encouraged amongst the people at large by a free market in the sale of drugs.

Fixated upon the symbolic importance of Coleridge, De Quincey and the Romantic imagination, standard histories of opium usually open their stories near the dawn of the nineteenth century.[97] This is understandable, for we still lack in-depth research on the history of the battery of medicaments prescribed by eighteenth-century physicians and bought over the counter by that highly self-dosing culture.

Abundant evidence, however, points to increasingly heavy consumption of opium long before. It was used as an analgesic, a sedative, a febrifuge and as a specific against gastro-intestinal disorders. Opiates were widely recommended, almost a panacea, by eminent physicians of the second half of the eighteenth century. Parssinen has claimed that 'it was not until the 1830s and 1840s that opium assumed a crucial therapeutic role in English medicine',[98] but this is certainly wrong, maybe by over a century. As early as the 1670s, Dr Thomas Sydenham had been praising opium to the skies ('medicine would be a cripple without it'). Sydenham's championship echoed down the eighteenth century in treatises such as Dr John Jones's *Mysteries of Opium Reveal'd* (1700),[99] George Young's *Treatise on Opium* (1753)[100] and Dr Samuel Crumpe's *Inquiry into the Nature and Properties of Opium* (1793),[101] all notably sanguine about the absence of serious risk attending the drug's medicinal use. Dosing with opium was also programmatic to 'Brunonianism', the therapeutic system adumbrated by John Brown in Edinburgh and mirrored by Benjamin Rush in Philadelphia, in which it was used both to calm but, above all, to stimulate.[102] Rush also prescribed opium as a universal sedative. In cases of grief and depression, for instance, he wrote, 'the first remedy . . . indicated . . . is opium. It should be given in liberal doses.'[103]

From the 1760s, Erasmus Darwin was prescribing opium in massive quantities to patients in his large Midlands practice. He advised it for many complaints (for instance, for sleepwalking: 'Opium in large doses'), and recommended to select patients half a grain a day 'as a habit'. His generous prescriptions may well have been responsible for the addiction of his friend and patient, Tom Wedgwood.[104] Moreover, with the emergence of a flourishing trade in potent patent and proprietary medicines, opiates were available in the form of nostrums such as the Solid Panacea, Dr Bate's Pacific Pill, Starkey's Pill, Matthews' Pill and, most popular of all, Dover's Powders (a mixture of opium and ipecacuanha) and Godfrey's Cordial.[105] A Nottingham chemist reported in 1808 that 'upwards of 200 lbs of opium and above 600 pints of

Godfrey's Cordial are retailed to the poorer class in the year'.[106]

Writing from Jamaica, the Revd William Jones noted that 'opium is greatly used in this Island, & in high esteem among the sons of sorrow to remove their Melancholy & solace their cares. Heard a person mentioned who always spent three quarters of his patrimony on *crude Opium*.'[107] He might almost have been writing about England. No small number of eighteenth-century figures – including Samuel Johnson's wife, Tetty – became little less reliant upon opiates than Coleridge or De Quincey later.

Under these circumstances, it is hardly surprising that numerous individuals, on their own initiative, swallowed heavy doses of such narcotics in their dying weeks or months: Sir Joshua Reynolds, for example. And many physicians prescribed liberal dosages to smooth the path to death.[108] Thus Parson Woodforde, watching his own father dying in 'acute' agony in 1771, noted 'Dr Clarke gives him liquid laudanum to compose him'.[109] Rather like heroic criminals *en route* to Tyburn, given Dutch courage with brandy to make a good end, people increasingly died insensible, stupefied with drugs (often medically prescribed), and thus conformed to the new model of the art of dying well. As Benjamin Rush put it, 'OPIUM has a wonderful effect in lessening the fear of death. I have seen patients cheerful in their last moments, from the operation of this medicine upon the body and mind.'[110] The doyen of the late eighteenth-century clinicians, William Heberden, was of a similar mind. Arguing that, when physicians could not vanquish it, they should 'try to disarm death of some of its terrors', he prescribed opium liberally so that life might 'be taken away in the most merciful manner'.[111]

Indeed, as with fatal overdoses nowadays, it is sometimes hard to tell with eighteenth-century deaths whether the pharmaceutical fix was intended to calm, stimulate or kill; for example, when Horace Walpole reported the end of Lord Crawford who 'died, as is supposed, by taking a large quantity of laudanum'.[112] As soon as he sensed he was near his end, Samuel Johnson deliberately left off his medically prescribed opiates, so that he could pass over in full possession of his faculties: 'I will take no more physic, not even my opiates; for I have prayed that I may render up my soul to God unclouded.'[113] Was Johnson by then in a minority? The increasing occurrence of 'insensible death' may well help explain late eighteenth-century fears about premature burial.[114]

In 1800 no less than in 1650, dying the 'good death' was critically important. Back in the seventeenth century, dying well meant meeting your maker with total vigilance. By 1800 a doctor-assisted peaceful death was becoming the norm and the ideal. From womb to tomb, the empire of medicine was steadily extending itself, thanks to growing 'demand' (itself, of course, a cultural artifact) for polite and professional services. In a milieu in which practitioners possessed little statutory power and few public openings, it was through persuading the public of, first, its indispensability, and, then, its authority, that medicine made its substantial inroads in the Georgian century. As in so many other fields, what began, in medicine, as a luxury, became a decency and eventually turned into a necessity.

9

Therapies

In the Georgian era the sick were attending doctors more frequently; yet there was no 'therapeutic revolution', at least till the nineteenth century.[1] This raises the issue of the efficacy of the treatments doctors meted out to patients. Did patients attend doctors because of – or was it in spite of – the therapies they received? The question of therapeutics was central to practical medicine, for, as John Ward described the true doctor: 'Four things make a practical physician; first, to have a materia medica in his head; second, pertinently to prescribe; third, exactly to judge of the disease; fourth, to have good prognosticks; the last is for his credit chiefly.'[2] The sick believed – maybe out of profound conviction, maybe out of sickness-induced desperation – that practitioners could activate procedures which would prove good for their health, or at least worth a try. Irked at being ill for more than a month with a dreadful cold, Charles Lamb begged his doctor for action; he was prescribed a scriptful of strong medicines – 'Spanish licorice, opium, ipecacuanha, paregoric, and tincture of foxglove'.[3] Sick people also looked to practical surgical skills. About to undergo surgery for his hydrocele, Gibbon sent his stepmother 'a short assurance of my health': 'You may justly reproach me with the long neglect of a growing complaint, but I am now in the hands of the most skilful physicians and surgeons who have given me immediate relief, and promise me safe and radical cure.'[4] (Ironically, his faith proved hardly justified in the event, for he was to die of post-operative sepsis.)

Certain kinds of professional interventions tackled problems unlikely to remit spontaneously and utterly beyond the capacity of even the most ingenious self-healer; and, if skilfully performed, they had a respectable measure of success. The layman might lance his own boils, but he would not attempt amputation on himself or his friends. Pepys gave up his barber and started shaving himself – it saved both time and money, but he got the best surgeon to remove his stone (he was luckier with that than Gibbon with his hydrocele.)[5] An adroit operator could successfully couch for cataract, thus sparing people loss of sight. It was a procedure not for the squeamish, and in an age in which oculists were typically itinerants, decked out in all the tinsel of quackery, sorting the capable operator from the rogue was a delicate business. The oculist, John ('Chevalier') Taylor, was widely abused as being little better than a charlatan, but he seems to have had a skilful hand (his foible, perhaps, being to extract fees from hopeless cases).[6]

At a more workaday level, people clearly had confidence in a surgeon's ability to set a fracture, and surgical dexterity with gunshot wounds also improved (vital in an age of escalating warfare).[7] As Samuel Johnson's case amply shows, even a truculent patient could appreciate the expertise of a good physician in managing potentially dangerous conditions such as dropsy.[8]

Doctors paraded spectacular cures. Early in his career, and doubtless with a view to advancing it, the Revd Dr Francis Willis got Robert James to insert in his *Dissertation on Fevers* one such case. It records the fate of 'one Isaac', dying of delirious fever, to whom Willis - both clergyman and doctor - was summoned 'to read the departing prayer'. He ordered the despairing wife 'to give him a clyster immediately, and apply a blister to his back and head', followed by 'a paper of Dr. James's Powder'. After 'convulsive twitchings' and vomiting, the patient spewed up 'three worms, one of which was upwards of a foot long'. Next day, further doses of James's Powders were given, causing him to bring up 'two more'. It worked: 'four days after, Mr. Willis saw him in a market, seven miles from home, very well, selling sheep.' Unsurprisingly Dr James, patentee of the powders, deemed this a 'very remarkable . . . case', which he 'desired to be made public'.[9]

With the possibility of such heroics at the back of their minds, doctors naturally liked to think of themselves as 'going to war against a fever' (as Erasmus Darwin put it), commandeering what John Fothergill called the 'pharmaceutical artillery' of 'Bleeding, blisters . . . boluses and draughts'.[10]

Yet it would be a mistake to assume that patients expected miracle cures, or even relief. For in many conditions, the doctor's action was known not to make much difference – as candid clinicians, such as William Heberden, were wont to admit. Joseph Farington reported a case in which Matthew Baillie asserted that 'fever must *have its way*; that medicine could do nothing against it, but that medicine might do good by counteracting some of the effects of fever.'[11] When he fell sick in 1798, put himself under doctors in Buxton and finally recovered,

William Hutton commented that he did not 'know whether *Time* was not the most skilful Doctor'.[12]

Indeed, the sick were often realists about what lay within medicine's power – as well as harbouring suspicions about the (in)competence of individual practitioners. Thus, in assessing what precisely patients *did* expect from their doctors, their instrument cases and medicine bags, we need to take many factors into account. The doctor played roles which were symbolic and psychological as well as scientific. Attending a physician lifted responsibility off one's own shoulders and displaced possible blame in the event of a baleful conclusion. Moreover, it reiterated acknowledgement of the paramount importance of experience. 'Any man may know drugs', was Buchan's axiom, 'but few know how to apply them.'[13] This chapter will hence explore what the doctors *did*, to gauge the importance of such procedures in cementing – or possibly corroding – patient/doctor relations.

DIAGNOSES AND PROGNOSES

In an earlier chapter we explored how a doctor arrived at a diagnosis, and the negotiating role of a patient in modifying or challenging it. This stage was crucial. A physician's reputation hinged upon the quality of his diagnoses. The top-rank physician was the age's detective. Such clinical mastery enabled Heberden to advance the understanding of angina,[14] just as, a little later, Matthew Baillie perceived the link between chronic heavy drinking and cirrhosis of the liver.[15]

The good diagnosis was accurate but acceptable; acuity had to be matched with tact in putting a judgement into words. The sick did not want to be deafened with jargon; but articulate patients were not prepared to be fobbed off with a few anodyne phrases. As we have seen, when the surgeon-apothecary Forbes hummed and hawed, Parson Holland fumed.[16] Patients wanted to be put in the picture. But they also needed diagnostic formulae conveying the right undertones. Some diagnostic terms sounded too grave; others stigmatizing. Thus not everyone was happy with the various compound terms involving 'nerves' (for example, 'nervous cholic'), for they could appear to hint at hypochondriasis. The touchiness of such delicate patients was rued early in the eighteenth century by Richard Blackmore, who claimed that a physician 'cannot ordinarily make his Court worse, than by suggesting to such patients [that is, difficult, hypochondriacal ones] the true Nature and Name of their Distemper.'[17]

These general concerns mattered in the individual case. Lady Louisa Conolly's niece, Charlotte, fell into a decline after a riding accident.

She took assorted medical advice. It was unclear whether her condition was merely a passing phase or was serious, presaging true consumption. Dr Quin was asked whether travelling for health would be desirable: 'Doctor Quin spoke in the most reasonable manner to us, to this purpose: that with regard to Charlotte going abroad to a southern climate, he could make no objection, provided she chose it and that her friends wished her to try it; but that there was no necessity, if Charlotte disliked it, or that it was inconvenient.'[18] The family obviously quizzed him at length as to the diagnostic basis for his equivocations. His deliberations were thus recorded:

> His reasons for being so undecided was that having lived long enough to see that going abroad was not an infallible remedy, *he* had resolved in *two* cases not to order people abroad. The *first*, in desperate cases, for that nothing could save the lungs once attacked and therefore it was cruel to send them off to die. The *next* was the *not* thinking a person's case desperate, for that, *if* the disorder *could* be removed, the helps procured at home were as likely to remove the disorder.[19]

Was there an eloquent silence as to which case Charlotte's resembled? The question of her travelling was not simply treated as a matter of 'doctor's orders'. 'Of course, this point cannot be settled by him', Louisa continued:

> and Charlotte is so averse to the idea of it that I should suppose it will be dropped. We then asked Doctor Quin his opinion of her, which he gave in a very plain manner, and told us (I believe) as much as he knew himself. He said that her pulse at present was good, but he could not say how long it might continue so; that the pain in her breast (if of a serious nature) would alter it soon, but that perhaps it might be removed; that the acuteness of the pain probably was nervous, and that he should endeavour to mix nervous medicines with what he should otherwise order, to try to remove the nervous complaint, which would then make the other disorder apparent (if totally removed). Charlotte is not alarmed about her life, and is so sure that it's nervous, that Doctor Quin agreed to call it so to her.[20]

Here it seems that, in a pious fraud perpetrated upon the patient, doctor and family agreed to call the fever 'nervous' so as to make it sound less grave than a 'hectic' fever, or consumption. Her mother, Emily, had little doubt, however, about its true gravity: '(in my opinion), there is an appearance of decay hardly to be mistaken; and I think it is plain that Doctor Quin apprehends it, though there are not as yet sufficient symptoms to pronounce it such.'[21] The astute diagnostician, now plain-speaking, now tactfully reticent, thus had to be alert to far more than mere pathophysiology.

Reaching an appropriate diagnosis, both realistic and reassuring, was the first indispensable task for the doctor. How far patients expected detailed *prognoses* is less clear. They probably did want to know if they were dying; but gloomy prophecies of chronic pain might be most unwelcome.[22]

The traditional humanist doctor of the sixteenth and seventeenth centuries had made this kind of medical prophecy an important string to his bow; 'prognosticks' formed Ward's fourth desideratum.[23] This applies especially to those astrologically inclined.[24] But such fortune-telling readily offered hostages to fortune: 'Mr Tho. Kempton dyed last Fryday', Lady Conway informed her husband in 1666, 'contrary to Dr Stubb his prognostick, who but the night before said he would not dye.'[25] The growing sensibility of the late-Georgian temper believed that prophecies of death were cruel, a gratuitous parade of medical vanity and (psychologically speaking) therapeutically counter-productive, for pessimistic prognoses readily became self-fulfilling. Better wait and watch, offering encouraging words, thought Georgian doctors, recovering the true spirit of Hippocratism.

PRESCRIBING AND MEDICATING

Obviously, diagnosis often ended in medication, as will shortly be discussed. But consultations could also issue in varied medical recommendations, including suggestions for radical changes in the patient's life. Not infrequently the doctor directed travel. Lady Duncannon was ailing in 1790, with 'spitting of blood' and an 'abominable cough'; her legs were so weak, she was on crutches. Everyone presumably thought it was consumption, although the term was not used. Her family consulted Sir Richard Warren. He was in no doubt: she must winter in the South of France; in fact she remained there three years. The doctor thus triggered a fundamental change of life-style.[26]

Yet doctors became ever more identified in the public eye with dispensing drugs (plate 7). Patients often groaned: 'my plague is physic', complained Lady Holland.[27] Yet patients and doctors seemingly colluded in multiplying the quantities of medication consumed. Patients sought relief from pain. They hoped for cures. They were willing to put a galaxy of medications to the trial.

Old-school doctors demurred from this trend towards exuberant medication. William Withering pronounced it the physician's duty to withstand the clamour, raised by the sick person and the apothecary, for a deluge of dosing. Patients had to be protected, he contended, from their own rather naïve assumption that the more medicine they took,

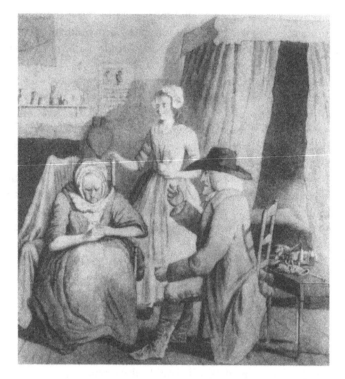

PLATE 7   Administering medicine

the more they were fighting their disorders.[28] In George Cheyne's lofty
view, automatic recourse to the prescription-pad was properly the give-
away of 'Country Apothecaries, ignorant Practitioners, much more
commonly, Quacks', 'who never dare order a Regimen, and who are
continually cramming their Patients with nauseous and loathsome
Potions, Pills and Bolus's, Electuaries, Powders and Juleps, and
plaistering every Pore of their Bodies.'[29] In Cheyne's eyes, heavy dosing
was a hazardous short-cut; regimen the royal road to health.

But events and preferences overtook this traditionalism, leading to a
bonanza of drugging. For one thing, a greater range of newer and
stronger drugs became available. From the mid-seventeenth century,
energetic trade with the New World and the Far East enormously
increased the variety of exotic drugs, such as Peruvian bark, being
imported. Supply rose, prices dropped and use spread. These exotica
were matched by a greater variety of laboratory-produced, artificial
drugs, thanks to the expanding skills of the chemist. First the Paracelsian
movement, then the 'new science' of the seventeenth century, helped to
bring chemical and mineral ingredients, such as aqua fortis, mercury,

antimony and calomel, into fashion. They were used to reduce fever or procure drastic purges. Poisonous in large quantities, such mineral and metallic medicines were typically more dramatic than the old herbal remedies.[30] The latter, however, did not lose their advocates. Herbalists in the Culpeper tradition continued to champion the use of 'simples' – vegetable remedies typically made of a single ingredient, distilled, crushed, dried, rubbed into the skin or whatever.[31] Physicians and apothecaries mainly used herbs in the form of 'galenicals' – complicated, compound remedies, commonly involving a multitude of ingredients. Often possessing the stamp of antiquity, these were made up according to formulae printed in the various official pharmacopoeias, such as the *London Dispensatory*, published under the imprimatur of the College of Physicians.[32] A glance at such a work indicates what a prolific pot-pourri of preparations was available to the Georgian doctor, ranging from exotica such as crabs' eyes, vipers' fat and coral, to mainstays such as opium, senna and sarsaparilla. (Unicorn's horn and spiders' webs did, however, disappear from the London pharmacopoeia, though powdered mummy still figured in the 1750 edition of the *Pharmacopoeia Universalis*.)

Thus the growing recourse to drugging was a consequence of greater availability. But it also directly reflected the economy of the medical profession. The great majority of professional practitioners in the eighteenth century had been trained as surgeon-apothecaries. During their apprenticeship, they spent long years rolling pills, distilling herbs and mixing boluses. Pharmacy was their stamping ground: their training familiarized them more with materia medica than with anatomy, physiology and diagnostics. In any case, in the eyes of the law, the apothecary, when acting as a general practitioner, was not permitted to bill for his time, trouble, travelling, attendence, experience and all the other rationales. He was allowed to charge only for medicines dispensed. No wonder apothecaries made sure they dispensed a goodly number.[33]

But the tendency towards heavier drugging also perhaps marks a shift in attitude, a growing demand for action, a tendency to associate remedy with medication and see the doctor's power embodied in the pills he dispensed. A 'progressive' culture that was accelerating the pace of life and pinning its faith on utility and instrumentality, business and technology, a society oriented upon food, drink and consumption and energized by the exchange of money and commodities was programmed to make this shift from regimen to dosing.[34] The Englishman's consuming passions encouraged a 'fast food' outlook upon drugs – the stomach was the heart of the matter. Enlightenment values[35] encouraged physicians such as Erasmus Darwin to be adventurously experimental in their dispensing habits.[36]

THE MEANING OF DRUGS

If therapeutics – prescribed medication, shop-bought nostrums and home-mixed medicines – entailed hefty druggings, what sorts of drugs were being taken in such large quantities? What results were expected? What did drugs mean to those who took them – what were their wider, symbolic associations?

The favourite treatments remained, as in earlier centuries, purges, vomits and sweats. Sydney Smith was sardonic about doctors' inordinate love of purging. Whence the reek of Auld Reekie? 'No smells were ever equal to Scotch Smells. It is the School of Physic; walk the Streets, and you would imagine that every Medical man had been administering Cathartics to every man woman and child in the Town.'[37] Yet patients were no less enamoured than their physicians, and the habitual, automatic self-purger became one of the stock figures of fun in the doctors' lay-medicine demonology.[38]

Doctors remained similarly faithful to the virtues of a vomit. George Cheyne thought emetics the finest medicines of all. He suggested to his patient, the novelist, Samuel Richardson, that 'Your short neck is rather an argument for a vomit now and then', and that he should take emetics because 'vomits are the best preservative from apoplexies'.[39] One of the favourite therapies for the lunatics at Bethlem was the 'smart vomit'.[40]

Such therapies as purging and vomiting had their rationales. Sickness, it was widely assumed, was due to 'peccant humours' or toxins in the gut. Expelling them upwards or downwards would rid the body of the source of irritation.[41] Medicine was thus aiding what Nature would do in any case. Moreover, such therapeutics gratified the desire of both doctors and the sick for visible effects. In contemporary medical parlance, purges 'wrought' or 'worked' – not necessarily in the sense of curing the distemper, but by producing the effect expected of the medicine itself.[42]

Why did the sick bother to consult doctors about conditions sure to be medicated with purges and vomits, when they could instigate these procedures themselves? After all, emetics and laxatives were composed of drugs – rhubarb, senna, etc. – readily available, often from the garden, and commonly handled by lay people.[43] Every medicine chest contained them. Proprietary medicines such as Dover's Powders were designed to produce precisely these effects.[44]

Doctors had their riposte ready. They emphasized that such purgatives should properly be regarded not as cures in themselves, but as a single item in a wider, balanced, carefully-structured, longer-term, therapeutic course. Dosage and frequency had to be tailored precisely to the needs of the individual patient, and possibly modified from day to day. This explained the practitioners' habit of prescribing only a few doses at a time but prescribing extremely frequently – a habit patients thought led to profiteering.[45]

Patients may or may not have believed all this. But they were fascinated by the elaborate rules, rituals and rationalizations surrounding their administration. His niece, Nancy, had a touch of 'ague' (perhaps malaria), so Parson Woodforde attended meticulously to the course proposed by Thorne, his general practitioner:

> Dr. Thorne's Method of treating the Ague and Fever or intermitting Fever is thus – To take a Vomit in the Evening not to drink more than 3 half Pints of Warm Water after it as it operates. The Morn' following a Rhubarb Draught – and then as soon as the Fever has left the Patient about an Hour or more, begin with the Bark taking it every two Hours till you have taken 12 Papers which contains one Ounce. The next oz. etc you take it 6. Powders the ensuing Day, 5 Powders the Day after, 4 Ditto the Day after, then 3 Powders the Day after that till the 3rd oz. is all taken, then 2 Powders the Day till the 4th oz. is all taken and then leave of. If at the beginning of taking the Bark it should happen to purge, put ten Dropps of Laudanum into the Bark you take next, then 4, then 3, then 2, then 1 and so leave of by degrees.[46]

He reported on the effects: 'Nancy continued brave but seemed Light in her head. The Bark at first taking it, rather purged her and she took 10 Drops of Laudanum which stopped it.'

Here we see a measured response towards purging. The initial purge would evacuate the system and thus prepare for the truly effectual medicine, the bark. But when that produced unnecessary and unwanted purgative effects, laudanum (that is, liquid opium) was employed to counteract it. (Often the reverse was the case: opium used as a pain-killer produced unwelcome constipation, needing to be countered with senna.) Thus, though Woodforde probably kept stocks of all the drugs deployed by Thorne, the secret – the medical mystique, even – lay in the art of dosing.[47]

In other words, doctors tried to convince their clients that drugs were not sufficient in themselves, but became efficacious within the framework of a wider regime, whose rationale only the doctor fully understood. Take, for example, Erasmus Darwin's treatment of James Watt's daughter, Janet (known as Jessy), who was wasting away.[48] Darwin energetically tried drug therapies, but he took care to explain to Watt the principles underlying their particular choice, mixture, timing and dosage. 'The principal thing, which can be done in these cases', he explained 'is by some stimulus a *little* greater than natural, and *uniformly* taken for months or years, to invigorate the digestive power.'[49] How might this be achieved?

> In some I have seen a great benefit by beginning with a pill of half a grain of opium taken at breakfast, and at going to bed (or tea in the afternoon) every day as a habit; and after a few weeks to increase it to a grain-pill twice a day - and after some months to a grain and a half twice a day. Pills are prefer'd to Laudanum.
>
> 30 drops of chalybeate wine in a glass of warm water along with 20 drops of tinctura cantharidum may be taken occasionally for a month, and then discontinued alternately.
>
> And extract of bark from 20 to 30 grains twice a day for a fortnight occasionally might be of service.[50]

Darwin acknowledged the opium, designed as a stimulant, would produce constipation: 'One stool daily or alternate days should be produced by rhubarb or by aloe'. But when more serious bouts of sickness supervened, other drugs were needed as reinforcements: 'When her fits come on, or threaten to come on, she should take 30 drops of mixture of equal parts tincture of castor and of laudanum, put into a two-ounce phial – besides the daily allowance of the opium in pills above recommended – ether may be used but is of less efficacy than the above – the same of assafoetida.'[51] Darwin then tossed in what was probably a bit of psychological humbug, emphasizing how one particular element of his medication was indispensable: 'The above is the general method, which is most likely to serve her; your surgeon will please to put the medicines in such forms as she can best take them. But the opiate I should wish to be given in a *very small pill* and *uniformly* persisted in.'[52] And he concluded with all those general philosophizings upon regimen that elevated the true physician above the mere quack-doser:

> In respect to diet, flesh-meat and small beer are recommended twice a day, but as her digestion is weak, her palate must be consulted in every thing both of what she eats and drinks. The young spring herbs, as asparagus, cabbages, etc are also recommended; and wine and water instead of small beer, if she prefers it.   She should go quite loose in her stays.
>
> And should lie down after her dinner for an hour if it be agreable to her and go to bed early.
>
> The drops of tincture of castor and laudanum must be repeated in 1/2 an hour, if the first dose does not remove the hysteric spasms.
>
> The medicines I last directed may be continued till you see if they are of advantage, but I wish her to begin the opiate pill immediately – and the drops of castor and laudanum.[53]

In other words, everyone had the drugs; only the doctor had the special prescribing skills. That is what Farington's friend, Sir Anthony Carlisle, had in mind when he praised a fellow practitioner: 'Dr Warren never killed in vain'. What did this apparently backhanded compliment mean? 'Warren', Carlisle explained, 'found that medicines which in certain cases were reputed to be specific, & did not produce the effect expected, He wd. not adhere to them as many Physicians do secundum artem, but wd. consider what might be more likely to meet the case with advantage.'[54] Thus Warren learnt from his apparent failures, and above all built up a profound understanding of how to match conditions, patients and drugs.

PAIN AND OPIATES

Georgian therapeutics did not proclaim there was a pill for every ill, that individual diseases could be overcome by specifics or 'magic bullets'.[55] After all, contemporary medicine did not view disease itself as 'specific', but as 'dis-ease' or 'dis-temper', marking a general imbalance of the humours, a disorder of the digestive system, nerves or blood. Hence, drugs were typically expected to perform indirect services. They might, as we have just seen, purge 'peccant humours'. Or they might fortify the body's own resources by cleansing, sweetening and purifying the blood, or toning up the nerves. 'Alterative medicines' were widely used to strengthen the constitution; tonics and bitters to brace the stomach. Some drugs would warm, others cool the system, important for counter-balancing the effects of chills and fevers.[56]

During the eighteenth century, a further use for drugs claimed greater attention: their role as pain-killers. Sick people in Antiquity, in the Middle Ages, and thereafter, had to bear pain to a degree hardly imaginable nowadays. In attempting to cope, they had recourse to religion and philosophy; alcohol, too.[57] But traditional medicine did not have a battery of effective pain-killers; indeed, pain-killing was not a primary part of its rationale.

Was the pain threshold of the pre-moderns in any objective sense different from ours? The question is probably circular and fruitless.[58] But the Georgians certainly began to argue that, as sensibility grew more refined, the endurance of excruciating pain was becoming more traumatic. Yet remedy was, providentially, to hand. For from the seventeenth century onwards, opium became more widely available. It was, and was recognized as being, a pain-killer and sedative without peer.[59] George Cheyne sang its praises:

Providence has been kind and gracious to us beyond all Expression, in furnishing us with a certain *Relief*, if not a Remedy, even to our most *intense Pains* and *extreme Miseries*. When our Patience can hold out no longer, and our Pains are at last come to be *insupportable*, we have always ready at Hand a Medicine, which is not only a present Relief, but, I may say, a standing and *constant Miracle*. Those only who have wanted it most, and have felt its friendly and kind Help in their Tortures, can best tell its *wonderful Effects*, and the great *Goodness* of Him who has bestowed it on us. I mean *Opium*, and its Solution *Laudanum*; which when properly prescribed, and prudently managed, is a most *certain* and *sudden* Relief in all *exquisite* and *intense* Pain.[60]

Commonly taken in the more palatable liquid forms of laudanum and paregoric, or in proprietary brews such as Godfrey's Cordial and the notorious Kendal Black Drop, opium became very widely used and was openly on sale. It was bought in halfpenny or penny paperfuls by common people to help cope with the routine pains of life – especially in fenland areas where it was used by chronic sufferers from 'marsh fever' (ague or malaria).[61] Thus opium became part of the self-dosers' repertoire. But it was most effective, argued doctors such as Thomas Trotter, when properly prescribed by experts: 'When pain and restlessness come to be urgent, and when common harmless remedies fail, there is no resource besides opium. We know its sovereign powers as an anodyne, and we must compound with its bad effects in the best manner we can.'[62] It could be taken in many forms, Trotter concluded, but 'I prefer the enema'. Doctors remained remarkably sanguine that, despite reports to the contrary, opium would not prove addictive. 'The End will be obtained, without any Fear of *Over-dosing*', argued Cheyne, for 'the Truth is, there is less Hazard of that, than Persons are aware. For those who die of an Over-dose of *Laudanum*, in the *Opinion of the World*, would have lived few Days without it. For there are those that, by Custom, have brought themselves to *Two Drams* of Solid, that is, near *six Ounces* of Liquid *Laudanum* a Day.'[63]

Thus opiates were prescribed with confidence by physicians. David Garrick's mother, who fell ill in 1734 with violent pains in her hip and a 'Fever on her Spirits', was treated by Dr Robert James. 'Nothing gives her ease but opium', her son reported, 'and she has been easy these three weeks.'[64] In 1791, the German technologist, Rudolf Erich Raspe, suffered 'tormenting nervous headaches'. He consulted his friend, Dr Joseph Black, who prescribed laudanum: 'that surely will lay the pain and make the Devil sleep'. Yet Raspe was not totally happy: 'will it not make me drowsy also?'[65] Unaccustomed to their materia medica possessing such power, doctors seized upon what seemed a wonder drug, experimenting with its possible uses for a multitude of conditions.

King-Hele has drawn attention to the diversity of Erasmus Darwin's recommendations, citing some instances from his *Zoonomia*:

Anorexia Want of appetite . . . Opium half a grain twice a day . . .
Impotency . . . he was advised to take a grain of opium before he went to bed . . .
Gallstones . . . Opium a grain and a half . . .
Painful epilepsy . . . Opium grain every half hour . . .
Sleepwalking . . . Opium in large doses . . .
Tetanus trismus . . . Opium in very large doses . . .

Darwin tried .out many of these therapies himself. When his first wife, Mary Howard, was dying of cirrhosis of the liver, Darwin 'relieved' her with 'great doses of opium'.[67] When three-year-old Milly Pole (soon to become his stepdaughter) lost flesh and spirits, he took her back with him to Lichfield for treatment with opium. He was soon pleased to report, 'She has now taken a grain of opium thrice a day for a month.'[68] Dying in agony, Mrs Wynne was heavily sedated with opiates, taking '120 drops of laudanum a day', which (her daughter recorded) 'convulses her in a shocking manner and at times deprives her of her senses.'[69]

THE PSYCHOLOGY OF DRUGGING

Some drugs – purges, above all – produced powerful effects, and opiates quelled pain. But the great majority of the ingredients in the most of the drugs the doctors prescribed were rather inert – as were many of the nostrums the sick bought by the gallon from empirics. Was this deluge of dosing, then, at best a soothing ritual, or at worst an exercise in cynical exploitation and profiteering orchestrated by the medicos?

Contemporaries certainly saw the potential for a beneficial placebo effect. Discussing the uncanny power of quacks to cure better than true physicians, Dr Peter Shaw contended that this was thanks to the patient's imagination, which quacks knew how to activate. People were often 'sick by Imagination', Shaw argued; in that case, it was perfectly proper that 'Physicians should endeavour to cure by Imagination. And, of such Cures, there have been so many remarkable Instances, as might afford sufficient Hints for ingenious Gentlemen to work upon.'[70] – and, he added, by so suggesting, 'I would not be suspected of endeavouring to degrade the Art of Physic'. Patients might be improved, partly through faith in the doctor's remedies, or faith in the doctor, somatized through his medicines, or even by a general wish to please him. In other words, prescribing medicine could impart a message which said 'I heal'. Little as patients might like medicines, they felt frustrated and nonplussed by the practitioner who would not prescribe them.   There were other ways in which special power seemed to be vested in the doctor's stewardship of drugs. One was the perception, fostered by the profession, that certain materia medica were dangerous and should be kept in the doctor's hands alone. Farington was told by his friend, Thompson, how he 'was much afflicted with fever during a visit to Italy': 'He also had the Ague, at Naples, for which he took *Bark* witht. it having the least effect, which caused a Neopolitan Physician to give Him two Pills which He took upon the symptoms of the *ague fit* commencing; and in a very short time He felt a *warmth* throughout, and the fit repelled & from that period He has never had a return of it.'[71] What was this sovereign medicine? 'The Physician afterwards told Him it was *Arsenick* . . . This remedy is known to our Physicians, but must be used with very great caution: & like other violent stimulants, may eventually bring on Paralysis.'[72] It is quite possible that many of the ailments of Shelley and of Charles Darwin were brought on by arsenical self-dosing.[73]

The faculty also claimed to possess certain specially potent compound medicines. Here they were skating on thin ice, since they themselves always calumniated secret remedies and panaceas as arrant quackery.[74] Regulars were not always lilywhite in this respect, however, and Sir Hans Sloane complained of 'some physicians of good morals and great reputation' who nevertheless made it their business to keep their remedies secret.[75] Hence it was believed important for regulars to publish the details of their darling cures. Thus Cheyne boasted the efficacy of what he called his 'universal remedy', valuable for all those suffering from their stomachs, but explained how to make it up:

> Take of simple *Camomile-Flower Water*, Six Ounces; *Compound Gentian*, and *Wormwood Waters*, each an Ounce and Half; Compound Spirit of *Lavender*, *Sal Volatile*, *Tincture of Castor* and *Gum Ammoniack* dissolved in some simple Water, each two Drams; Tincture of the *Species Diambrae*, each a Dram; the *Chymical Oils* of *Lavender*, *Juniper*, and *Nutmeg*, each ten Drops, mix'd with a Bit of the Yolk of an Egg, to make the whole uniform; *Assafoetida* and *Camphire* in a Rag, each half a Dram: But these may be left out by Those to whom they are disagreeable.[76]

How seriously did Cheyne intend this 'universal' claim to be taken? Was he engaging in a harmless psychological bluff?

During the course of the century, however, doctors took it upon themselves to pioneer new drug treatments. Sloane was one of the leading popularizers of bark (quinine).[77] William Withering pioneered digitalis, extracted from foxglove, which was beneficial in cases of dropsy and asthma (that is, what we would see as heart disease).[78] Numerous doctors championed ether.[79] Some, most notably Thomas Beddoes, Erasmus Darwin and their circle, tested factitious airs, such as carbon dioxide and nitrous oxide, and experimented with soda-water for the cure of scurvy. Beddoes imaginatively speculated on the use of foxglove, combined with artificial airs, to conquer consumption, whereby multitudes would be 'preserved from premature death'.[80] Therapeutic optimism and innovation were in the air.

At the very least, the association of doctors' reputations with particular concoctions provided an endless topic of society conversation. One day, a certain 'Eau Medicinale' was mentioned. Farington's physician friend, Hayes, identified it as the 'celebrated medicine which in gouty complaints produces extraordinary effects. He said it has not been yet ascertained what this medicine consists of, but it has no mineral in it, & its quality is of a vegetable nature.'[81] Here further medical opinion weighed in, only to heighten the mixture's mystique: 'Dr. Clarke informed Hayes that Sir Henry Halford had assured Him that He had given it in 18 instances in each of which it was successful. Hayes gave it to a patient lame with the gout on whom it operated so quickly that in three Hours He was able to run up stairs.'[82] (Echoes of quack puffery here!) But if the Eau was hot stuff, the doctors nevertheless immediately dissociated themselves from its possibly quackish abuses: 'When further experience of it has been had Hayes thinks it may become a medicine of very great value; at present, as no medicine will suit all constitutions, objections have been made to it on acct. of unfavourable effects having been produced in some instances: but He observed that similar objections might be made to that most valuable medicine *Opium* & to the no less sovereign remedy *Mercury*, when injudiciously given.'[83]

SURGERY

Drugs formed a vital exchange between the sick and their physicians, indeed, the main currency passing to the patient in return for the fees accruing to the doctor. And yet, as we have seen, they were a slightly dubious coinage. Patients worried whether they were counterfeit (almost literally, since apothecaries were always being accused, by patients and physicians alike, of adulterating medicaments for the sake of profit). At best, there was the fear that drugs constituted sleight of hand, rather in the manner of Catholic transubstantiation.

The services provided by surgeons were far more tangible and appreciated (even where dangerous), thus constituting a better bond between the patient and professional. Partly because the quality of surgical training and skills improved during the century, surgery rose in esteem.[84] At a pinch, the patient could make do without a physician; but when need arose, the surgeon was indispensable. Of course, there was a great deal of home surgery, first-aid in case of emergency. It was a boozy harvest in 1790: 'This afternoon Briton cut off part of his left hand Thumb with a Sickle', lamented Parson Woodforde, 'owing in a great Measure to his making too free with Liquor at Norwich to day, having met his Uncle Scurl there who treated him with Wine. It bled very much.'[85] Woodforde to the rescue: 'I put some Friars Balsam to it and had it bound up, he almost fainted.'

Yet all the signs point to a general extension of surgery carried out by professionals, and with the growing confidence of the laity. The surgeon-apothecary's bag became a sophisticated item of equipment during the eighteenth century (all too often, we think only of the strong knots of Dr Slop). One of the key topics in the Weekes correspondence comprised the orders for medico-surgical supplies of the latest design, which Hampton Weekes was to obtain in London for his family's Sussex practice.[86]

There was much need for surgery in the pre-modern world: accidents were common at work, on the road, in the home; life-events such as childbirth often led to lesions that needed patching up. The Weekes letters reveal the kinds of surgery routinely being performed in Sussex at the close of the eighteenth century:

Crural hernia which Hampton thought was probably an aneurism
Hand shattered by a bursting gun, amputated
Hydrocele injected
Cut for the stone, and the bill of £15 was thought too much, but the parish eventually paid
Forming a new anus in a girl of 14 months
Injection of hydrocele with an apparatus Hampton sent from London
Reference to strangulated hernia that Richard Weekes had operated on previously
Congenital hernia that became irreducible after the truss broke, strangulated and operation offered, but refused by the patient
Fistula in ano operated on by Dick [Richard Weekes's younger son], during which the bistory broke
Reference to previous lithotomy at Patcham
Dick sent to draw a tooth. 'Should get half a guinea at least'
Reference to previous lithotomy at Withdean
Carcinoma of the breast referred to Blizard for operation
Opening of abscess in thigh. One quart of curdled pus evacuated
Two scrophulous hip abscesses
Carcinoma of the rectum
Bleeding from haemorrhoidal vessels[87]

Pre-modern surgery was undoubtedly hazardous, and greatly feared – not without good reason. A compound fracture of a leg, common in those days of horse transport, usually meant an amputation, and amputees often died of trauma, blood loss or sepsis. People held back from major surgery when they could. For example, William Windham, Pitt the Younger's one-time secretary for war, underwent an operation which had proved utterly terrifying. According to Carlisle, as reported by Farington: 'abt. 3 weeks before the operation was performed upon Him, he asked His [Carlisle's] opinion respecting an operation. Carlisle's answer was for the negative. He then told me that Mr. Windham was in reality a very nervous man; and that when the persons who were to perform the operation & to superintend it were assembled, viz: Messrs. Home, Lind & the Apothecary; Mr. Windham was for sometime very irresolute.'[88] We might not be surprised; yet, by the standards of 1800, Windham's behaviour was thought pretty unmanly: 'He walked about His room in His night gown, & told them, that though He had sent for them to perform the operation He now felt Himself not to be ready to submit to it, that He found He was not a Man constituted for such a purpose.'[89] He was presumably shamed into action: 'At last, however, He determined to have it performed. Lind performed the operation, & the *Cutting* part lasted 20 *minutes*, during which Mr. Windham occasionally spoke to them . . . After it was over He said He "should never recover from it".'[90] Almost as if to prove himself right, 'he continued to think so till his Death.'

Yet it is remarkable how few Windhams there were. Contemporary documents reveal a stalwart preparedness to submit to the surgeon for all manner of treatments. Suffering from his eyes, Thomas Turner had Snelling, his surgeon, open one of his temples (the rationale: letting blood would release pressure upon the vessels): 'The artery lying deep, the operation was obliged to be performed with a dissecting knife. The first cut did not hurt greatly, but the incision not being big enough at the 1st cut, he was obliged to cut a second time, which hurt me very much . . . My wife very ill.'[91] Turner was proud of his own resolution: 'I asked several people to assist Mr. Snelling in doing it, but could get none till I asked Dame Durrant, who assisted in doing it.'[92]

Perhaps the knife actually held out the allure of radical, instant relief from atrocious, chronic conditions, and so possessed an attractive simplicity. Becoming dropsical once again late in life, Samuel Johnson wanted to be tapped. His surgeon proceeded cautiously. Johnson was furious, retorting that he wanted life, whereas the surgeon was afraid of giving him pain. On another occasion, Johnson reportedly said he would be prepared to have a limb amputated if it would relieve him of his melancholy.[93]

Thus surgery made sense because it promised action, and its advances were eagerly followed. Early in the seventeenth century, John Manningham bubbled over about a 'cure by cutting' which was 'a newe invention, a kinde of practise not knowne to former ages'. What he described was a new lithotomy technique: 'There is seame in the passage of the yard neere the fundament, which the surgeons searche with a crooked instrument concaved at the one end (called a catheter) whereinto they make incision and then grope for the stone with an other toole which they call a duckes bill, Yf the stone be greater.'[94] Although lithotomy remained dangerous, most of the operations performed by surgeons were small-scale and relatively safe. Blood-letting was the epitome. It had many rationales appreciated no less by the laity than by the profession. It would evacuate stale blood and provide vital relief to a patient suffering from a plethora. Sometimes phlebotomy was used as a routine prophylactic, rather like a purge.[95] Lady Louisa Conolly's niece, Charlotte, had, as we saw above, a fall from her horse. The surgeon, Mr Poole, was called in, and she was 'blooded by way of precaution'.[96] She was confined to bed, and bled again a fortnight later, and, as a result of these measures, seemed to recover. Her mother was pleased to have gone in for the bleeding; the episode 'proves the necessity of being over-cautious'.[97]

Historians commonly depict blood-letting as barbaric and bizarre, evidence surely of the primitive nature of pre-modern medicine. Yet it was clearly popular amongst the public. 'There were not a few, especially among the country working-people, who deemed bleeding once or twice a year a great safeguard, or a help to health', was Sir James Paget's recollection of popular feeling in early-Victorian East Anglia:

> [Countryfolk] came frequently on market-days at the times of spring and fall, and generally did their work in the market and then walked to the surgery. There they were at once bled, and usually were bled till they fainted, or felt very faint and became pale; then a pad was put over the wounded vein, and a bandage round the elbow; and they went home, often driving three or four miles into the country. I have no recollection of any evidence that either good or harm was ever done by this practice.[98]

It was not just Suffolk yokels who had faith in regular blood-letting: it had its devotees across the social spectrum. Thomas Turner sometimes had his blood let on his birthday. Dr Taylor, Boswell reported, had a nose-bleed. Taylor explained that it was 'because he had omitted four days to have himself blooded after a quarter of a year's interval'.[99] Obviously he thought he had simply filled up with too much blood. Through the operation, bad blood would be removed and the body would feel cleansed. Elizabeth Iremonger was troubled in the summer of 1800 with headaches and 'Plethora'. She 'submitted to be blooded', and it 'gave me immediate relief'. She also 'had leeches applied' to her temples.[100] These were operations which could be done at home, by oneself, a servant or a friend; yet they could most conveniently be performed by a dextrous surgeon.

Bleeding is the best example of the enduring popularity of an ancient surgical procedure; the best instance of a new one is inoculation. This was a folk practice, widely used in the Levant, where it was traditionally administered by old women.[101] Once brought to England, doctors significantly took it over (though occasionally it was performed by lay people). Medical practitioners tried to make a mystique of it, advising careful pre-inoculation preparation and medication, post-inoculation rest and the need for appropriate physical isolation. What might have been the work of a few minutes was turned into an elaborate fortnight's ritual for those with money to spare and time on their hands.[102]

The enlargement of surgical interventions perhaps marks the first signs of a new medical Prometheanism, the belief that mechanical means could fix the misfunctioning body. The spread of medical electricity epitomized this vision. Many Georgian surgeons made much of the potential of electric fields, sparks and currents, particularly for overcoming nervous conditions and revivifying the debilitated. Erasmus Darwin was an enthusiast. He had a patient, 'Mr S., a gentleman between 40 and 50 years of age, [who] had had the jaundice about six weeks, without pain, sickness, or fever; and had taken emetics, cathartics, mercurials, bitters, chalybeates, essential oils, and ether, without apparent advantage.' He tried electrification:

> On a supposition that the obstruction of the bile might be owing to paralysis or torpid action of the common bile-duct, and the stimulants taken into the stomach seeming to have no effect, I directed half a score smart electric shocks from a coated bottle, which held about a quart, to be passed through the liver, and along the course of the common gallduct, as near as could be guessed, and on that very day the stools became yellow; he continued the electric shocks a few days more, and his skin gradually became clear.[103]

Patients themselves were eager for electrical treatment. John Baker underwent electrification, directed by his surgeon, for his multiple arthritic pains. The benefits were not lasting.[104]

The new science began to unfold promising vistas for doctors with a technological bent. Eighteenth-century pneumatic chemistry stressed the medicinal virtues of air. Thomas Beddoes set up his Pneumatic Institution in Bristol to experiment with airs as putative consumption cures.[105] In correspondence with Beddoes, Erasmus Darwin became similarly fascinated with the powers of aerated waters to overcome bilious conditions. Writing to his friend, Matthew Boulton, he inquired where Jacob Schweppe's admirable waters could be obtained, outlining their splendid powers: 'Now I have a patient, who has I think a small stone in his bladder, left after having frequently made bloody urine, and I am giving him aerated water, with half an ounce of sal soda to the pint -

but could wish to have it better impregnated with the carbonic acid gas.'[106] After experimental trials, Darwin became a warm advocate of aerated seltzer waters, recommending them in his *Zoonomia* and to individual patients, particularly for use against the stone.

If there was no revolution in therapeutics in the Georgian age, there was at least a bubbling ferment, which helped to buoy up the status of medical practitioners. On the one hand, claims to therapeutic skills enhanced that element of personal mystique which (as we saw in the previous chapter) practitioners were deploying with considerable aplomb. On the other, a culture increasingly investing significance in the possession and power of material objects was disposed to treat the doctor's armoury of drugs with expectancy, though hardly implicit trust. Increasingly, drugs provided the medium of exchange which cemented the implicit contract between patients and practitioners.

10

Doctors and Women

It has been widely contended that the long eighteenth century was of decisive importance in reorienting the relative gender identities of men and women, and thereby transforming the place and role of women within English society. Feminist scholars have argued that the development of new forms of professional authority made no small contribution to such processes. The power of all-male professions (the law and medicine, above all) was conscripted to underwrite patriarchalist hegemony, legitimating prejudices through the mystiques of science, reason, nature, law, etc. In this brief chapter, we ask how, and how far, changing kinds of interaction between women and doctors in the Georgian era square with such interpretations. Does evidence deriving from letters, diaries, etc., support the view that professional authority was serving to put women in their place as the 'weaker vessel'?[1]

Two radically contradictory interpretations have, in fact, been put forward as to the significance of medicine and medical practitioners in shaping the broader social destiny of women. One, which may be called 'optimistic', is largely associated with the work of Edward Shorter.[2] This argues that the subordinate place of women in the pre-modern social order was fixed by a combination of biological and social factors. Above all, pregnancy and childbirth massively disadvantaged women, in ways poignantly summed up on a gravestone for a young widow: 'Nineteen years a maiden, – One year a wife, – One hour a mother – And so I lost my life.'[3] A succession of pregnancies tied the great majority of women in the prime of life to childbearing, motherhood and household management; in the late eighteenth and early nineteenth centuries, what had always been necessity was turned increasingly into an ideal ('the angel in the home').[4] The mother of Edward Gibbon was married for 127 months before she died in childbed. She was pregnant for at least sixty-three of these months, bearing six children. Only her eldest child survived her.[5]

Being a fertile married woman in pre-contraceptive age, when most married couples did not practise what Malthus called 'moral restraint', was perhaps the highest-risk occupation of all. Many women, such as Mary Wollstonecraft, died in childbed itself. Countless thousands more suffered both the short-term sicknesses associated with pregnancy and birth, and their attendant long-term disabilities, including disfigurement and diseases of the womb and genitals.

Men forced this lot upon women by subjecting them to many pregnancies. It was exacerbated by the upholding of certain traditional practices, such as the collective women-only ritual of childbirth orchestrated by the midwife. For, Shorter argues, excluded from a proper medical-anatomical education, the traditional midwife was not particularly skilful, especially when faced with abnormal deliveries. Moreover, midwives enjoyed exercising their own authority over mothers, and ostentating their own virtuosity. They were 'interventionist' by disposition, and their petty ways – above all, their eagerness to pluck out the baby, by force if necessary, at the earliest opportunity – was often dangerous, even fatal, for mother and baby alike. Such perils of childbirth helped perpetuate a culture in which women's conditions (menstruation, parturition, suckling, etc.) and women's diseases were seen as manifestations of the 'polluted' nature of women's biological bodies. In turn, this underlined a sexual division of labour in which the medical care of women, especially in pregnancy, was kept exclusive to women.[6]

Women were thus virtually segregated, but were accomplices in the perpetuation of the process. They began to make progress towards social integration and equality only, Shorter argues, when they left this women-only ghetto and joined the wider world of men. This could not happen before they ceased to be chained to careers of endless childbirth and childcare, and before childbearing itself ceased to be so hazardous. Such transformations have come about essentially within the last century, thanks to advances in modern scientific medicine, the development of effective contraception, the widespread practice of safe abortion and the emergence of obstetric techniques safe for mothers and babies alike. All these might be seen as gifts to women from the largely male-dominated medical profession.[7]

Some harbingers of these processes, however, can be traced during the long eighteenth century, above all in the development of man-midwifery. For increasingly, amongst affluent, polite society at least, the old 'granny midwife' was being abandoned in favour of regularly-trained medical men specializing in obstetrics.

These men-midwives or accoucheurs as some liked to call themselves, were well trained in anatomy. They had typically attended one of the Scottish universities or the midwifery courses run by experts such as William Smellie or William Hunter in London.[8] They were thus better able to cope successfully with abnormal births involving malpresentations; they could, for example, perform podalic version. Following the lead of William Hunter, they were far more apt to let Nature take her course, condemning the excessive, officious interference of the traditional midwife: this, in itself, proved safer. And not least, when childbirth went amiss, they were skilled in the handling of forceps – quite a recent innovation – and other surgical instruments, from the use of which midwives were debarred. Thus to a certain degree, one of the most traumatic events of a woman's life was becoming medicalized, placed in the hands of a male practitioner and all-male expertise. As Shorter has argued, this represented a small progressive step.

Feminist scholars have put a far more pessimistic reading on the developments just outlined. They have argued that the effects upon women's well-being of this drift towards medicalizing the crucial events of their lives – menarche, menstruation, pregnancy, birth, infant-feeding, child-rearing, menopause, etc. – have been ambiguous, to say the least. They have characterized the new Georgian accoucheurs as 'forceps-happy', and it has been argued that by their invasive, aggressive and unnecessary deployment of surgical instruments they did far more harm than good. Above all, dirty instruments spreaded post-partum sepsis, particularly in the new lying-in hospitals set up for poor women. Worse still, this march of medicalization invaded and appropriated an area of traditional female support and expertise, displacing midwives from what always had been women's work.[9]

By way of parallel, it has been claimed that the hounding of witches similarly resulted in the exclusion of women from the practice of healing. All such developments were part of a wider movement whereby medicine, operating as the mouthpiece of patriarchy, wedged women firmly in their (inferior) place. In proposing marriage to Rebecca Smith, Benjamin Rush, America's leading late eighteenth-century physician, made the situation perfectly plain: 'Don't be offended when I add that from the day you marry you must have no will of your own. The subordination of your sex to ours is enforced by nature, by reason, and by revelation.'[10]

The authority of doctors, educators and moralists thus joined (feminists claim) to induct women even more rigidly into a culture of domesticity and femininity, demarcated by 'separate spheres': public life for men, the home and children for women.[11] It was a role women themselves internalized, often with some exultation at their own superiority. Seeing her sick father in 1815, Georgina Capel wrote: 'Papa's illness makes me more than ever pity *Batchelors*; for after all what miserable helpless wretches men are without [wives], if they require any sort of comfort or attendance.'[12]

The domesticity of women was, in turn, enforced (it is argued) by the formulation by medicine and science of a highly convenient physiological theory, which emphasized with renewed force how women were fundamentally anatomically and physiologically – and hence psychologically – different from men. Being governed by their reproductive system, women were weaker, supersensitive, highly nervous by nature. Properly to fulfil their biological role as childbearers and mothers, it was essential that women did not intellectually over-exert themselves through educational ambition or attempt to emulate men in public life. Increasingly in the nineteenth century, it was further emphasized that virtuous and healthy women should also experience only the most attenuated sexual desires and needs. Women who attempted to break out of this mould of innocent domesticity would become sickly, overstrained and, indeed, hysterical – would suffer from what Elaine Showalter has called 'the female malady'.[13] It tickled Byron to contemplate the absurd contortions involved in the idea that to be interesting and attractive a woman had to be ultra-delicate. He told Lady Melbourne about the wife of 'my friend Webster': 'His bride Lady Frances is a pretty pleasing woman – but in delicate health & I fear going – if not gone – into a decline – Stanhope & his wife – pretty & pleasant too but not at all consumptive – left us today – leaving only ye. family – another single gentlemen and your slave.'[14]

This chapter cannot pretend to resolve the debate just outlined. One reason for this is that we have found that the type of evidence upon which our book is based affords only rather few signs that contemporary women were particularly conscious of their gender as a prime factor in general health differentials or in shaping patient/doctor relations. Without a doubt, medical treatises throughout the long eighteenth century were endlessly laying down the law as to the special biomedical nature of women, and the social duties and moral prescriptions inexorably following from it. Sex-advice literature was for ever instructing women (and men, too) in their proper sexual attitudes and practices; a multitude of pamphleteers argued the case *pro* and *con* male and female midwives. The rights and wrongs of women were debated in the political arena, and numerous novels discussed the 'women question'.[15] The importance of such general writings for forming individuals' attitudes cannot be gainsaid. Nevertheless, we have encountered relatively few signs that the attitudes and actions of women, when actually sick and confronted with making medical choices, were coloured by sexual politics, by wider questions relating the rights and duties of women to the rights and duties of doctors.

The research that would afford a true profile of the extent of healing as a female occupation in Georgian England has not yet been done. The extent of female practice should not be underestimated. Many women healers advertised in newspapers, for example, Mrs Plunkett Edgcumbe, the cancer-curer, who touted her services widely in Bath newspapers late in the eighteenth century.[16] When Henry Fielding's wife was racked with toothache, he looked for 'the best tooth-drawer' available, and ended up with 'a female of great eminence in the art'.[17] Some women achieved fame and fortune, such as Joanna Stephens with her stone-dissolving nostrum.[18] Sally Mapp of Epsom became the most eminent bone-setter of her day. Large numbers of other women dabbled in the art. At Kingston Grammar School, to which Gibbon was sent, a Mrs Wooddesdon was said, by a male detractor to have 'a dangerous propensity to dabble in medicine, and thought herself perfectly able, with the aid of an ignorant apothecary, to manage the most formidable disorders'.[19] Records such as Ralph Josselin's diary show local women being widely called upon to treat children, servants, family, friends and neighbours alike. Early in the eighteenth century, the Blundell family used a local woman, Betty Morice or Morris, to let blood and perform minor surgery on wounds. 'My wife took Phisick from Mrs Meginnis', wrote Nicholas Blundell in 1713.[20]

The employment of women healers was normal. Is there any evidence that sick women wished to be treated exclusively by women? We have found none. Indeed, the radical author, Maria Hays, asserted that the idea of women being handled by women was disgusting.[21]

Women were prominent in domestic healing. It might be assumed, moreover, that with the development of the reality and ideology of separate spheres for men and women, the dispensing of domestic physic might become left almost entirely in the hands of women, or monopolized by them, as being beneath the attention of the superior sex. But this surmise is not supported by the evidence. From the mid-seventeenth century right through to the mid-nineteenth, men and women, husbands and wives, fathers and mothers were both more or less equally involved in the practice of 'medicine without doctors'. There is no discernible trend to the feminization of the domestic healing role. Perhaps medical self-care was so important – and the need for first aid so common – that no individual could afford to abandon the field, even to his or her spouse. Writers of health-care manuals conspicuously addressed them to both sexes. The lay meddlers of whom Dr Adair so vociferously complained were 'gentlemen and lady doctors'.[22] It was certainly not the case that men read the medical books and women made use of the oral lore. In his *Virgin Unmasked*, Bernard Mandeville's character, Lucinda, boasts, 'I have read several Books of Physick'.[23]

The different sexes may have had a tendency to specialize in different fields. Women perhaps knew kitchen ingredients better – they would certainly be more familiar with common abortifacient herbs such as savin, thyme and marjoram.[24] Possibly it was the man who was more likely to use instruments – for pulling teeth or lancing boils. But if domestic physic was not left to the ladies, it may be significant that it was widely argued that it should certainly not be left to the menials. It should no more be beneath the dignity of the lady of the house to exercise medical skill, argued Lady Pennington, than to breastfeed her own babies: 'The management of all domestic affairs is certainly the proper business of women – and, unfashionably rustic as such an assertion may be thought, it is not beneath the dignity of any lady, however high her rank, to know how to educate children, to govern her servants, how to order an elegant table with economy and to manage her whole family with prudence, regularity, and method.'[25]

BODIES, WOMEN, DISEASES

It has been argued that during the long eighteenth century in particular, a new medical conception of women was formulated. The traditional notion that women were simply feebler versions of men was increasingly replaced by the claim, emanating chiefly from medical men, that women were anatomically quite distinct from men, above all, possessing far more delicate nervous systems.[26] This rendered them more susceptible to disease, and liable to disorders which men seldom, if ever, suffered from, especially hysteria.[27] In the long run, mental and emotional disease increasingly came to be associated with the female of the species.[28]

This had repercussions for sexuality. It was claimed in medical tracts that female sexuality was by its very nature passive.[29] By the Victorian age, extremists were contending that active sexuality in a woman was something pathological, leading both to physical and mental disease.[30]

Ideas of this kind are extremely common in medical tracts and advice literature, not to mention comic novels. But they are remarkable by their absence from the letters and journals of men and women faced with the actual circumstances of sickness. The age of sensibility produced a great crop of hysterical women, but only between the covers of novels.

The classic female invalid (of the stamp of Florence Nightingale) is a product not of the Georgian but of the Victorian era. In the eighteenth century, preoccupation with being ill, weak and delicate was arguably more of a worry to men than to women. Male hypochondriacs perhaps outnumbered female hysterics. Medical pundits such as Thomas Trotter, anxious about what they saw as the disposition of the age to nervous diseases warned against the tendency for 'many of our fair countrywomen [to] carry laudanum about with them, and take it freely when under low spirits'.[31] Such authors were, however, perhaps more alarmed at the 'feminization' of men than at invalidism amongst women.

WOMEN AND DOCTORS

It is easy to find examples of the doctor reinforcing male authority in a patriarchal society. Thus Patrick Blair, treating a married woman who had become mildly distracted and opted out of her marital and parental duties, showing 'dislike to her husband', went in for appallingly sadistic punitive treatment:

> I ordered her to be blindfolded. Her nurse and other women stript her. She was lifted up by force, plac'd in and fixt to the Chair in the bathing Tub. All this put her in an unexpressable terrour especially when the water was let down. I kept her under the fall 30 minutes, stopping the pipe now and then and enquiring whether she would take to her husband.[32]

The lady was not for turning:

> She still obstinately deny'd till at last being much fatigu'd with the pressure of the water she promised she would do what I desired on which I desisted, let her go to bed, gave her a Sudorifick as usual. She slept well that night but was still obstinate. I repeated the Tryal by adding a smaller pipe so that when the one let the water fall on top of her head the other squirted it in her face or any other part of her head neck or breast I thought proper. Being still very strong I gave her 60 minutes at this time when she still kept so obstinate that she was laid a bed as formerly but next day she was still obstinate.[33]

At last she broke under the physical and mental torture:

> Evacuations being endeavoured for 90 minutes under it, promised obedience as before but she was as sullen and obstinate as ever the next day. Being upon resentment why I should treat her so, after 2 or 3 dayes I threatned her with the fourth Tryal, took her out of bed, had her stript, blindfolded and ready to be put in the Chair, when being terrify'd with what she was to undergo she kneeld submissively that I would spare her and she would become a Loving obedient and dutiful Wife for ever thereafter. I granted her request provided she would go to bed with her husband that night, which she did with great chearfullness.[34]

Blair was pleased to report a happy ending: 'About 1 month afterwards I went to pay her a visit, saw every thing in good order.'

The general picture, however, is very different. The evidence of the correspondence of hundreds of women indicates that their relations to professional doctors were primarily shaped not by gender but by class. We have found no evidence of women correspondents complaining that doctors mistreated or abused them, or even condescended to them, because of their sex; nor, indeed, any sign that women of the middling and upper classes were unwilling to consult doctors because that would involve unacceptably demeaning or dangerous relations. When Anne Lister in early nineteenth-century Halifax suspected that she had caught venereal disease from her girl-friend, she appears to have felt no embarrassment in taking her condition to her local practitioner. Likewise, when the Duchess of Grafton summoned a man-midwife (William Hunter) and instructed him to handle with utter discretion the clandestine delivery of her illegitimate child, it was with the imperious authority of one used to command. The Duchess expected – and got – no moral lectures from the unctuous Scot. Doctors knew their place, and had an eye to their careers.[35]

Does this apply to childbirth at large? As scholars such as Jean Donnison, Adrian Wilson, Edward Shorter, Audrey Eccles, Margaret Versluysen and Judith Lewis have very amply documented, the man-midwife increasingly became the normal recourse for those who could afford his services.[36] In the seventeenth century, the male accoucheur seems to have been used almost solely for difficult and abnormal deliveries.[37] By contrast, increasingly during the Georgian age, women drew upon the service of male operators for routine deliveries. Over a period of some eighteen months, the Weekes partnership at Hurstpierpoint in Sussex left record of the following obstetrical work:

Puerperal fever

Peforator used last week, 'The woman is brave'

Went to Ditchling and finding Mrs Godly not likely to be delivered Mrs Hannington brought abed

Four labours from five in the afternoon until next morning

Richard Weekes used the perforator

Richard Weekes at Poynings six hours before delivery

Mrs Burt in labour just before she developed smallpox. Child unmarked

Two or three labours a week

An abortion

Used the perforator for face to pubis presentation. Waters had broken previously, so would not chance turning the large baby. He had used the instrument ten times and only the first [mother] died

Mrs Dennett delivered. Paid five guineas. Father [Richard Weekes] goes every
day
Six labours this week. One to Dick [Richard Weekes jun.]
Dick at three labours in four days
Eleven labours in twelve days, of which Dick attended six
Mrs. Wood brought abed
Two deaths from puerperal fever last year
Patient with scarlet fever three days post partum. Initially thought to be fever
Mrs P [?Payne] brought abed
Dick attended five more labours lately and will have attended fifty to sixty by
the time he gets to London[38]

During twenty-eight years in practice, Richard Weekes attended some
three thousand labours.

How do we explain this growing female recourse to male operators
and the decline in the fortunes of the traditional female midwife (already
referred to above)? It marked a transition of deep significance for
our wider understanding of the consolidation of medical authority.
Traditional medical historians explained the emergence of the man-
midwife as a function of their monopoly on forceps and other
instruments. Some feminists have built upon this, suggesting that the
typical accoucheur was more aggressive than the traditional midwife.[39]
Men-midwives were forceps-happy, abandoning the old, safe natural
childbirth. Mary Daly has claimed that men midwives were part of a
'gynaecidal' campaign by men to destroy women's health.[40]

But the evidence hardly supports this. For forceps and other
instruments were, in fact, rarely deployed. The public face of fashionable
man-midwifery, on the contrary, emphasized gentleness, patience and
the importance of allowing nature to take its course. Childbirth, argued
luminaries such as William Hunter and Erasmus Darwin, should, above
all, be *natural*.[41] Dismissing the old midwives' habits of dosing mothers
with alcoholic caudle, etc., Darwin insisted 'As Parturition is a natural,
not a morbid process, no medicine should be given, where there is no
appearance of a disease. The absurd custom of giving a powerful opiate
without indication to all women, as soon as they are delivered, is, I
make no doubt, frequently attended with injurious, and sometimes with
fatal consequences.'[42] The march of medicine clearly aimed to win the
confidence of women (and presumably their husbands) by appeal to
cultural values (nature, ease, expertise), carrying powerful resonances in
the age of the Enlightenment. Mothers-to-be seem to have looked to
practitioners who were smooth, polite and confident, in place of the
traditional lower-class and uncouth woman.[43]

From all quarters, complaints arose about the unsatisfactoriness of
traditional midwives. The eminent midwife, Jane Sharp, opened her

Midwives' Book (1671) with this very plea: 'I have often sate down sad
in the Consideration of the many Miseries Women endure in the Hands
of unskilful Midwives; many profess the Art (without any skill in
Anatomy, which is the principal part effectually necessary for a
Midwife).'[44] Fashionable ladies took up the complaint, and increasingly
abandoned the all-women childbirth ritual, adopting instead the new
recommendations for childbirth practice advocated by male practitioners.
Increasingly, the husband was present in the birth room, whereas the
gossips were dismissed. Daylight replaced the darkened room; ventilation
was introduced. At a later stage, maternal breast-feeding replaced the
old wet-nurse.[45] Thomas Withers thus spelt out the optimal conditions
for birth:

> During labor the patient should be kept agreeably warm, but the imprudent
> application of heat should be industriously avoided. The curtains should
> be open, the air cool and pure, and the circulation of it continually
> promoted. The attendants in the room should be few, and they should
> in general keep at a distance from the bed. If they be numerous, and
> croud about the patient, they heat the air and render it impure. By this
> means the woman is weakened, and the birth of the child is necessarily
> retarded. If the labor be severe and difficult, and the patient naturally of
> a relaxed constitution, an impure confined air, together with an imprudent
> application of heat, proves often dangerous, or even fatal in its
> consequences. For by such treatment the patient at last becomes exhausted;
> the natural labor is at a stand; violent measures are adopted; fevers,
> floodings, and inflamations ensue. A pure and temperate air to a woman
> in labor is extremely refreshing.
>
> The general use of caudle should be abolished, as being unnatural and
> pernicious. The period during labor, as well as for some time after
> delivery, is critical, and not very convenient for beginning to acquire the
> habit of drinking wine and spirits . . . The common caudle given during
> labor, heats the patient quickens the pulse, and produces pains in the
> head, with obstinate sickness and depression of strength. It hardly agrees
> even with those women, who at other times are unfortunately accustomed
> to the liberal use of fermented liquors. – The operations of midwifery
> should be performed with the greatest caution and judgment. During
> natural labor, the practitioner should give the necessary assistance, but
> he should not injure the health of the woman, nor increase her misery,
> by his too great officiousness under the specious pretence of relieving
> nature, when nature rejects his aid.[46]

Midwives protested against the emergence of the male operator; but
the most vociferous opposition was voiced by traditionalist men, afraid
that the new male accoucheurs would debauch their wives.[47] William
Cobbett fulminated that to expose one's wife to the ministrations of

such men was 'no small evil'.[48] Wives and mothers, by contrast, seem to have accepted the new development with alacrity.[49]

The emergence of the man-midwife had profound repercussions for the development of the medical profession. In general, the rise of midwifery practice amongst country and small-town practitioners completed the range of skills possessed by the old surgeon-apothecary, who thereby turned into the fully 'general' practitioner. Midwifery could be a kind of 'loss leader'. The local practitioner might find delivering babies gruelling and hardly profitable; but the family that used him to deliver its babies would retain his services for treating infant and childhood sickness and for the whole range of family medicine, from cradle to grave.[50]

THE EMERGENCE OF PAEDIATRICS

In one field in particular, this represented a significant departure, for it was bound up with the emergence of paediatrics. Much evidence suggests that before the eighteenth century it was relatively rare for physicians to be called in to treat young children. Parents seem to have thought of that as their own responsibility, and doctors were not eager to meddle with such precarious lives, in particular with patients who could not helpfully relate their own histories. There is evidence to corroborate this point. In the seventeenth century, the Verney children would not let the doctor near them:

> Molly and Ralph continue as they were, very ill of a feaver & pains with a short Cough very fast, they will not tell where their paines are, nor will they take anything but small Beare, nor that if anything be mingled with it, that we have trouble enough. Those things that they love so very well when in health as Sugar, Candy, Pruines etc. they will not now touch, nor will they let the Doctors touch theire hands, but pray that neither their Unkle Dr. nor Mr. Gelthorpe the Apothecary may not come to 'em.[51]

'God be theire Phisitian', wrote the distracted father, '& spare their lives.'

All this changed, doubtless because of the 'new world of the children in the eighteenth century'.[52] The Georgian age set particular store by the health and growth of the youngster. The boom in manuals on child care and education testifies to a new interest in childhood.[53] Increasingly, doctors themselves contended that it was crucially important that professional practitioners be summoned in case of sickness, instead of ignorant women with their foolish reliance on cordials and juleps. 'Health is a nice Affair', James Nelson argued,

and Life precious to every Individual. The best Advice then I can give
to Parents is, that they do not, where these are at Stake, hazard either
one or the other by Indolence, or an illtim'd Frugality. Those who are
rich, let them at once send for the Physician, especially if it be a Matter
of Moment; and surely Prudence points out this to us: so those who
cannot reach the best, let them take the next best; that is, where calling
in a Physician would too sensibly affect their Circumstances, Prudence
demands, that they employ a good Apothecary first.[54]

In his advice to families, William Buchan confessed that the prejudice
against doctors being called in to treat children still ran strong, not least
amongst old-style doctors themselves:

I know very well in how unbeaten and almost unknown a Path I am
treading; for sick Children, and especially Infants, give no other Light
into the Knowledge of their Diseases, than what we are able to discover
from their uneasy Cries, and the uncertain Tokens of their Crossness;
for which Reason, several Physicians of the first Rank have openly
declared to me, that they go very unwillingly to take care of the Diseases
of Children, especially of such as are newly born, as if they were to
unravel some strange Mystery, or cure some incurable Distemper.[55]

The result, Buchan confessed, was that all too often doctors ignored
young children and left them to unskilled nurses:

Even physicians themselves have not been sufficiently attentive to the
management of children: That has been generally considered as the sole
province of old women while men of the first character in physic have
refused to visit infants even when sick. Such conduct in the faculty has
not only caused this branch of medicine to be neglected, but has also
encouraged the other sex to assume an absolute title to prescribe for
children in the most dangerous diseases. The consequence is, that a
physician is seldom called till the good women have exhausted all their
skill; when his attendance can only serve to divide the blame and appease
the disconsolate parents.[56]

Buchan wanted all this to change. 'Nurses should do all in their power
to prevent diseases; but, when a child is taken ill, some person of skill
ought immediately to be consulted.' This was because the 'diseases of
children are generally acute and the least delay is dangerous'.[57]

What Buchan called for, was beginning to happen. During the
Georgian century, a few physicians actually began to specialize in the
treatment of children, above all the Armstrong brothers.[58] The evidence
of parental letters and diaries registers this new 'aggressive' stance of
doctors towards child diseases, though it marks considerable ambiguity
on their behalf as to whether the 'doctor in the nursery' was a desirable
development. It seems that mothers tended to accept a subordinate role

as the lieutenants implementing regimes for their children's health as instructed by the newly present doctor. If, as we have suggested, there is little sign that middle- and upper-class women were themselves subordinated to the medical profession in the Georgian age, they may well have increasingly deferred to doctors in respect of their children.

PART IV

Medicine, Ideology and Society

11

Medical Knowledge

Samuel Johnson penned an introduction to his friend, Robert James's monumental *Medicinal Dictionary*. Yet he was also critical of James's much-vaunted fever powders: 'I never thought well of Dr James's compounded medicines. His ingredients appeared to me sometimes inefficacious and trifling, sometimes heterogeneous, and destructive of each other.' Could a layman nowadays so confidently[1] evaluate pharmaceuticals? Johnson, as Hester Thrale emphasized, had made medicine his study and his hobby.[2] Yet he clearly believed it the right and duty of every man not to swallow everything on trust, and to conduct a never-ceasing dialogue with his doctors. Many agreed, seeing medicine not as an arcane mystery fit only for the faculty but as central to the arena of open public discourse. The domain of medical knowledge was mapped differently then, and it is the aim of this chapter to offer a sketch map of the distribution of medical awareness in Georgian consciousness, the barriers marking off its separate spheres and the channels through which it percolated.

Many issues emerge. To what degree was medicine open, or rather did some groups have far greater access to it, even monopolize its circulation? Was there a single, unitary medical discourse? Or were there many modes of medicine, mutually coexisting, overlapping and competing for attention and authority within a mental market-place characterized by cognitive pluralism? Indeed, to return to the historiographical questions mooted in part I of this book, was a single privileged form of medicine – 'scientific', print-culture knowledge, as endorsed by the profession – driving other types of medical beliefs (popular, folk, oral, female or whatever) to the margins or, indeed, to the wall?[3]

The rich, variegated and open-ended relationships negotiated between the sick, their relations and friends and their medical practitioners, as analysed in earlier chapters, could never have existed had lay people not felt competent to hold forth about their disorders and their preferred treatments. Individual, personal 'knowledge' – the term is used purely descriptively – was the indispensable prerequisite for devising strategies and making choices.[4] But people reached their knowledge of matters medical through many media. These may be worth teasing out, before assessing the interactions between its diverse spacial sectors and hierarchical layers.

SUBJECTIVE KNOWLEDGE

The most direct and authoritative knowledge of sickness was personal experience of pains, diseases and remedies. 'We all have our own hospital within', noted Smollett, who trained as a doctor. Doctors often indulged in this autobiographical mode, being the living union of both patient and practitioner. 'I have consulted nothing but my own Experience', boasted George Cheyne, writing his 'history', 'and Observation on my own crazy Carcase, and the Infirmities of others I have treated.'[5]

Personal knowledge of this kind was not without its problems. Enlightenment culture was undecided about pure subjectivity. The *philosophes'* scientific quest and commitment to destroying error distrusted merely intuitive dogmatism. Yet the legacy of Locke formulated an empiricist psychology privileging experience, and accepting that reality had to be mediated through the sense organs, and thereby enregistered as pleasures and pains. Despite the heroic endeavours of Benthamite utilitarianism to provide a rational, objective calculus of the feelings, most acknowledged that the individual's experience of pain was irreducibly personal.[6]

In turn, the notion of the primal ineffability of the individual response ('*la maladie, c'est moi*') was codified by traditional humoralism, which presupposed that each individual's internal fluid balance was unique: no two constitutions were precisely identical.[7] And such a perception was, in the social sphere, incorporated into the structure of the patient/physician duo, which set such store by 'taking the history', by personal advice-giving and by the precisely-tailored regimen. 'Off-the-peg' quack nostrums, by contrast, could not possibly 'fit'.[8]

The sick were not shy in advancing impressively educated accounts of what ailed them. 'I understand my own disease well enough to know that I cannot be reliev'd by any remedies this Country affords', Mrs Isabella Duke informed her physician, John Locke, 'or at this distance from my Physitian, unless it be by mending the Habit of my Body in general, and sweetening my Blood, which doubtless is Scorbutical in a high degree, as appears by the swelling and Bleeding of my Gums, a frequent Lassitude of my whole Body; inward Convulsions, and a mighty faintness, and dispiritedness, with a trembling of my Heart, and all my Nerves; much the same complaints I have formerly laboured under, only the swelling and bleeding of my Gums is new.'[9] Mrs Duke feared that because she had already tried everything herself, the physician was unlikely actually to prove of much use; however, 'if you can substitute any thing in the room of Waters, for this Year; or any way help me, you will do a great piece of Charity, for i am at a non plus, and can have no further recourse to any thing but Castle Cary Waters.'[10]

People meditated deeply upon their own pangs and pains. But they also inquired after and collected other people's experiences. No data might be too insignificant to hoard, as is evident from, say, John Aubrey's or Oliver Heywood's miscellaneous scrapbooks bulging with information about deaths and diseases, or from Joseph Farington's tireless buttonholing of acquaintances about the equilibrium of their health.[11] Was such collecting merely rampant, prurient curiosity, or was it true empirical inquiry? A female quack from Hungerford, so the newspapers reported, cured cancer with live toads. Did it work? The Revd Gilbert White wanted to know the truth, so, being one day 'not far from Hungerford', he 'did not forget to make some inquiries concerning the wonderful method of curing cancers by means of toads':

> Several intelligent persons, both gentry and clergy, do, I find, give a great deal of credit to what was asserted in the papers: and I myself dined with a clergyman who seemed to be persuaded that what is related is matter of fact; but, when I came to attend to his account, I thought I discerned circumstances which did not a little invalidate the woman's story of the manner in which she came by her skill.[12]

Hence that non-pareil natural history observer checked out the healer with his own eyes:

> She says of herself 'that, labouring under a virulent cancer, she went to some church where there was a vast crowd: on going into a pew, she was accosted by a strange clergyman; who, after expressing compassion for her situation, told her that if she would make such an application of living toads as is mentioned she would be well'. Now is it likely that this unknown gentleman should express so much tenderness for this single sufferer, and not feel any for the many thousands that daily languish under this terrible disorder? Would he not have made use of this invaluable nostrum for his own emolument; or, at least, by some means of publication or other, have found a method of making it public for the good of mankind? In short, this woman (as it appears to me) having set up for a cancer-doctress, finds it expedient to amuse the country with this dark and mysterious relation.[13]

ORAL LORE

Everyone had his own feelings and theories about health and sickness. But these individual globules of experience typically derived from, and merged into a common stream of wisdom, circulated by word of mouth down the generations, from nurse to mistress and mother to daughter, across tavern floors and over the tea-cups. Such lore was most likely to be preserved for posterity when memorialized in the form of proverbs. 'Prevention is better than cure', dates back at least to the seventeenth century, as do such gems as:

Ague in the spring is physic for a king.
Agues come on horseback, but go away on foot.
A bit in the morning is better than nothing all day.
You eat and eat, but you do not drink to fill you.
At forty a man is either a fool or a physician.
After dinner sit a while, after supper walk a mile.
After dinner sleep a while, after supper go to bed.
A good surgeon must have an eagle's eye, a lion's heart, and a lady's hand.
Good kale is half a meal.
If you wish to live for ever, you must wash milk from your liver.[14]

When we examine this pass-me-down medical wisdom, we encounter a gigantic irony. All strata of society retailed oral lore about health and healing. But what the more educated classes learned about medicine at their mother's knee is, paradoxically, harder to recover than the beliefs pervasive amongst people at large. The educated were always chattering about health and discussing their pet theories and remedies. For example, on 11 September 1677, in Garaway's coffee-house, Robert Hooke was told of a man who had been 'recoverd of a bad memory and severall other distempers by carrying a small box of very fine filings of the best refined silver and now and then licking of it with his finger and swallowing it'.[15] But – unlike Hooke! – most people in polite society did not record every bit of tittle-tattle, every superstition or quaint saying they believed or heard about healthy and unhealthy foods, about why bones ached, feet sweated, piss stank and hair fell out, about fate and fortune at large. By contrast, at least from the seventeenth century, and much more so later, preserving in amber every little health saw of ploughman and milkmaids became the avocation of swarms of marauding folklorists. There is no need to dilate here upon the gross distortions introduced, wilfully or inadvertently, by such zealously theorizing and commonly prudish parson and gentleman antiquarians, often anxious to demonstrate the exotic irrationality of such popular beliefs.[16] Even so, the everyday health culture of the illiterate or semi-literate may, ironically, be better documented than the ideas lodged deep in the brains of the educated.

Obviously the elite – above all, the folklorists amongst them – believed they were free from the taint of such superstitions. In reality, they had become deaf to their own superstitions, which remain as a consequence largely hidden from history. The yokel folklore of health was widely, though not wisely, studied by Victorian folklorists; the lore of educated folk has never attracted such backyard anthropology.[17] A potential optical illusion is thereby created: the appearance of a chasm between 'plebeian' medical 'lore' and 'patrician' medical 'knowledge'. Recorders of popular beliefs certainly fostered such a myth. Thus Alpheus Smith noted a lower-class deathbed scene in 1820:

> Whilst the woman was dying I was standing at the foot of the bed, when a woman desired me to remove, saying, 'You should never stand at the foot of a bed when a person is dying'. The reason, I ascertained, was because it would stop the spirit in its departure to the unknown world.
>
> Immediately after the woman was dead, I was requested by the persons in attendance to go with them into the garden to awake the bees, saying it was a thing which ought always to be done when a person died after sunset . . .[18]

All this nonsense was too much for the antiquarian: 'I reasoned with them on the absurdity of the practice, but it was in vain, for they actually went out at midnight and did awake them.' Modern cultural anthropologists of medicine such as Cecil Helman argue, by contrast, that we should discount such distinctions between reason and absurdity, and alert ourselves instead to the features common to high and low, advanced and primitive belief systems.[19] This book is not about folk beliefs, and there is no room to explore their finer texture here; but a few features should be pointed out, because they are significant in assessing differential strategies of self-healing and of consulting with doctors.

During the long eighteenth century, popular health and sickness lore in the 'low' or 'little' tradition seems increasingly to have come adrift from its traditional cosmological moorings. In Tudor and Stuart England, sickness and injury (human and animal) had been widely attributed to witchcraft, and witchcraft beliefs were governed by a theological framework, underwritten by the churches, giving prominence to the Devil, possession and Hell. 'Vervain and dill Hinder witches from their will', jingled Aubrey. In Georgian times demonology and witchcraft beliefs steadily lost their cultural legitimacy. Visitations of sickness were less widely ascribed and anchored to spiritual and satanic forces, or indeed to witches themselves.[20]

A similar tale may be told for magic. Of course, magical medicine remained popular in many circles throughout pre-modern England, if by 'magical' we allude loosely to remedies lacking or transcending the explanatory sanction of approved medical science (the laws of physiology, etc.), but rather drawing upon such mechanisms as charms, spells, talismans, object displacement, correspondences and numerology, and invoking supernatural powers or cosmic properties.[21] Many very common healing practices in pre-modern England smacked of magic. For instance, a sapling would be spliced and a sickly child passed through it. The tree would then be bound together once more. As the tree grew whole, so would the child. That ritual, evoking natural sympathies, common in the seventeenth century, was still sometimes being practised in the nineteenth. By a rather similar thought symbolism, the touch of a dead man's hand was widely believed to bear disease away.[22]

Magical means were commonly used in the seventeenth century, and not merely amongst the vulgar. 'This night about one a Clock', recorded the astrologer, Elias Ashmole: 'I fell ill of a Surfett, occasioned by drinking water after Venison. I was greatly opprest in my Stomack, & next day Mr Saunders the Atrologian sent me a peece of Bryony Root to hold in my hand.'[23] The intrinsic properties of the root, or the ritual it encompassed, worked: 'within a quarter of an houre, my stomack was freed of that great oppression, which nothing which I tooke from Dr: Wharton could doe before.'

Yet, by contrast at least to many tribal cultures, medical magic in England did not espouse – it certainly did not express – an articulate cosmology, challenging Christian orthodoxy and public reason.[24] Magic rather manifested itself primarily through investing particular curative objects and healing rituals with intrinsic powers: a herb – like Ashmole's bryony root; a formula, repeated to the letter; ceremonial gestures involving displacement, expulsion, sympathy and so forth. By thus empowering objects and actions, magic was not radically different from everyday and indeed, professionally authorized patterns of healing and items of materia medica. Both shared the desperation of the powerless in the teeth of cosmic disaster. The English, educated and uneducated alike, were less afraid of other-worldly ghosts, spirits and bogeymen than of the weather, miasmatic exhalations, old age, infertility and all the other natural hazards of existence.

In other words, no impenetrable 'great wall' divided plebeian magic from progressive medicine. For example, in 1771 Dr Richard Brookes advised, 'when there is a Pain in the Head with a Delirium, cut open a live Chicken or Pigeon, and apply it to the Head': was this a medical therapy or a sacrifice?[25] The aura of magic was to provide an endorsement of regular herbalism and kitchen physic. For popular medical lore dictated, above all, a familiar therapeutic battery of medicaments, each to be tried under appropriate circumstances. Many herbal remedies would clearly produce an effect (that is, they genuinely acted as diuretics, diaphoretics, emetics, etc.); in that sense, they possessed an empirical authenticity.[26] Yet many had some further identifiable rationale – for example they were authorized by the doctrine of signatures. Thus the fact that eyebright (*Euphrasia officinalis*) had a bloom so marked as to resemble an eye, demonstrated it to be a specific for eye disease. As the dozens of plants used to cure warts show, it would be quite artificial and anachronistic to seek to demarcate rigidly between herbal remedies used 'magically', and those deployed on scientific or rational authority. For, in the whole range of recommendations, the medicinal object itself (the cure) tended to become invested with mystique.[27]

Of course, mocking the primitive medical beliefs of the vulgar and the credulous remained an elite sport.[28] Early in the seventeenth century, Bishop Hall drew the character of the superstitious man: 'Old Wives and Starres are his Counsellors: his Night-spell is his Guard, and Charms his Physicians.'[28] A century and a half later, William Buchan suggested that, amongst the uneducated, all medicines tended to be revered and used in the manner of charms.[30] Throughout the eighteenth century, medical men were for ever denouncing the ignorant folly of the people – those who, for example, paid no heed to the laws of hygiene. They would cluster in overcrowded quarters, wear filthy clothes, sleep several to a bed and fasten all windows in order to keep warm – small wonder they created a polluted, miasmatic atmosphere and fell prey to putrid fevers and the like![31]

Thus enlightened medical opinion tended to discredit popular lore and berate vulgar hygienic errors; yet a powerful cross-current was also at work: a preparedness to be fascinated by, and even open-minded towards, traditional beliefs and practices. Robert Burton candidly recalled that he had always poohpoohed his mother's quaint herbal lore as nothing better than old wives' tales, until he discovered similar ideas expressed in the great classical herbalist, Theophrastus.[32]

As this instance shows, the medical wisdom of the 'great' and 'little' traditions converged no less than they diverged. 'It being near Full Moon I cut my Wives Hair off.'[33] This was written in 1717, the high noon of the Enlightenment: was this some hempen homespun? No, it was a Lancashire gentleman, Nicholas Blundell. For Blundell, belief in the medical significance of the full moon was not some bizarre rustic absurdity, but a rational fact. And in attributing to the moon a regulating meaning for the human body, he was far from unusual amongst the educated men of his time. It was a subject to which no less a luminary than Richard Mead devoted a whole treatise, though cast not as magical formula but as scientific inquiry. Many mad-doctors still believed in links between the moon and lunacy.[34]

Similarly, to soothe a stye in his eye, Parson Woodforde stroked it with his black Tom cat's tail. Did he see the requirement that the cat be *black* as a magical vestige?[35] Did Blundell know the rationale for his belief about cutting hair? And would they have justified their practices in scientific terms if called upon? In such matters, we must remain frustrated, because what tends to be recorded is the deed and not its underlying legitimation.

'I took early in the morning a good dose of Elixir', wrote Elias Ashmole on 11 April 1681, 'and hung three Spiders about my neck, and they drove my Ague away. Deo Gratias.'[36] The highly-educated Ashmole unambiguously endorsed the cure; how far he or others would have called it 'magic', and what precisely that would have meant, is a trickier matter. Often it is unclear whether similar cures, prognostications, omens, etc., were merely being recorded, positively endorsed, or treated with an open mind. John Aubrey preserved in vast quantities the oral medical lore of his times. 'To make a man Gunne-proofe', he said, 'write these characters + Zada + Zadash + Zadathan + Abira + in virgin paper [I beleeve parchment] carry it always with you, and no gun-shott can hurt you.'[37] He often gave a source for such beliefs and the cures they supposedly wrought. Through citing such authority, he perhaps simultaneously underwrote their credit, yet distanced himself from having to stake his own reputation upon them. But with Aubrey, the doubt remains how far his collections were the unique expression of his own magpie mind, or were representative of the times.

Similar problems face interpretation of the many surviving family recipe books, mainly of gentry origin. Their jumbled profusion of juxtaposed cures, healing salves, prophylactics, remedial practices, and the like commonly includes items – the use of dead toads or vipers' blood, for example – whose roots surely lie in the occult.[38] But the practice has equally surely become disengaged from its original rationale. Moreover, the recording of a curative practice in such compilations is no proof that it was actually believed in and used. The hotch-potch of remedies – some deriving from lords and ladies, some from kitchen-maids and stable-lads, others from newspapers and *Culpeper's Herbal* – found higgledy-piggledy in such receipt books probably authentically registers the enduring pluralism of medical authority.

MEDICINAL LITERATURE FOR THE LAYMAN

Lady Caroline Fox worried that her son, Stephen, suffered from St Vitus's dance. She consulted a gaggle of doctors over his case.[39] Some years earlier, someone with a similar problem had tried another tack, by writing to the general advice magazine, the *British Apollo*, asking what caused the condition. '*Chorea Sancti Viti*, or *St Vitus's Dance*', replied the editor, 'seems to proceed from a Disorder of the Animal Spirits, by an Heterogeneous *Copula*, which becoming fierce and unbridled, it is necessary they should be so Exercised and Fatigued, that they themselves might be tamed, and the Offending Matter dissipated.'[40] Whether or not the questioner felt any the wiser, the case points to an important development during the long eighteenth century. The literate public could increasingly gain its medical information – indeed, even have its medical problems settled – by reading books, pamphlets and magazines.[41]

Different sorts of reading matter purveyed different types of medical knowledge to different readerships. Some popular, non-specialist works provided snippets of general information. Amongst the big-sale periodicals, almanacs offered simple medical directives. The *British Merlin*, for example, carried seasonable advice about what sorts of clothes and medication to use at various times of the year – as well as carrying patent medicine advertisements.[42]

General periodicals pitched at a rather more elevated readership performed similar services. Many of the monthly magazines flourishing in the wake of the *Spectator* carried medical features and ran reviews of medical books. When Sophie von la Roche visited London in 1786, she: 'bought the September and October numbers of the *Lady's Magazine*, and was sorry I had not procured them all, as they contained very nice essays, most useful for the information of my sex, as, for example, An idea of true philosophy and wisdom; On the spirit of contradiction; Educational institutes; Medical notes for women; Blind delusions of love [etc.].'[43]

The biggest circulation journal for the educated public, the *Gentleman's Magazine*, boasted the most impressive medical coverage of all. It regularly contained insertions contributed by readers seeking information about diseases and their cures or detailing favourite home remedies; it published short articles by medical practitioners, informing the public of medical dangers and health hints ('altruism' thus mingled here with self-publicizing 'interest'); and not least it specifically encouraged 'medical correspondence', leading to the exchange of ideas and occasionally to controversies over epidemics, local remedies, the identification of diseases, etc. Items of broad public medical concern were printed, including reviews of medical books, the annual reports and financial accounts of the new general hospitals being founded throughout the provinces and, on one occasion, a list of standard prices for materia medica with addresses of reputable retailers in London. It was axiomatic for the *Gentleman's Magazine* that health was everyone's business, and that educated readers and medical practitioners would be able to communicate in the give-and-take of the correspondence columns.[44]

As Virginia Smith in particular has shown, the long eighteenth century also multiplied the range of literature devoted to health education and domestic medicine, directed to the lay reader.[45] Some was written by laymen, an increasing proportion by medical practitioners and some was put out by entrepreneurs puffing nostrums behind the innocent face of a family medicine instructor.

One genre of such works concentrated on dispensing broad health-care information: the management of diet, cleanliness and hygiene, the pursuit of temperance and moderation – in fact, a golden mean in life as dictated by the age-old medical teaching of the 'non-naturals'. Others focused chiefly on domestic physic, occasionally explaining, but more commonly merely specifying, cures for assorted ills and listing the properties of various pills and plasters, electuaries and enemas.

Such works were targeted at different sectors of the market, whose life-styles and pockets dictated different approaches to coping with sickness. For the poor and possibly autodidact reader, John Wesley's *Primitive Physick* (1747) proved the favourite, going through scores of editions. Wesley essentially offered instructions in the most direct and simple form, organizing his cures, illness by illness. He kept his materia medica simple and within the compass of potential readers, making much use of honey, onions, garlic, cold water and other freely-available ingredients, and drawing on traditional lore. In all instances, the founder of Methodism trusted to Providence and the healing power of Nature rather than recommending complex drug cocktails or quack remedies. The implicit assumption of Wesley's recipe book is that his readers, when sick, would need to medicate themselves as best they could, by way of running repairs, because they simply could not afford to take to their beds and be unable to work.[46]

The craftsmen, tradesmen, bourgeoisie and clerics of Georgian England found their vade-mecum in William Buchan's *Domestic Medicine* (1769). Regularly trained in Edinburgh, Buchan, a general practitioner, pitched his appeal at those who notionally had the time, money and disposition to take some preventive care of their health, to control their life-style and order their domestic environment – people able to take to their beds when sick. Buchan distanced himself from the gross medical superstitions of the uneducated, the impositions of the quacks and the restrictive practices of regular medicine alike. In taking this stance, he doubtless struck a chord with thousands of sturdy, independent-minded, self-help readers – his followers were dubbed 'Buchaneers' – anxious to maintain and maximize control, wherever possible, over the fate of their own bodies. Like Wesley, Buchan made great play of simple treatments, deeming diet did more for health than drugs. Unlike Wesley, he went beyond mere dos-and-don'ts, explaining the nature of disease, the signs and symptoms of particular disorders and a general philosophy of positive health through temperance and hygiene.[47]

The favourite manual with polite society was undoubtedly George Cheyne's *Essay of Health and Long Life* (1724). This had relatively little to say about the cure of sickness (presumably its readers were educated enough to know what to do in such a contingency, or were more likely to be in close contact with medical practitioners). But it offered immensely detailed instructions for the patterning of a healthy life-style, organized around the classic grid of the non-naturals. It was a tactful work, side-stepping the rather extreme dietary recommendations (vegetarianism, a milk and seed diet, no alcohol) that Cheyne occasionally expressed elsewhere. Rather, it encouraged readers to cut out gourmandizing, guzzling and toping, and to curb the other inordinacies of the fashionable fast lane (late nights, sedentary occupations, tight lacing, etc.). Thereby, the diseases of civilization could be avoided, and a truly refined mode of living facilitated.[48]

The inflections of these works – and of dozens of other carbon copies of them – differed, yet their message was basically similar. Wesley actually cited Cheyne's general health advice. All assumed that much fell within the common man's power, but that there were times when professional medical aid should be summoned. (Wesley was emphatic that the doctor must be a good Christian.)[49]

Works targeted at a lay readership were practical rather than theoretical. Thus John Archer's *Every Man His Own Doctor* claimed to show

> How every one may know his own Constitution and Complection, by certain Signs. Also the Nature and Facilities of all Food as well Meats, as drinks. Whereby every Man and Woman may understand what is good or hurtful to them. Treating also, of Air, Passions of Mind, Exercise of Body, Sleep, Venery and Tobacco etc.
> The Second part shews the full knowledge and Cure of the Pox, and Running of the Reins, Gout, Dropsie, Scurvy, Consumptions, and Obstructions, Agues. Shewing their causes and Signs, and what danger any are in, little or much and perfect Cure with small cost and no danger of Reputation.[50]

It was quite unnecessary, Archer insisted, 'that every particular Person should be able to read an Anatomy Lecture upon the parts of his own Body, nor study the Nature, differences, causes of Diseases.' It was enough to know the rules of health – which he set out under the headings of the non-naturals – and some simple self-help therapeutical measures.[51] Action was the keynote. Such books were commonly indexed in alphabetical order, by disease, for ease of reference. Occasionally an attempt was made to make them more appetizing reading. For instance, Bernard Mandeville's *Treatise on the Hypochondriack and Hysterick Diseases* and John Profily's *Easy and Exact Method of Curing the Venereal Disease* were both couched in dialogue form. In Profily's work in particular, the patient was exemplarily forthcoming and obedient; the doctor, wise and humane. Clearly readers were expected to take the hint.[52]

Noticeably absent from all such eighteenth-century popular medical texts was anything resembling the systems of alternative medicine – for example, homoeopathy – which achieved such a surge of popularity amongst the self-improving laity during the Victorian era.[53] Despite Wesley's and Buchan's ambivalence towards the profession, neither they nor any other influential authors recommended secession from professional services, or proposed their own physiologies and pathologies. The same even applied to the lectures and pamphlets of quacks. Georgian quacks typically cashed in on the names of the luminaries of professional medicine for intellectual authority, whereas in the nineteenth century such nostrum-mongers as James Morison were more likely to advance their own alternative hypotheses.[54] Thus in the 1780s the 'sex therapist', James Graham, built his crusade for national sexual regeneration upon an impeccably orthodox commitment to temperance and moderation derived from Cheyne.

Health-care books were bought by the thousand. But were they read and their recommendations implemented? Abundant evidence shows the answer is 'yes'. As we have seen above, contemporary diaries and letters contain plenty of explicit references to following their suggestions.[56] Reading Cheyne may have helped launch the Bristol clerk, William Dyer, upon his energetic spare-time healing activities.[57] In the nineteenth century, the artisan, Joseph Gutteridge, began with the herbals and ended up a lay healer. 'My father gave me an old edition of Culpeper, with coloured plates', he explained:

> By the aid of this book I soon found out not only the common names of plants but their uses and medical properties. The boys of the first and second forms were allowed by the master to sketch in pencil and to use water colours, and availing myself of this privilege, I experienced great delight in delineating the forms and colours of plants and flowers. The ability to do this proved to me in after times a ready means of fixing in

my mind the peculiar characteristics of plants that otherwise might slip my memory. . . . I made quite a collection of these leaf impressions with the name attached to each and a record of the locality where it was found – its habitat.[58]

This initiation proved crucial in setting Gutteridge on the road to abandoning the doctors altogether, in the more common Victorian artisan manner. When his eldest son fell sick, and he could not afford a doctor,

We were obliged to fall back upon our own resources. To succeed in this I procured by loan or purchase all the medical and physiological works I possibly could, especially books treating on the eyes, including Fyfe's 'Anatomy', Grainger's 'Elements of Anatomy', Southwood Smith's 'Philosophy of Health', and two or three Dictionaries of Medicine, but the work most suited to my wants was Gray's Supplement to the Pharmacopoea.'[59]

Gutteridge offered some reflections upon how being a medical autodidact was the epistemological foundation for a much wider grasp of the terrain of knowledge:

It is said that 'A little knowledge is a dangerous thing'. The sentiment would perhaps be more accurate if it read '*Too* little knowledge, or knowledge mis-applied, is a dangerous thing'. Certainly, in my own case, the study of these works laid the foundation for a more intimate knowledge in succeeding years of those abstruse questions relating to chemical affinities and to natural cause and effect, which in these more modern times have revolutionised the world. It was a great drawback that I could not – owing to illness when young – commit to memory the details of matters of importance, but could only remember general results.[60]

He felt an ethical scrupulosity towards the practice of his skills that seems characteristic of the Victorian, but not of the Georgian age: 'I did not feel at liberty to use this knowledge as a means of profit, though great demands were made upon it by sufferers amongst our friends and neighbours. It was a source of pleasure to be able, by relieving pain and suffering, and sometimes even curing deep-rooted diseases, to earn the gratitude of those benefited.'[61]

CROSS-FERTILIZATION

Alongside the avalanche of works written by doctors for doctors (this was the period which saw the launching of medical journalism),[62] many publications were thus appearing, aimed at lay readers, mainly offering simplifications of approved regular medicines, interlarded with ideological bracers commending moral improvement and social discipline. Medical knowledge was not an exclusive arcana. The climate of the times – the meliorism of the Enlightenment – favoured the diffusion of knowledge. Market opportunities encouraged doctors to write for a wider readership. Prima facie, the picture was one of fluidity, pluralism, and intermingling. Medical knowledge was perceived to be no respecter of traditional educational and class barriers. John Aubrey remarked, with evident approval, that the great humanist doctor, Platerus, confessed 'that many of his rare receipts he had from old women'; and numerous medical men followed his practice. 'The ancients have writt their hippiatria and veterinarias', noted John Ward, 'and why should not wee in these days collect the experiments of old women and farriers as well as they did formerly?'[63] Inoculation was classically a folk remedy that became medicalized.[64] Jennerian vaccination codified the rural awareness that those who had suffered cowpox did not subsequently catch smallpox.[65] William Withering derived his knowledge of digitalis from countryfolk:

> In the year 1775 my opinion was asked concerning a family receipt for the cure of dropsy. I was told that it had been kept a secret by an old woman from Shropshire who had sometimes made cures after the more regular practitioners had failed. I was informed also that the effects produced were violent vomiting and purging, for the diuretic effects seem to have been overlooked. This medicine was composed of 20 or more different herbs; but it was not very difficult for one conversant in these matters to perceive that the active herb could be no other than foxglove.[66]

In some cases it is difficult to tell whether true arrows of influence are pointing from the 'little' to the 'great' tradition[67] or vice versa, or whether parallel beliefs were flourishing independently amongst different groups. A popular folk notion of humours coexisted alongside the learned one:[68] did the one underpin the other, or were they essentially autonomous? Popular wisdom held that getting drunk was a certain cure for fever. A similar idea seems implicit in the Brunonian advocacy of cure by alcoholic stimulus. Did John Brown here borrow, perhaps unconsciously, from popular practice – from his own peasant roots?[69] Assimilation and borrowings were going on all the time, in all directions. In the 1760s William Heberden identified and named angina pectoris. John Wesley alerted himself to this important discovery, and in subsequent editions of his *Primitive Physick*, makes mention of the condition under the title of 'Quinsy of the Breast'.[70]

Doctors learned from medical beliefs which were 'in the air'. But the laity equally learned from doctors. Edward Gibbon and Adam Smith attended William Hunter's courses at his private anatomy school.[71] Medical entrepreneurs such as the hygienist, James Graham, and the oculist, John ('Chevalier') Taylor, attracted large (and sometimes fashionable) lecture audiences.[72]

The public read not only the works of home physic but sometimes more specialized tomes as well. Thomas Turner studied surgical and anatomical tracts: Thursday, 9 November 1758 found him engrossed in 'Wiseman's Chyrurgery', just a few days after he had read 'a poor empty piece of tautology' called *A Serious Advice to the Public to Avoid the Danger of Inoculation*.[73] In his diary, Turner would commonly use such technical medical phrases as 'the inner process of the tibia', which he surely picked up from books or from conversing with doctors[74] (thereby calling to mind Walter Shandy, anxious that every well-informed man should have read his 'Hippocrates, or Dr James Mackenzie').[75]

Libraries played an important part in the percolation of information from the profession to the laity. Even popular circulating libraries often carried a fair number of medical works. For example, around 1789 Palmer and Merrick's Circulating Library in Oxford possessed the following medical books:

Anatomy of Melancholy
Boerhaave's Chemistry
Keil's Anatomy
Cheselden's Anatomy
Drake's Anatomy
Arbuthnot's Works
Elaboratory Laid Open or the Secrets of Modern Chemistry
Hartmann's Perserver of Health
Manningham on Nature and Cure of the Little Fever
Materia Medica
Buchan's Domestic Medicine
Monchy's Essays on the Cure of Diseases
Nelson's Essay on the Government of Children
Primitive Physic (Wesley)
Profily's Easy & Exact Method of Curing the Venereal Disease[76]

(It is noteworthy that works on venereal disease were not believed too offensive to stock.) Booksellers' advertisements in newspapers commonly gave prominence to newly issued medical works, and, as noted earlier, libraries, booksellers and newspaper agents doubled in the sale of pharmaceutical preparations.[77] All such medical texts were clearly believed to be proper reading matter for educated folks. 'I have plenty of books for you, my loves', remarked Lady Maclaughlan in Susan Ferrier's novel, *Marriage*:

> All the books that should ever have been published are here. Read these and you need read no more: all the world's in these books – humph! Here's the Bible, great and small, with apocrypha and concordance! Here's Floyer's Medicina Gerocomica, or, the Galenic Art of preserving

Old Men's Health; – Love's Art of Surveying and Measuring Land; – Transactions of the Highland Society; – Glass' Cookery; – Flavel's Fountain of Life Opened; – Fencing Familiarized; – Observations on the use of Bath Waters; – Cure for Soul Sores; – De Blondt's Military Memoirs; – MacGhie's Book-keeping; – Mead on Pestilence; – Astenthology, or the Art of preserving Feeble Life![78]

The good lady's circle evidently agreed, for they were always airing their own pet theories about health. Writing about the death of a friend, Duncan M'Dunsmuir, another character, Grizzel Douglas, explained:

> What renders his death Particularly distressing, is, that Lady Maclaughlan is of opinion it was entirely owing to eating Raw oysters, and damp feet. This ought to be a warning to all Young people to take care of Wet feet, and Especially eating Raw oysters, which are certainly Highly dangerous, particularly where there is any Tendency to Gout. I hope, my dear Niece, you have got a pair of Stout walking shoes, and that both Henry and you remember to Change your feet after Walking. I am told Raw Oysters are much the fashion in London at present; but when this Fatal Event comes to be Known, it will of course Alarm people very much, and put them on their guard both as to Damp Feet, and Raw oysters.[79]

Medico-sexological works proliferated during the Georgian age, in particular that evergreen favourite, *Aristotle's Master-Piece*, which went through scores of editions in several different versions.[80] 'Amongst the many books I delighted in I got Aristotles Masterpiece wch cost two shillings', recorded the early eighteenth-century Taunton apprentice, John Cannon. He confessed that it spurred him to acts of lewdness ('to watch the Servant Maid when Nature directed her to do her Occasions'), culminating in masturbation.[81]

Were girls and women more shielded from medical accounts of the facts of life? The evidence is contradictory. Parson Woodforde's niece, Nancy, read *Aristotle's Master-Piece*, and surviving eighteenth-century copies are not uncommonly inscribed with female names. When, however, in the 1820s, Charles Tennyson's wife, Fanny, was told by her doctor that she had something wrong with her uterus, she wrote to her husband 'of the meaning of this word I am ignorant and want you to tell me'.[82]

IDEOLOGIES IN CONFLICT

Thus different levels and kinds of medical knowledge interacted. Did they also conflict? Was there a power struggle between different discourses? And if so, what was the outcome?

The gobblydegook of professional terminology provided one perennial grumble amongst the laity. 'One of the constant butts of ridicule, both in the old comedies and novels', noted William Hazlitt,

> is the professional jargon of the medical tribe. Yet it cannot be denied that this jargon, however affected it may seem, is the natural language of apothecaries and physicians, the mother-tongue of pharmacy! It is that by which their knowledge first comes to them, that with which they have the most obstinate associations, that in which they can express themselves the most readily and with the best effect upon their hearers; and though there may be some assumption of superiority in all this, yet it is only by an effort of circumlocution that they could condescend to explain themselves in ordinary language.[83]

For their part, doctors fretted over the seemingly impenetrable ignorance and wrong-headedness of old midwives, nurses and countryfolk in general. The story was endlessly told of the sick rustic who was given a prescription by a doctor, and when asked a week later how he was, replied that he had indeed eaten the prescription and had quite recovered.

In other words, there were spheres at which lay and professional knowledge and outlooks were incommensurable. Yet there was much common ground too. It was an exceedingly frequent belief amongst the Georgian laity that gout was a salutary disease; it allegedly kept other diseases at bay, and thereby betokened long life.[84] 'Lady Hesketh in her last Letter mention'd your having lately had a fit of the Gout', William Cowper wrote to his friend Joseph Hill, 'I will not congratulate you on an acquisition not very desireable perhaps in any case to Him who makes it, but your friends, and among them myself in particular, I will congratulate, because it seems to promise us that we shall keep you long.'[85] This may seem an outlandish conceit, but in reality it was widely endorsed by professionals as well.[86]

If doctors often found lay beliefs wrong-headed, ordinary people returned the compliment. John Wesley read M'Bride's *Practice of Physic*: 'Undoubtedly it is an ingenious book; yet it did not answer my expectations. Several things I could contradict from my own experience; e.g. he says, 'All fevers are attended with thirst and vigilia'. Nay, in two violent fevers I had no thirst at all, and slept rather more than when I was in health.'[87] The ultimate test, Wesley was convinced, was personal experience.

It would be far too simple, therefore, to propose the presence of simple demarcations and struggles between professional and lay knowledge. Medical ideas and information are better envisaged as one vast continuous ocean, partially divided up here and there into seas, bays and straits. A maid in Eliza Pierce's household contracted small-pox. Luckily the other maid had been inoculated, so Eliza felt confident it would spread no further. Not so the stupid maid: 'she had taken it into her Head that she should have the disorder, tho' she was inocculated about three years ago, and had them very thick.'[88] The poor mistress was infuriated: 'this has provoked me & done me more harm then any thing else, as she wou'd sit like a dead thing, and no reasons had any effect on her. [I] am convinced that had she had the least real complaint, or any feverish disorder that the College of Physicians could not have saved her Life, so strongly was she preposessed she would have the small Pox.'[89]

A RECEPTIVE SOCIETY?

What then was the quality of the transmission of medical knowledge in England during the long eighteenth century? Was it a closed world? Or was it open to innovation and cross-fertilization? The spread of knowledge and ideas brought rapid change in certain respects. Styles of childbirth and baby-rearing changed amongst the educated; inoculation was popularized faster than in any other European nation. These developments happened precisely because of the effectiveness of joint medical and lay initiatives. Innovations were not restricted to narrow, professional elites at court, in the metropolis or the universities. Inoculation was pre-eminently a provincial, even rural, innovation.

Above all, there was a great thirst for medical information. 'As I am very curious in the nature and process of all diseases, and like the theory, though not the practice of physic', Lady Hervey told Mrs Howard in 1724, seeking information about the effectiveness of bathing in the waters at Bath:

> I should be very much obliged to you, if you would give me some account of those invalids who are most distempered, with the observations you have made on the nature and symptoms of their several maladies, and what medicines you think would prove efficatious to those who are absolutely incurable. There is a poor lady [Lady Bristol] that went there a little while ago, who, I fear is of the last class. She abounds with peccant humours, and has a complication of distempers, for she has frequently had ruptures, is subject to inflammations, false conceptions, to diseases of the tongue, and is hardly ever free from a fistula lachrymalis; indeed I believe there is no hopes of her ever being better, and in my opinion the best things that can be given her are repeated quieting draughts.[90]

Some people satisfied themselves with discussing such matters. Others, by contrast, were fired with the empirical spirit of the age and were prepared to give all possibilities a try. Elizabeth Montagu suffered badly from headaches. She consulted her doctor, Sandys, who recommended cold bathing: 'The Duchess went with me the first time, and was frightened out of her wits, but I behaved much to my honour. Mrs Verney went to learn to go in of me. Mrs Pendarves went with me to-day, and was as pale as a ghost with the fear of my being drowned, which you know is impossible. I go in everyday and have found benefit already.'[91]

Mrs Montagu's 'dip' may serve as an emblem for medical knowledge in the long eighteenth century. The pool of information was not only large and deep, but undivided. Rigid barriers did not exist – they perhaps became more pronounced later – between lay and profession, 'high' and 'low' cultural knowledge. In many theatres of the arts and life, the Georgian age saw increasingly rigid cultural stratification. Perhaps because of its more urgent demands and its ultimate 'empiricism' (the experience of sickness was radically personal), medical knowledge remained a pool relatively open to all to bathe in.

12

Survey and Conclusion

This book may be read almost as a gloss upon Frank Wedgwood's late-Victorian apothegm: 'No doubt the final cause of patients *is* the doctor.'[1] The patient/doctor relationship assumed great importance in Georgian England – as a personal tie, as a social expression and as a nodal point of occupational growth. Under the biological *ancien régime*, sickness continued to be endemic and death an ever-present threat. Yet sickness does not automatically create patients and doctors. Many conditions have to be satisfied before the sick become patients. There must be doctors available under whom they can place themselves; but doctors will never emerge in any number till there are enough sick people to draw upon, and to afford medical services. Hence the teleological, symbiotic yoking put forward by Wedgwood.

We have argued that relations between the sick and their doctors during the long eighteenth century were in the broadest terms defined by the state-society orientation of post-Civil War England. The prospect of all-embracing corporate control of medicine – on a scale and in a manner comparable to that developing in the Continental absolutist states – slipped through the profession's fingers with the defeat of 'absolutism' after the mid-seventeenth century. Thereafter, quasi-monopolistic professional control did not become effective until the second half of the nineteenth century. In the two-centuries' interim, what was tantamount to a free market flowered, allowing any kind of healer to peddle his wares and all sick people to choose their own practitioners. The medical market-place was eclectic and open, being determined chiefly by ability to pay. Doctors would sink or swim as individuals; the professional life-raft lay in the future. In the absence of revolutionary changes in medical knowledge, pharmacology and medical technology (and in the absence of a radical transformation in the healing power of doctors) practitioners needed to make their services marketable, palatable and indispensable.

They had no captive audience. For although people were sick more often than today, the sick were not locked into relations with the medical profession as they have latterly become, thanks to the rise of state-backed compulsory medical insurance, medical examinations, medical certificates and so forth. It was not mandatory upon the sick to hire the services of doctors. Above all, there was no compulsion for them to draw upon the services of *regular* practitioners, as distinct from the kaleidoscopic variety of other healers who sold or gave their services in that free-range medical world.

Above all, doctors were competing with the sick themselves for the treatment of illness. Necessity, traditions of sturdy independence and the dictates of Protestant, and then Enlightenment, individualism all conspired to create, and to continue to breathe life into, a self-help medical culture. He who experienced sickness developed the resources – religious and philosophical – for coming to terms with it emotionally, personally and socially, and then, often enough, also treated it himself. Doctors themselves fostered (even as, in various ways, they deplored) this self-help culture by choosing to broadcast medical knowledge and know-how to the literate book-buying and pamphlet-reading public.

We have contended that this lay medical self-help culture did not lose its vitality during the long eighteenth century. But we have also argued that the sick in fact increasingly, at the same time, also drew upon the medical services offered by regular practitioners. Lady Mary Wortley Montagu thus cynically expressed it: 'the English are easier than any other infatuated by the prospect of universal medicines . . . we run . . . after recipes and physicians.'[2] In part, this may simply register growing affluence; it is undoubtedly integral to and indicative of a wider trend in an emergent 'consumer' society for people to transform services into commodities and to buy on the market rather than making shift within the domestic, household economy. Not least, the use of purchased drugs increased dramatically. 'I think amazing quantities are consumed every year', wrote John Ball about opium in 1796: 'and am of opinion, that there is twenty times more opium use now in England only, than there was fifteen or twenty years since, as great quantities are used in outward applications, and it is continually advancing in price.'[3] People drew more heavily and frequently upon the market for their medicine because practitioners became better able to provide medical services sufficiently satisfying to the customer. Style may have counted in this at least as much as efficacy. Medical self-help and consumerism did not compete against each other; they proved mutually reinforcing.

It is a moot point whether the doctor of 1830 saved notably more lives than his great-grandfather, But the sick did not judge this the principal criterion of medical success. As Edward Shorter has rightly stressed, only within living memory have patients developed high expectations of the powers of the general practitioner specifically to cure disease. Disappointment over medical failure has only recently begun to play a key role in attitudes.[4] Taking his examples from early nineteenth-century America, Shorter suggests that people had grown inured to medicine being as brutal as life itself; not until the latter part of the nineteenth century did the trusted, gentle, avuncular family doctor come into his own. Our English evidence suggests a somewhat different chronology. There are considerable signs of cordial, if complex and contested relations developing between the sick and their practitioners in England during the long eighteenth century.

We have adduced evidence to show that the sick commonly valued the advice, recommendations and support doctors afforded, even where (as we have equally commonly seen) they had not the power to heal. The failures of medicine – however much lampooned by satirists – did not discredit the profession. In fact there are signs of a general improvement in medical standards. William Heberden offered some pointers of this, towards the close of the eighteenth century:

> There has lately been established, in several of the London hospitals, a plan of courses of lectures in all the branches of knowledge useful to a student in physic. Such plans, if rightly executed, as I have no reason to doubt they will be, must make London a school of physic, superior to most in Europe. The experience afforded in an hospital, will keep down the luxuriance of plausible theories. Many such have been delivered in lectures, by celebrated teachers, with great applause; but the students, though perfectly masters of them, not having corrected them with what nature exibits in an hospital, have found themselves more at a loss in the cure of a patient, than an elder apprentice of an apothecary.[5]

Heberden dilated upon the general benefits of this spread of medical education:

> I please myself with thinking, that the method of teaching the art of healing, is becoming every day more conformable to what reason and nature require; that the errors introduced by superstition and false philosophy are gradually retreating; and that medical knowledge, as well as all other dependent upon observation and experience, is continually increasing in the world. The present race of physicians are possessed of several most important rules of practice, utterly unknown to the ablest in former ages, not excepting Hippocrates himself, or even Aesculapius.[6]

The experiences of men such as Richard Kay and Hampton Weekes bore out Heberden's remarks. Increasingly the sick could feel they were cared for by responsible experts, who also observed the norms of politeness valued in a progressive, confident, affluent society.

But everything was fluid; face-to-face relations were crucial. To the sick person, medicine was only as good as his current practitioner (who, in the worst possible case, possessed the power to destroy him entirely). The sick did not solicit the aid of 'medicine' (that amorphous, faceless, intricately intertwined gigantic network of mutually supporting knowledges and practices we know today), they went to William Pulsford, Sally Mapp or Sir Richard Warren (and if, as we have seen, he did not please, they then tried Sir Lucas Pepys).

For this reason, we have focused primarily upon the interplay between individual sick people and the particular practitioners they hired. Their relationship needed to be mutually supportive and reciprocal if it was to survive and thrive. Indeed, as Jewson has emphasized, unless the doctor could conscript the sick person as a partner, he remained in a state of abject diagnostic ignorance.[7] But the relationship was subject to all manner of ambiguities and jockeyings for power and authority. It was necessarily overshadowed by the ultimate threat of mortality. These tensions and negotiations have been discussed in several of our chapters. Looking from the patient's point of view, we have seen the lay person exerting greater overt control over the shaping of medical relations than we are familiar with nowadays. Looking from the doctor's viewpoint, we saw, in chapter 8 in particular, the development of psychological stratagems, management techniques and a gentle tide of medicalization, which enabled him to control the patient.

People saw medicine and the doctor becoming more integral to the new way of life. There was, indeed, an old way, which was perhaps disappearing, perhaps mythical. As a character in Jane Austen's *Sanditon*, put it:

> 'Here have I lived seventy good years in the world and never took physick above twice – and never saw the face of a doctor in all my life, on my own account. – And I verily believe if my poor dear Sir Harry had never seen one neither, he would have been alive now. – Ten fees, one after another, did the man take who sent him out of the world. – I beseech you Mr Parker, no doctors here.'[8]

The Georgian perception was, however, that doctors were playing an increasing role in people's lives and in society at large. Robert Campbell inserted this view into a comprehensive conjectural historical mythology. 'In the first Ages of the World', he suggested:

> Mankind subsisted without this Species of Men: Their Diseases were few, and Nature taught them the Use of Simples, to assist her when in Extremity: Temperance, Sobriety and moderate Excercise, supplied the Place of Physicians to the Patriarchal Age, and every Field spontaneously

furnished them with Restoratives more potent than are to be found in all our modern Dispensatories, or most celebrated Apothecaries Shops; but as Vice and Immorality gained Ground, as Luxury and Laziness prevailed, and Men became Slaves to their own Appetites, new Affections grew up in their depraved Natures, new Diseases, and till then unheard of Distempers, both chronick and acute, assaulted their vitiated Blood, and baffled the Force of their former natural Catholicons.[9]

Slowly but inexorably all had changed:

> Then Physicians became necessary; Nature grew weak, and sunk under the Load of various Evils, with which Vice, Lust, and Intemperance had loaded her; her Faculties became numbed, the Frame of the Human Constitution was shaken, and her Natural Powers debilitated: The Stamina Vitae, the first Principles of Life, were infected, and the whole Mass of Fluids contaminated with the deadly poison: This produced new Phaenomena, uncommon Symptoms, and expiring Nature must be helped by Art to recover her lost Tone, and restore her to her former Functions. The most sagacious observed the Struggles of fainting Nature, guessed the Causes by the outward Symptoms, and administered to her Relief with such Remedies as were most likely to effect a Cure by removing the Cause of the Malady.[10]

Doctors came to play extended roles in new situations such as childbirth and death. According to Cobbett, the arrival of the man-midwife 'brought the "doctor" into *every family* in the kingdom'.[11] People grew more doctor-dependent, and to that degree medicalization proceeded.

Spokesmen for the old order deplored these developments, seeing their ultimate embodiment in the figure of the *malade imaginaire*. We may dispute whether modern civilization was or was not making people objectively less healthy. It was certainly believed that they were growing more sensitive to pain; less willing to bear it stoically; more hypochondriacal, rather like Peacock's satirical character, in *Melincourt*: 'Humphrey Hippy, Esquire, of Hypocon House . . . a singular compound of kind-heartedness, spleen and melancholy'.[12] Analyses of these developments often carried a tone of disapproval. Thus Willich argued, at the beginning of the nineteenth century, that sickness had become *à la mode*, and 'fashionable complaints' were proliferating:

> The greater number of our fashionable complaints and affections are nearly related to each other. The gout, formerly a regular but uncommon disease, which attacked only the external parts of persons advanced in years, has now become a constitutional indisposition, a juvenile complaint, torturing the patient in a thousand different forms. The famous Podagra and Chiragra of our ancestors are now nearly obsolete, and instead of the gout in the feet or hands, we hear every day of the nervous gout, the

gout in the *head*, and even the fatal gout in the *stomach*. No rank, age, or mode of life seems to be exempt from this fashionable enemy. – The next and still more general malady of the times, is an extreme sensibility to every change of the atmosphere; or rather, constantly sensible relation to its influence.[13]

From the doctor's point of view, Thomas Trotter enlarged upon such developments. Commercial, polite society was subjecting people to excessive strains; they resorted to stimulants (tea, alcohol, medicinal and leisure-time drugs); they grew more dependent, and civilization risked plunging in a descending cycle of utter corruption.[14] Trotter's diagnosis was largely endorsed by his contemporary, Thomas Beddoes. Beddoes deplored the pretensions of the laity in matters medical:

There are a number of nurses, I know, who will laugh you in the face, if they hear you express any anxiety about an infant's taking cold. But these ladies do not appear to have been favoured with any peculiar illumination as to the latent causes or remote consequences of indisposition. And I have known contemners of petty cautions, whose success in rearing children could not be said to add particular weight to their sentiments.[15]

Beddoes advanced this gloomy view to confirm a socio-political critique of the evils of the times, while calling upon the medical profession to put matters to rights. Only a well-informed elite of active, public-spirited doctors could, he argued, save society from the misinformed but dogmatic lay know-alls whose bad habits and false ideas were ruinous to health, both public and private. Their contemporary, William Buchan, by contrast, took a more optimistic view. Foolish self-medicators could be turned into enlightened ones by making constructive use of widespread literacy and the free trade in information. Writing immediately after the French Revolution he contended that the blessed dawn of the rights of man had emancipated man the self-medicator:

For a long while air, water, and even the light of the sun, were dealt out by physicians to their patients with a sparing hand. They possessed for several centuries the same monopoly over many artificial remedies. But a new order of things is rising in medicine, as well as in government. Air, water, and light, are taken without the advice of a physician, and Bark and Laudanum are now prescribed every where by nurses and mistresses of families, with safety and advantage. Human reason cannot be stationary on these subjects. The time must, and will come, when, in addition to the above remedies, the general use of Calomel, Jalap and the lancet, shall be considered among the most essential articles of knowledge of men.[16]

All such diagnoses of society's evils and its remedies regarded the relations between the public and the profession as essentially fluid, capable of alteration and determined by the broader weave of socio-cultural ties. They were not the inevitable product of sickness and medicine.

For overall it was a society more energetic about seeking remedy. In any case, people could simply afford those greater services and medicaments that were more readily available. Consciousness of health grew, possibly as concern with the soul became less tangible in a culture growing more secular. Above all, self-medication and professional medicine complemented and supplemented each other. There was not a 'zero-sum game' between them. All kinds of medicine formed a growth sector, mutually supportive.

It is here that a contrast with *ancien régime* France – and, by implication, much of continental Europe – may be hazarded. For it would seem as if, for a variety of social and cultural factors, effective demand for medicine remained rather contained in France, and the professional sector, at least, was not aggressive in trying to extend its pitch throughout the entire market, or in attempting to whip up new medical demand. The more limited articulation of capitalist relations appears to have inhibited the growth of commercial practices in medicine. Folk, irregular and orthodox healers kept rather more to their own separate spheres. In England, on the other hand, the mobilizing of greater effective demand and supply led to a much more open-ended development of medical consumerism on the one hand and medical entrepreneurship on the other.

Doctors such as Trotter feared the rise of dependence; yet what is more in evidence is deployment. That is why phrases such as the 'expropriation of health', frequently bandied around today, would be inappropriate.[17] English medicine grew in a market society which gave the consumer considerable choice. No effective 'medical police' emerged in England. We might more appropriately speak of a 'moral economy of health'.

Notes

CHAPTER 1   FACING SICKNESS

1   A note on terms is necessary. The book is primarily concerned with the span roughly from the Restoration to the Regency. There is no brief, precise phrase for this period current in historians' terminology. We shall often call it 'the long eighteenth century,' with echoes of '*la longue durée*', the term employed by *Annales* historians to evoke relative changelessness over time. When we use words such as 'Georgian' they are intended in an elastic sense, stretching both backwards and forwards, for we see no sharp breaks between the seventeenth and the eighteenth centuries; and if there are turning-points in the nineteenth, they come in the second half of the century. In respect to medicine, the 'pre-modern' era runs to approximately the age of bacteriology and antiseptic surgery (*c*.1870s).

    When referring to people at large of either gender, we have chosen not to use the cumbersome locution 'his or her'. The male pronoun should, where relevant, be taken to include the female gender. We have used the word 'doctor' rather anachronistically as a generic term for any kind of professional healer.

2   For the history of diseases and epidemics in this period see Dobson, 'Chronology of epidemic disease'; Clarkson, *Death, Disease and Famine*; Imhof, 'Methodological problems in modern urban history writing'.

3   Ford (ed.), *Medical Student at St Thomas's*, 11.

4   Ibid.

5   Burton (ed.), *Letters of Mary Wordsworth*, 147.

6   Braithwaite (ed.), *Memoirs of Anna Braithwaite*, 168.

7   Bagley (ed.), *Great Diurnal of Nicholas Blundell*, III, 145.

8   Miller, *Adoption of Inoculation for Smallpox*; Razzell, *Conquest of Smallpox*; J. R. Smith, *Speckled Monster*; Hopkins, *Princes and Peasants*.

9   Stevenson, 'New diseases'; Durey, *Return of the Plague*.

10   Brockbank and Kenworthy (eds), *Diary of Richard Kay*, 4.

11   Verney and Verney (eds), *Memoirs*, III, 389; Bynum and Nutton (eds), *Theories of Fever from Antiquity to the Enlightenment*; Pelling, *Cholera, Fever and English Medicine*.

12   Verney (ed.), *Verney Letters*, I, 44.

13   Porter, 'Medicine and the decline of magic'.

14   These matters form the main discussion in Porter and Porter, *In Sickness and in Health*. See also Fissell, 'Physic of charity', 20f.

15   Nicolson (ed.), *Conway Letters*, 39ff.

16   Crawfurd, *Last Days of Charles II*; Sedgwick (ed.), *Lord Hervey's Memoirs*; Woolf, 'On being ill', 193–203.

17   For example, leg ulcers proved extremely serious at this time, exacerbated by dietary deficiency. See Loudon, 'Leg ulcers'.

18   Hillam, 'Development of dental practice in the Provinces'; Woodforde, *Strange Story of False Teeth*; Kanner, *Folklore of Teeth*. Mintz, *Sweetness and Power*, discusses the impact of the growing use of sugar on dental health.

19   Fitzgerald (ed.), *Correspondence of Emily, Duchess of Leinster*, I, 100.

20   Slack, *Impact of the Plague*; Farr, 'Medical developments and religious belief'.

21   Chapman (ed.), *Letters of Samuel Johnson*, II, 334.

22   Porter, 'Enlightenment in England'; Holmes, *Augustan England*.

23   Himmelfarb, *Idea of Poverty*; Oxley, *Poor Relief*.

24   For both the emancipatory and the repressive dimensions of individualism see Macfarlane, *Origins of English Individualism*.

25   Idem, *Marriage and Love in England*; Laslett, *World We Have Lost*.

26   Owen, *English Philanthropy*; Rodgers, *Cloak of Charity*.

27   Thomas, 'Old Poor Law and medicine'; Loudon, '"I'd rather have been a Parish surgeon than a Union one"'; idem, *Medical Care and the General Practitioner*; Lane, 'Provincial practitioner and his services to the poor'.

28   Porter, *English Society in the Eighteenth Century*, ch. 7, emphasizes the potential for brutality in the individualistic, pre-Benthamite world of Old Corruption; cf. for the implications of liberalism for health, Porter and Porter, 'The enforcement of health'. Weindling (ed.), *Social History of Occupational Diseases*.

29   Halévy, *Growth of Philosophical Radicalism*.

30   Weindling (ed.), *Social History of Occupational Diseases*.

31   Appleby, *Famine in Tudor and Stuart England*.

32   Campbell, *Romantic Ethic*, 17f.; McKendrick, Brewer and Plumb, *Birth of a Consumer Society*; Marland, *Medicine and Society in Wakefield and Huddersfield*; Weatherill, *Consumer Behaviour*.

33   Holmes, *Augustan England*; for buying medical services, see Weatherill, *Consumer Behaviour*, 121, 127.

34   Feather, *Provincial Book Trade*; Slack, 'Mirrors of health'; V. S. Smith, 'Cleanliness'; idem, 'Prescribing the rules of health'. See for example Maynwaring, *Method and Means of Enjoying Health*; Smythson, *Compleat*

Family Physician; Family Companion to Health; Family Guide to Health; Modern Family Physician; Faust, *Catechism of Health.*

35 Porter, 'Enlightenment in England'.

36 Burke, *Popular Culture in Early Modern Europe;* idem, 'Revolution in popular culture'.

37 Cf. Marshall (ed.), *Autobiography of William Stout.* Stout was a Quaker from Lancaster, flourishing around the turn of the eighteenth century.

38 Ayres, *Paupers and Pig Killers,* 24.

39 See Porter and Porter, *In Sickness and in Health.* Many of these questions are admirably dealt with as regards the seventeenth century in Beier, *Sufferers and Healers;* in a broader context in Herzlich and Pierret, *Illness and Self in Society.*

40 Porter, 'Patient's view'.

41 For today see Cartwright, *Patients and their Doctors;* Kleinman, *The Illness Narratives;* Balint, *Doctor, the Patient and his Illness;* Cassell, *Talking with Patients;* Parsons, *Social System;* and the discussion in Turner, *Medical Power and Social Knowledge.*

42 Jewson, 'Medical knowledge and the patronage system'; idem, 'Disappearance of the sick man'; Brody, *Stories of Sickness.*

43 Rosen and Rosen, *400 Years of a Doctor's Life.*

44 For a doctor's case-book see Dewhurst (ed.), *Willis's Oxford Casebook;* or see the case-book of the Leeds General Infirmary (Anning, 'A medical case book'), which shows copious details of patients' injuries and diseases but no account of their experiences.

45 Throughout this period many patients corresponded with physicians by post, sometimes without ever meeting the doctor in person. These letters are a fascinating genre of clinical encounter interesting in its own right, but not necessarily revealing about the general relations between patients and their doctors.

46 This people-centred history may be taken as an alternative to radically different ways of conceiving the non-Whiggish, non-doctor-oriented history of medicine, for instance Foucault, *Birth of the Clinic,* where the thrust is upon the patient as a construct of the medical gaze. For evaluation see Wright and Treacher (eds), *Problem of Medical Knowledge,* 'Introduction'; Wright, 'Radical sociology of medicine'; Figlio, 'Sinister medicine?'; Jordanova, 'Social sciences and history of science and medicine'.

47 Poynter (ed.), *Evolution of Medical Education;* C. Lawrence, 'Medicine as culture'.

48 Cook, *Decline of the Old Medical Regime;* Webster (ed.), *Health, Medicine and Mortality;* Beier, *Sufferers and Healers,* esp. ch. 2; Porter, *Disease, Medicine and Society.*

49 Elias, *Civilizing Process;* Vigarello, *Corps Redressé;* Gallagher and Laqueur (eds), *Making of the Modern Body;* Barker, *Tremulous Private Body.* And for discussion and bibliography, Porter, 'Body politics'; and idem, 'Barely touching'.

50 Porter, 'A touch of danger'.

51 Rosenberg, 'Therapeutic revolution', suggests change. C. Lawrence, 'Incommunicable knowledge', shows how slowly change came about in England.
52 Szasz, *Myth of Mental Illness*; Goffman, *Presentation of Self in Everyday Life*.
53 Wedgwood and Wedgwood, *Wedgwood Family Circle*, 329.

CHAPTER 2   HEALING IN SOCIETY

1 Obviously distance and difficulties of travelling could be a major consideration. On 4 December 1724, Nicholas Blundell was sick. He set out to go to see Dr Worthington in Wigan, but *en route* 'the Coach was overturned, and when we came near Wigan it was laid fast the Rode being so deep, so we left it in the Laine all night, and went with our Horses to Wigan'. Three days later, perhaps not surprisingly, he was 'somthing Aguish': Bagley (ed.), *Great Diurnal of Nicholas Blundell*, III, 145.
2 See the discussion in Burke, *Popular Culture in Early Modern Europe*; idem, 'Revolution in popular culture'.
3 Bushaway, *By Rite*; Brand, *Observations on Popular Antiquities*.
4 An instance of this older view is Chaplin, *Medicine in England during the Reign of George III*. For a corrective survey see Porter, *Disease, Medicine and Society*.
5 Cook, *Decline of the Old Medical Regime*.
6 Clark, *History of the Royal College of Physicians*, II, 427f.
7 See the discussion in Porter, 'William Hunter'.
8 Barbeau (ed.), *Life and Letters at Bath*, 92; Schnorrenberg, 'Medical men of Bath'.
9 Quoted in Pinkus, *Grub Street*, 205.
10 Percival, *Medical Ethics*.
11 Burton, *Anatomy of Melancholy*, 390.
12 Pelling, 'Apothecaries and other medical practitioners in Norwich'; idem, 'Healing the sick poor'; Pelling and Webster, 'Medical practitioners', 235; Fissell, 'Physic of charity', 31f. for Bristol.
13 Loudon, *Medical Care and the General Practitioner*; Lane, 'Medical practitioners of provincial England'.
14 Cook, *Decline of the Old Medical Regime*, 210f.; Clark, *History of the Royal College of Physicians* II, 490f.
15 These are well evoked in Holmes, *Augustan England*; Loudon, *Medical Care and the General Practitioner*; Lane, 'Role of apprenticeship'.
16 Discussed in Loudon, *Medical Care and the General Practitioner*; Waddington, *Medical Profession in the Industrial Revolution*.
17 Loudon, 'Nature of provincial medical practice'.
18 Brockbank and Kenworthy (eds), *Diary of Richard Kay*, 112.
19 Holmes, *Augustan England*; Brockbank and Kenworthy (eds), *Diary of Richard Kay*; S. Lawrence, 'Science and medicine at the London hospitals'; Porter, 'Medical education in England before the Teaching Hospital'; C. Lawrence, 'Medicine as culture'. George Crabbe's account of his

apprenticeship as an apothecary and his attendance at lectures in London is wonderfully instructive. Bound to a country apothecary, he said 'I read romances and learned to Bleed'. Faulkner (ed.), *Selected Letters and Journals of George Crabbe*, 11.

20 Loudon, *Medical Care and the General Practitioner*, chs 2–4; idem, 'A doctor's cash book'; Brock, 'Happiness of riches'; Singer and Holloway, 'Early medical education in England'.

21 Percival, *Medical Ethics*, 115; Loudon, 'Origin of the general practitioner'; idem, 'Concept of the family doctor'.

22 Porter and Porter, 'Rise of the English drug industry'.

23 Loudon, *Medical Care and the General Practitioner*, 65f.; Poynter (ed.), *Evolution of Pharmacy*.

24 Lewis, *In the Family Way*, esp. 85f.; Schnorrenberg, 'Is childbirth any place for a woman?'; Versluysen, 'Midwives, medical men'; Donnison, *Midwives and Medical Men*; Porter, 'A touch of danger'.

25 Inoculation was often performed by the medically untrained. Thus Woodforde noted that John Bowles's wife was 'under inoculation' by 'one Drake, formerly a serjeant in the Militia': Beresford (ed.), *Diary of a Country Parson*, I, 192. And note this advertisement in the *Oxford Journal*, 11 February 1758:

> I George Ridler near Stroud in the County of Gloster Broadweaver at the desier of peepel hereabout do give betweene 2 and 300 for the Smale Pox, and but too or three of them died –. A Mainy peepel be a feard of the thing but evaith it is No More than Scrattin a bit of a haul in theier Yarm A pushin in a peece of Skraped rag dipt in Sum of the pocky Matter of a Child Under the distemper – That Everybody in the Nashion may be sarved. I will God Willin undertake to Inockilate them with the pervizer that they will take too Purges before hand and loose a little blood away, for half a Crown a head; and I will be bould to say Noo body goes beyond Me.
> N.B. Poor Volk at a Shilling a head, but all Must pay for the Purgin.

26 Zwanenberg, 'The Suttons'; J.R. Smith, *Speckled Monster*, 68f.; Beresford (ed.), *Diary of a Country Parson*, I, 40.

27 Eccles, *Obstetrics and Gynaecology*; Wilson, 'Participant or patient?'; idem, 'William Hunter'; Donnison, *Midwives and Medical Men*.

28 Beresford (ed.), *Diary of a Country Parson*, I, 184–5.

29 Sprott (ed.), *1784*, 48–9.

30 Hillam, 'Development of dental practice in the provinces'. For specialists in treating the deaf see Hughes, *North Country Life*, II, 85.

31 Porter, 'Lay medical knowledge'; G. Smith, 'Prescribing the rules of health'.

32 Hone, *Life of John Radcliffe*, 71.

33 Porter, 'Language of quackery'.

34 Porter, 'Before the fringe'; Hambridge, *Empiriconomy*.

35 Porter, *Health for Sale*.

36 Porter, 'Sexual politics of James Graham'; idem, 'Sex and the singular man'; idem, *Health for Sale*, ch.2.

37 Marland, *Medicine and Society in Wakefield and Huddersfield*, 234f.

38   Berridge and Edwards, *Opium and the People*, 21f.; Looney, 'Advertising and society in England'.
39   Cooter, 'Bones of contention?'; West, *Taylors of Lancashire*.
40   Richardson, *Death, Dissection and the Destitute*, 3f.
41   Verney (ed.), *Verney Letters*, I, 26. There was a smallpox epidemic.
42   Hall and Hall (eds), *Oldenburg Correspondence*, XIII, 70.
43   Adair, *Essays on Fashionable Diseases*, 73f.
44   Quoted in Bottrall, *Every Man a Phoenix*, 130.
45   Dick (ed.), *Aubrey's Brief Lives*, 161.
46   Ibid.
47   Guthrie, 'Lady Sedley's receipt book'.
48   In England there were fewer 'miracle curers', religious healers, and the like than in more rural France, partly, because neither the Church of England nor any other denomination positively encouraged those kinds of religious manifestations. See Devlin, *Superstitious Mind*, 43f.; Ramsey, *Professional and Popular Medicine in France*.
49   Cope, *William Cheselden*.
50   Porter, 'Before the fringe'.
51   Matthews, *History of Pharmacy in Britain*.
52   Porter, '"I think ye both quacks"'.
53   Cobbett, *Advice to Young Men*.
54   Of course, that is to some degree true, since Poor Law medical services were exclusively for paupers, and hospitals exclusively for the labouring poor: see Thomas, 'The Old Poor Law and medicine'; Woodward, *To Do the Sick No Harm*, 17f. For provision under the Old Poor Law, see Bell, 'Early health care in Luton and Dunstable', 229–35.
55   Nicolson (ed.), *Conway Letters*, 244f.
56   Porter, 'Medicine and the decline of magic'.
57   Williams, *Age of Agony*.
58   Bynum, 'Health, disease and medical care'; King, *Medical World of the Eighteenth Century*; idem, *Road to Medical Enlightenment*; idem, *Philosophy of Medicine*.
59   Buchan, *Domestic Medicine*, xxi. Buchan argued that those pursuing the regular 'trade' of medicine had to be conformists. It was outsiders only who had the incentives to innovate. 'Very few improvements are to be expected from a man who might ruin his character and family by even the smallest deviation from an established rule.'
60   Percival, *Medical Ethics*.
61   Quoted in Oppenheimer, *New Aspects of John Hunter*, 115.
62   Trotter, *View of the Nervous Temperament*, 109.
63   Loudon, *Medical Care and General Practice*, 189; Waddington, *Medical Profession in the Industrial Revolution*, 96f. Ramsey, 'Property rights and the right to health'; idem, *Professional and Popular Medicine in France*.
64   Cave (ed.) *Diary of Joseph Farington*, X, 3812.
65   Verney and Verney (eds), *Memoirs*, III, 419–20.

CHAPTER 3   SELF-MEDICATION

1 Eliot, *Middlemarch*, 116–17.
2 Cf. Beier, *Sufferers and Healers*, 154f., for a seventeenth-century perspective.
3 G. Smith, 'Prescribing the rules of health'.
4 Smythson, *Compleat Family Physician*, vi.
5 Burton (ed.), *Letters of Mary Wordsworth*, 22.
6 Clark, *Benjamin Franklin*, 213.
7 This and subsequent quotations from Cooke are contained in J. Heyden, *The English Physicians Guide* ('for the use and benefit of the meanest capacities'), copy in the Library of the Wellcome Institute for the History of Medicine, London. We have not been able to ascertain the identity of Cooke, though it is thought he might have been the hack writer and journalist (1703–56), who, the *DNB* notes, spent his life in chronic debt; or the 'eccentric divine' (1722–83) who had a spell in Bédlam: *DNB*, IV, 1020–22. See also Porter, 'Drinking man's disease'.
8 Climenson (ed.), *Diary of Lybbe Powys*, 230. Cf. Porter and Porter, *In Sickness and in Health*, ch. 2.
9 Herbert (ed.), *Pembroke Papers*, II, 216.
10 Ibid.
11 Ibid., 217. Robert, Lord Pembroke was a great champion of vomits, especially for jaundice: 'Experto crede Roberto', he wrote (ibid., 357). He believed clysters also worked well.
12 Ibid., 217. For ipecacuanha, see Dewhurst, *Quicksilver Doctor*, 154f.
13 Herbert (ed.), *Pembroke Papers*, II, 218.
14 For discussion of hypochondria, see Fischer-Homberger, 'Hypochondriasis'; Baur, *Hypochondria*, 11f; Porter and Porter, *In Sickness and in Health*, ch. 12.
15 Silverman, *Life and Times of Cotton Mather*.
16 Fitzgerald (ed.), *Correspondence of Emily, Duchess of Leinster*, I, 341.
17 Ibid., 331.
18 Hemlow (ed.), *Journals and Letters of Fanny Burney*, VI, 560.
19 Wesley, *Primitive Physick*, 'Introduction'.
20 See the discussion in Knox, *Enthusiasm*, 425–31.
21 Buchan, *Domestic Medicine*, xix.
22 Quoted in Turner, *Taking the Cure*, 88.
23 Slack, 'Mirrors of health'; V. S. Smith, 'Cleanliness'; idem, 'Prescribing the rules of health'.
24 Porter, 'Lay medical knowledge'.
25 Vaisey (ed), *Diary of Thomas Turner*, 105.
26 Ibid. Turner felt no compunction about contradicting Lind. He also noted a recipe for the Duke of Portland's powder for the gout.
27 Matthews (ed.), *Diary of Dudley Ryder*, 227–8.
28 North, *Life of John North*, 155.
29 Ibid.
30 Quoted in Wedgwood and Wedgwood, *Wedgwood Circle*, 57.

31 Posner, 'Josiah Wedgwood's doctors'.
32 Little and Kahrl (eds), *Letters of David Garrick*, III, 1098. Garrick widely urged tar-water on his friends. See ibid., I, 406. For Myersbach, see Porter, '"I think ye both quacks"'.
33 Chapman (ed.), *Letters of Samuel Johnson*, III, 58.
34 Ibid., 34.
35 Hone, *Table Book*, 41.
36 Cobbett, *Advice to Young Men*, 230. cf. Porter, 'A touch of danger'.
37 Cf. Davidoff and Hall, *Family Fortunes*.
38 Matthews (ed.), *Diary of Dudley Ryder*, 288.
39 Toynbee and Whibley (eds), *Correspondence of Thomas Gray*, III, 903.
40 Chapman (ed.), *Letters of Samuel Johnson*, I, 82; Mulhallen and Wright, 'Samuel Johnson: amateur physician'.
41 See discussion in Porter, *Social History of Madness*, ch. 3.
42 Thomas, *Religion and the Decline of Magic*, 14.
43 Robinson (ed.), *Clare's Autobiographical Writings*, 41.
44 Verney and Verney (eds), *Memoirs*, IV, 256.
45 Hone, *Life of John Radcliffe*, 61.
46 Hemlow (ed.), *Journals and Letters of Fanny Burney*, VI, 490.
47 Ibid.
48 Fitzgerald (ed.), *Correspondence of Emily, Duchess of Leinster*, II, 224–5.
49 Ibid.
50 Ibid.
51 Ibid.
52 Lewis (ed.), *Letters of Lady Brilliana Harley*, 119.
53 LeFanu (ed.), *Betsy Sheridan's Journal*, 85. In his final illness in Russia, John Howard dosed himself with James's Powders. These possibly precipitated his death.
54 Stein, *Ada*, 26. A great household doser in the earlier mould was Lady Hoby. See Mead (ed.), *Diary of Lady Hoby*, 104 ff.; Beier, *Sufferers and Healers*, 218.
55 Cf. Hultin, 'Medicine and magic'.
56 Beresford (ed.), *Diary of a Country Parson*, I, 192–3.
57 Gibson (ed.), *Parson in the Vale of the White Horse*, 129. 'Sangrado' was a fictional doctor notorious for his blood-letting.
58 Beresford (ed.), *Diary of a Country Parson*, I, 81.
59 Spence, *Anecdotes*, I, 399.
60 Little and Kahrl (eds), *Letters of David Garrick*, II, 743.
61 Ibid.
62 Hemlow (ed.), *Journals and Letters of Fanny Burney*, VI, 470.
63 Ibid.
64 Chapman (ed.), *Letters of Samuel Johnson*, III, 498–9.
65 Nicolson (ed.), *Conway Letters*, *passim*. See also Porter and Porter, *In Sickness and in Health*, ch. 4.
66 Garlick and Macintyre (eds), *Diary of Joseph Farington*, III, 815–16.
67 Ibid.

68 Ibid.
69 Ibid.
70 Chapman (ed.), *Letters of Samuel Johnson*, III, 106.
71 Beresford (ed.), *Diary of a Country Parson*, II, 9. The recipe came from Buchan's *Domestic Medicine*.
72 Bagley (ed.), *Great Diurnal of Nicholas Blundell*, II, 3. See also ibid., III, 28. Blundell seems to have specialized in ague remedies.
73 Ross (ed.), *Diary of Henry Yeonge*, 32.
74 Bishop, *Short History of the Royal Humane Society*.
75 Vaisey (ed.), *Diary of Thomas Turner*, 105.
76 Jeaffreson, *Book about Doctors*, 148.
77 Quoted in Nicolson and Rousseau, *This Long Disease My Life*, 32.
78 Toynbee and Whibley (eds), *Correspondence of Thomas Gray*, III, 903. cf. Toynbee (ed.), *Letters of Horace Walpole* IV, 351.
79 Verney (ed.), *Verney Letters*, II, 126.
80 Paston, *Mrs Delany*, 133.
81 Franklin, *Autobiography*, 28
82 Spence, *Observations*, I, 438–9.
83 Ibid.
84 Ibid.
85 Yorke (ed.), *Diary of John Baker*, 133.
86 Romilly, *Memoirs*, III, 235. From the nineteenth century, people widely medicated themselves with leeches. See William Macready's diary for 20 October 1838: 'Put leeches on my throat, and whilst they were adhering read the romantic play translated by Mrs Sloman, which promises very well.' Toynbee (ed.), *Diaries of William Charles Macready*.
87 Griggs, *Green Pharmacy*, 88f.
88 Quennell (ed.), *Private Letters of Princess Lieven*, 137. 'We are always well stocked . . . with all the common remedies for sprains and bruises': Mr Heywood in Jane Austen, *Sanditon*, 158.
89 Quoted in Chamberlain, *Old Wives' Tales*, 184.
90 Ayres (ed.), *Paupers and Pig Killers*, 49.
91 Fitzgerald (ed.), *Correspondence of Emily, Duchess of Leinster*, I, 80; Nicolson, 'Ward's Pill and Drop'.
92 Solomon, *A Guide to Health*; Brodum, *Guide to Old Age*; Collins, 'Two Jewish quacks'; Porter, 'Language of quackery'.
93 Berridge and Edwards, *Opium and the People*, 14f.
94 Gosse, *Dr. Viper*, 287.
95 Dewhurst, *Quicksilver Doctor*.
96 Crellin, 'Dr James's fever powders'; [Heathcote], *Sylva, or the Wood*, Essay XXI, 'An apology for Dr James's Fever Powder'. Heathcote says that, motivated by envy, the physicians either maligned or counterfeited it.
97 Quoted in Welsh, *Bookseller of the Last Century*, 26. Christopher Smart dedicated his 'Hymn to the Supreme Being' to James. For another occasion

on which Walpole urged the virtues of James's Powders see Toynbee (ed.), *Letters of Horace Walpole*, XI, 275.

98 Welsh, *Bookseller of the Last Century*, 22.
99 King and Ryskamp (eds), *Letters and Prose Writings of William Cowper*, IV, 89.
100 Ibid., 80, 113, 101.
101 Thale (ed.), *Diary of Francis Place*, 233.
102 Ibid.
103 Gillow and Hewitson (eds), *Tyldesley Diary*, 84.
104 Aldington, *Strange Life of Charles Waterton*.
105 King and Ryskamp (eds), *Letters and Prose Writings of William Cowper*, III, 73.
106 Jeaffreson, *Book about Doctors*, 201.
107 Buchan, *Domestic Medicine*, viii.
108 Burkhardt and Smith (eds), *Correspondence of Charles Darwin*, I, 75. Darwin's father warned him against it. Colp, *To Be an Invalid*.
109 Colvin (ed.), *Correspondence of Maria Edgeworth*, 21.
110 Cave (ed.), *Diary of Joseph Farington*, VIII, 2929–30.
111 Fitzgerald (ed.), *Correspondence of Emily, Duchess of Leinster*, II, 354.
112 Saunders, *Edward Jenner*, 49.
113 Dewhurst (ed.), *Willis's Oxford Case Book*, 121.
114 Ilchester (ed.), *Lady Holland's Journal*, 213.
115 Baur, *Hypochondria*; Fischer-Homberger, 'Hypochondriasis'.
116 Willich, *Lectures on Diet*, 2.
117 Ibid.

CHAPTER 4   ATTITUDES TOWARDS DOCTORS

1 Herbert (ed.), *Pembroke Papers*, II, 318. Percivall Pott was the most eminent surgeon of the day.
2 Bourne (ed.), *Palmerston Letters*, 146.
3 The next chapter will investigate these clinical encounters. Chapter 8 below will examine what the doctors thought of their patients. The general theme of this chapter is admirably covered in Lane, '"The doctor scolds me"'.
4 Quoted by Thomas, *Religion and the Decline of Magic*, 17.
5 Franklin, *Poor Richard's Almanack*, 1744.
6 LaCasce, 'Swift on medical extremism'.
7 Severn (ed.), *Diary of the Revd John Ward*, 119.
8 Griggs (ed.), *Collected Letters of Samuel Taylor Coleridge*, I, 154, 256.
9 Bond (ed.), *Spectator*, I, 88–90. Cf. LaCasce, 'Swift on medical extremism'.
10 Jeaffreson, *Book About Doctors*, 199. 'Dover' was Dr Dover's Powders, a nostrum designed to purge. Cf. Dewhurst, *Quicksilver Doctor*, 141.
11 Mandeville, *Fable of the Bees*, 65.
12 Keynes (ed.), *Complete Writings of William Blake*, 51. Blake gives a

capsule account of the death of Chatterton: 'he took Fissic or somethink, – & so died!': 49.

13 Pope, *Moral Essays*, Epistle iii, line 1, in Butt (ed.), *Poems of Alexander Pope*, 570.

14 Marchand (ed.), *Byron's Letters and Journals*, II, 18–19. There are dozens of political satires in which scheming ministers are portrayed as slashing surgeons dissecting the body politic. See George, *English Political Caricature* 14, 51, 61ff.

15 Garlick and Macintyre (eds), *Diary of Joseph Farington*, II, 477.

16 Hughes, *North Country Life*, I, 95.

17 Buchan, *Domestic Medicine*, xxiv; cf. [Glyster], *Dose for the Doctors*.

18 Wesley, *Primitive Physick*; Rousseau, 'John Wesley's *Primitive Physick*'.

19 Prior, *Alma*, canto iii, line 97. 'Bill' has the double sense of prescription and demand for money.

20 Ward, *London Spy*, 129.

21 Ponsonby (ed.), *More English Diaries*, 166.

22 Barrett (ed.), *Diary and Letters of Madame D'Arblay*, I, 292.

23 Prest (ed.), *Professions in Early Modern England*.

24 Bamford (ed.), *Dear Miss Heber*, 168.

25 Toynbee and Whibley (eds), *Correspondence of Thomas Gray*, III, 951.

26 Home (ed.), *Letters and Journals of Lady Mary Coke*, III, 273.

27 Cave (ed.), *Diary of Joseph Farington*, VII, 2726–7.

28 Herbert (ed.), *Pembroke Papers*, II, 225.

29 Ibid., 228

30 Greig (ed.), *Letters of David Hume*, II, 319–20.

31 Ibid.

32 Ibid.

33 Ibid.

34 Ibid., 324–5.

35 Ibid., 319–20.

36 Ibid., 325.

37 Garlick and Macintyre (eds), *Diary of Joseph Farington*, III, 819.

38 Fremantle (ed.), *Wynne Diaries*, III, 1. Compare William Holland's comment on the ailing Mr Rich: the doctors 'will wear him out with their Physick'. Ayres (ed.), *Paupers and Pig Killers*, 22.

39 Herbert (ed.), *Pembroke Papers*, II, 169.

40 Chapman (ed.), *Letters of Samuel Johnson*, II, 388.

41 Pottle (ed.), *Boswell's London Journal*, 172.

42 Ibid.

43 Matthews (ed.), *Diary of Dudley Ryder*, 227.

44 N. C. Smith (ed.), *Selected Letters of Sydney Smith*, 223.

45 Brady and Pottle (eds), *Boswell in Search of a Wife*, 60; Pottle (ed.), *Boswell's London Journal*, 158. Cf. Ober, 'Boswell's Clap'.

46 Toynbee (ed.), *Letters of Horace Walpole*, IX, 164.

47 Gazley, *Life of Arthur Young*, 365. Bobbin writes, 'having so much physic

I am right down tired of it'. 367. For long, Young chid his daughter about not taking all her medicines.

48 F. B. Smith, *Retreat of Tuberculosis*; Bryder, *Below the Magic Mountain*.
49 Bamford (ed.), *Dear Miss Heber*, 12.
50 Hartshorne (ed.), *Memoirs of a Royal Chaplain*, 104.
51 Cave (ed.), *Diary of Joseph Farington*, X, 3806–7.
52 Ayres (ed.), *Paupers and Pig Killers*, 260.
53 Ibid., 173f.
54 Cope, *William Cheselden*, 25.
55 Verney (ed.), *Verney Letters*, II, 84.
56 Pope's couplet is discussed in Nicolson and Rousseau, *This Long Disease My Life*, 9f.
57 Zuckerman, 'Dr. Richard Mead'; Cope, *William Cheselden*, 31f.
58 Lane, '"The doctor scolds me"'.
59 Cumberland, *Memoirs*, 280.
60 Baird and Ryskamp (eds), *Poems of William Cowper*, I, 385. Compare Cowper's similar paean to Dr Nathaniel Cotton, keeper of the madhouse in which he was temporarily confined: ibid., 322.
61 Lustig and Pottle (eds), *Boswell: English Experiment*, 196–7.
62 *Gentleman's Magazine*, 70 (1800), 373.
63 King and Ryskamp (eds), *Letters and Prose Writings of William Cowper*, II, 537.
64 Nicolson (ed.), *Conway Letters*, 31.
65 Percival, *Medical Ethics*.
66 Porter, 'Touch of danger'.
67 Christie (ed.), *Diary of Revd William Jones*, 273. For the tragedy see Lewis, *In the Family Way*, 182f.
68 Christie (ed.), *Diary of Revd William Jones*, 273.
69 Ford (ed.), *Medical Student at St Thomas's*, 12.
70 Home (ed.), *Letters and Journal of Lady Mary Coke*, III, 288.
71 Ibid.
72 The phrase is Joseph Gutteridge's: Chancellor (ed.), *Master and Artisan*, 143.
73 Toynbee and Whibley (eds), *Correspondence of Thomas Gray*, II, 842.
74 Ibid., 512.
75 Gosse, *Dr. Viper*, 284.
76 Quoted in Ober, 'Boswell's Clap'.
77 Ellis (ed.), *Early Diary of Frances Burney*, 256. Burney appends the following wry observation:

> Nevertheless, this old prig sometimes affects something bordering upon gallantry. The first time he came, after he had been with Mrs Allen to the bedside, and spoken to mama, – and then written her prescription; he stalked up to me, and endeavouring to arrange his rigid features to something which resembled a smile; 'And what', cried he, 'must we do for this young lady's cough?' Then he insisted on feeling my pulse, and with a kind of dry pleasantry, said, 'Well, we will wait till to-morrow; we wont lose any blood to-night'.

78 Wyndham (ed.), *Chronicles of the Eighteenth Century*, 170.
79 LeFanu (ed.), *Betsy Sheridan's Journal*, 138. On doctors disagreeing, see Mandeville, *Treatise of the Hypochondriack and Hysterick Diseases*, 31f.
80 Price (ed.), *Letters of Sheridan*, 107.
81 Barrett (ed.), *Diary and Letters of Madame D'Arblay*, II, 109.
82 Cobbett, *Advice to Young Men*, 251.

CHAPTER 5   CONSULTATIONS

1 Fitzgerald (ed.), *Correspondence of Emily, Duchess of Leinster*, II, 295.
2 See Beier, 'In sickness and in health'.
3 Beresford (ed.), *Diary of a Country Parson*, IV, 143–52, 180–90.
4 Macdonald (ed.), *Letters of Eliza Pierce*, 67.
5 Hospital and other charity patients were not accorded the same rights and privileges as private patients. See Risse, *Hospital Life in Enlightenment Scotland*, 21. It was, for example, widely acknowledged that hospital patients were proper subjects of medical experimentation.
6 Blythe (ed.), *William Hazlitt, Selected Writings*, 249.
7 For some contemporary sociological perspectives see Strong, *Ceremonial Order of the Clinic*; Balint, *The Doctor, the Patient and his Illness*.
8 King-Hele, *Erasmus Darwin*, 106.
9 King-Hele, *Doctor of Revolution*, 29.
10 For a Christmas Day call, see King-Hele (ed.), *Essential Writings of Erasmus Darwin*, 81.
11 Verney (ed.), *Verney Letters*, II, 81.
12 Cf. Brody, *Stories of Sickness*; Kleinman, *The Illness Narratives*; Fissell, 'Physic of charity'.
13 Reiser, *Medicine and the Reign of Technology*, 1f.; Bynum and Porter (eds), *Medicine and the Five Senses*.
14 C. Lawrence, 'Incommunicable knowledge'; Reiser, *Medicine and the Reign of Technology*, 40.
15 See Nicolson, 'Stethoscopy in Edinburgh in the nineteenth century'.
16 Porter, 'Rise of physical examination'; idem, 'A touch of danger'; Shorter, *Bedside Manners*; Porter and Porter, *In Sickness and in Health*.
17 See ch. 4 above.
18 Cf. Risse, 'Dr William Cullen'.
19 MS letters of Hallett Turner to James Jurin, 29 May 1726, in Jurin MSS, Wellcome Institute for the History of Medicine, London. There are many similar items in this collection.
20 Ibid.
21 Ibid.
22 De Beer (ed.), *Correspondence of John Locke*, IV, 157, 3 November 1690.
23 King-Hele (ed.) *Letters of Erasmus Darwin*, 81.
24 Ibid.
25 For a good seventeenth-century example, the practice of Dr Nathaniel Johnston of Pontefract, see Oakley, 'Letters to a seventeenth-century

Yorkshire physician'. Some of the letters sent to Johnston included physical specimens ('I have sent by my man some phleagme that my wife spit this last night, also her water wich you may please to look upon'). John Locke's letters give ample evidence of postal diagnosis, as, nearly a century later, do Cullen's and Erasmus Darwin's. Various physicians, such as Dr William Cole, corresponded with Locke asking him for opinions on their own patients. See, for example, De Beer (ed.), *Correspondence of John Locke*, IV, 73. Cf. Risse, 'Dr William Cullen'.

26 De Beer (ed.), *Correspondence of John Locke*, IV, 104.
27 Lustig and Pottle (eds), *Boswell: the Applause of the Jury*, 191. All the physicians replied, and Boswell reported the more optimistic aspects of their findings to Johnson.
28 Percival, *Medical Ethics*, 102.
29 Porter and Porter, *In Sickness and in Health*, ch. 8.
30 Chapman (ed.), *Letters of Samuel Johnson*, III, 850; cf. II, 476. Mulhallen and Wright, 'Samuel Johnson: amateur physician'.
31 Mandeville, *Treatise of the Hypochondriack and Hysterick Diseases*, 8.
32 Bagley (ed.), *Great Diurnal of Nicholas Blundell*, II, 198.
33 Hobhouse (ed.), *Diary of a West Country Physician*, 99.
34 Fitzgerald (ed.), *Correspondence of Emily, Duchess of Leinster*, I, 199. She was herself taking seltzer water and vitriol drops for her nerves.
35 Ibid.
36 Little and Kahrl (ed.), *Letters of David Garrick*, II, 451.
37 Mulhallen and Wright, 'Samuel Johnson: amateur physician'.
38 De Beer (ed.), *Correspondence of John Locke*, V, 274.
39 Percival, *Medical Ethics*.
40 Ibid.
41 Barrett (ed.), *Diary and Letters of Madame D'Arblay*, IV, 136–42. See Macalpine and Hunter, *George III and the Mad Business*; Porter, *Social History of Madness*, ch. 3.
42 Arbuthnot, *History of John Bull*, 67.
43 Harley, 'Honour and property'.
44 De Beer (ed.), *Correspondence of John Locke*, V, 354. See also Harley, 'Honour and property'. For Dr. John Woodward's duel with Richard Mead, see Levine, *Dr Woodward's Shield*.
45 Cave (ed.), *Diary of Joseph Farington*, VIII, 3010–11.
46 Ibid.
47 Ibid.
48 Nicolson (ed.), *Conway Letters*, 25.
49 Ibid., 62.
50 Ibid.
51 Curwen (ed.), *Journal of Gideon Mantell*, 163. Mantell entertained a low opinion of his own profession: ibid., 152: 'My excellent friend the Earl of Munster shot himself in paroxysm of insanity. The stupid phyicians who attended him were unaware of the danger, and no precautions were taken! He was an excellent man, and one from whom I have received much

kindness and attention! It is a sad affair.'

52 Ibid.
53 Mandeville, *Treatise of the Hypochondriack and Hysterick Diseases*, 31.
54 Colvin (ed.), *Correspondence of Maria Edgeworth*, 499.
55 See Niebyl, 'Non-naturals'; Rather, '"Six things non-natural"'.
56 Lewis (ed.), *Letters of Lady Brilliana Harley*, 1; Burton, *Anatomy of Melancholy*, 391.
57 Climenson (ed.), *Passages from the Diary of Lybbe Powys*, 220–2.
58 Carroll (ed.), *Letters of Richardson*, 110.
59 Ibid.
60 Porter, *Health for Sale*.
61 Porter and Porter, *Sickness and Self*, Ch. 2.
62 Beresford (ed.), *Diary of a Country Parson*, IV, 154.
63 Jeaffreson, *Book about Doctors*.
64 See the discussion in Shorter, *Bedside Manners*.
65 *Anecdotes, Professional, or Ana of Medical Literature*, I, 153.
66 Ibid.
67 Cf. Percival, *Medical Ethics*.
68 Johnson (ed.), *Letters from Lady Mary Wortley Montagu*, 8–9.
69 Verney and Verney (eds), *Verney Memoirs*, IV, 421.
70 Christie (ed.), *Diary of the Revd William Jones*, 128.
71 King and Ryskamp (eds), *Letters and Prose Writings of William Cowper*, IV, 201.
72 Percival, *Medical Ethics*, 103.
73 Coburn (ed.), *Letters of Sara Hutchinson*, 272.
74 Ibid.
75 Bessborough and Aspinall (eds), *Lady Bessborough*, 62.
76 Lewis (ed.), *Letters of Lady Brilliana Harley*, 79.
77 LeFanu (ed.), *Betsy Sheridan's Journal*, 67.
78 J. M., *Letters to a Sick Friend*, 126–7.
79 Ibid.
80 Ibid.
81 Ibid.
82 Mandeville (ed.), *Retrospections of Dorothea Herbert*, I, 25.
83 Ibid. The doctor was presumably Maxwell Garthshore.
84 Hughes (ed.), *North Country Life*, I, 97.
85 Ibid.
86 Mitchell and Penrose (eds), *Letters from Bath*, 35.
87 Ibid.
88 Herbert (ed.), *Pembroke Papers*, II, 235.
89 Ibid.
90 Ilchester (ed.), *Lady Holland's Journal*, II, 203.
91 Chapman (ed.), *Jane Austen's Letters*, 426.
92 Bamford (ed.), *Dear Miss Heber*, 128–9.
93 Johnson (ed.), *Letters from Lady Mary Wortley Montagu*, 432.
94 Ibid.

95 Paston, *Mrs Delany*, 272.
96 Ibid., 273.
97 Cave (ed.), *Diary of Joseph Farington*, IX, 3221.
98 Ibid.
99 Verney (ed.), *Letters*, I, 186.
100 Quoted in Fox, *Fothergill*, 32. Burney had her own favourites, including John Armstrong, whose 'very sight' was 'medicinal'. 'This medical Aesculapius succeeded in dethroning and extirpating the raging fever' threatening her father's life. Quoted in Maloney, *George and John Armstrong*, 34.
101 Severn (ed.), *Diary of the Rev. John Ward*, 259–60.
102 Ibid.
103 Ibid.
104 Little and Kahrl (eds), *Letters of David Garrick*, II, 640.
105 Fitzgerald (ed.), *Correspondence of Emily, Duchess of Leinster*, II, 202.
106 Lewis (ed.), *Extracts from the Journals and Correspondence of Miss Berry*, II, 333.
107 Ponsonby, *Call a Dog Hervey*, 48.
108 Ibid.
109 Chapman (ed.), *Letters of Samuel Johnson*, II, 290. In the end she chose Heberden.
110 Burkhardt and Smith (eds), *Correspondence of Charles Darwin*, II, 13. Darwin had some tips for handling patients: ibid., 17.

CHAPTER 6   IRREGULARS

1 See ch. 2 above.
2 See ch. 3 above.
3 For a lengthy bibliography on eighteenth-century quackery, see Porter, 'Language of quackery'; idem, *Health for Sale*.
4 Porter, '"I think ye both quacks"'.
5 Ward, *London Spy*, 131.
6 Ibid.
7 Looney, 'Advertising and society'.
8 Sprott, *1784*, 161.
9 Ibid.
10 Ibid., 26–7. For patent medicines advertised in East Anglia, see Goodwyn, *Selections from Norwich Newspapers*, 31; and, more generally, Porter, 'Newspapers as resources for social historians'; Feather, *Provincial Book Trade*.
11 Tring, 'Influence of Victorian "patent medicines"'.
12 Cf. McKendrick, Brewer and Plumb, *Birth of a Consumer Society*, 9f.
13 Bagley (ed.), *Gregt Diurnal of Nicolas Blundell*, II, 92; II, 100.
14 Verney (ed.), *Verney Letters*, II, 93.
15 Erhenreich and English, *Witches, Midwives and Nurses*; Viseltear, 'Joanna Stephens'; Wyman, 'The surgeoness'.

16 Bynum and Porter (eds), *Medical Fringe and Medical Orthodoxy*, 2f.
17 Stansfield, *Thomas Beddoes*; cf Porter, '"I think ye both quacks"'.
18 Porter, 'Before the fringe'; for James Graham as an instance, see idem, 'Sex and the singular man'.
19 Crellin, 'Dr. James's Fever Powder'.
20 Porter, 'Language of Quackery'.
21 Hone, *Life of John Radcliffe*, 71.
22 Cf. Porter, 'Before the fringe'.
23 Buchan, *Domestic Medicine*, xix.
24 Trotter, *View of the Nervous Temperament*, 218–19.
25 Stern, *Medical Advice*. It is ironical that Stern himself vended a nostrum, Dr Stern's Balsamic Aether, as a consumption cure. Stern is discussed in Porter, 'Laymen, doctors, and medical knowledge', 304.
26 Stern, *Medical Advice*.
27 Buchan, *Domestic Medicine*, 471. Trotter, *View of the Nervous Temperament*, 122; he likewise condemned the quack use of mercury: ibid., 127.
28 Vaisey (ed.), *Diary of Thomas Turner*, 208; see also Barry, 'Publicity and the public good'.
29 Ward, *London Spy*, 129.
30 Porter, 'Language of quackery'; idem, '"I think ye both quacks"'.
31 Buchan, *Domestic Medicine*, xxi.
32 Porter, '"I think ye both quacks"'.
33 Vaisey (ed.), *Diary of Thomas Turner*, 208.
34 Matthews, *History of Pharmacy*; Poynter (ed.), *Evolution of Pharmacy*, 25; cf., Porter and Porter, 'Rise of the English Drug industry'.
35 Berliner, 'Medical modes of production'.
36 McKendrick, Brewer and Plumb, *Birth of a Consumer Society*, 27.
37 G. Smith, 'The popularization of medical knowledge'; Marland, *Medicine and Society in Wakefield and Huddersfield*, 234f.
38 LeFanu (ed.), *Betsy Sheridan's Journal*, 123; for De Mainauduc, see Porter, 'Under the influence'.
39 Bessborough and Aspinall (eds), *Lady Bessborough*, 40.
40 Lustig and Pottle (eds), *Boswell: The English Experiment*, 195.
41 Ober, '*Boswell's Clap*'.
42 Lustig and Pottle (eds), *Boswell: The English Experiment*, 195.
43 Ibid.
44 Cozens-Hardy (ed.), *Diary of Sylas Neville*, 24.
45 Fielding, *Journal of a Voyage to Lisbon*, 209.
46 King and Ryskamp (eds), *Letters and Prose Writings of William Cowper*, IV, 288, 299; Nicolson and Rousseau, 'Berkeley and tar-water'.
47 Sedgwick (ed.) *Lord Hervey's Memoirs*, 314. Hervey also persuaded Princess Caroline to take Ward's Pill:

> The Princess Caroline had been extremely ill all this summer at Hampton Court of rheumatic pains, and growing every day worse, notwithstanding all the medicines that had been given her in what the physicians call a regular way, Lord Hervey upon her coming to town had persuaded her to take Ward's Pill, a nostrum belonging to one Ward, an excellent medicine not only in rheumatism

but in several cases, which, for being so, all the physicians and surgeons endeavoured to decry.

Princess Caroline, persuaded by Lord Hervey, had taken this medicine since her arrival in London, with the privity rather than consent of the King and Queen, and keeping it a secret to everybody else; but in four times taking only she had found such benefit that, notwithstanding she had been unable to walk or get up from her chair without help when she began it.

48 Ibid.
49 Ibid.
50 Ibid.
51 Hartshorne (ed.), *Memoirs of a Royal Chaplain*, 299. cf. Viseltear, 'Joanna Stephens'.
52 Hartshorne (ed.), *Memoirs of a Royal Chaplain*, 299.
53 Wadd, *Mems., Maxims and Memoirs*, 65–6.
54 Moore, quoted in Hunter and Macalpine, *Three Hundred Years of Psychiatry*, 498.
55 Ibid.
56 Ibid.
57 Ibid.
58 Wadd, *Mems., Maxims and Memoirs*, 66.
59 Spilsbury (ed.), *Free Thoughts on Quacks*; Spinke, *Quackery Unmask'd*.
60 Crellin, 'Dr James's Fever Powder'.
61 Hemlow (ed.), *Journals and Letters of Fanny Burney*, VI, 477.
62 Ibid.
63 Dewhurst, *Dr Quicksilver*, 150–2; Arthur (ed.), *Medicine in Wisbech*, 62; Berridge and Edwards, *Opium and the People*, 19.
64 Bynum, 'Treating the wages of sin', 11–12.
65 Buchan, *Venereal Disease*, 22.
66 Ibid.
67 Looney, 'Advertising and society in England'.
68 Bynum, 'Treating the wages of sin'.
69 Ober, '*Boswell's Clap*'.
70 Ibid., 11.
71 Brady and Pottle (eds), *Boswell in Search of a Wife*, 286.
72 Buchan, *Venereal Disease*, iv.
73 Ibid. See also Porter, 'Before the fringe'.
74 Ober, '*Boswell's Clap*', 7.
75 Ibid., 18.
76 Ibid., 21.
77 Buchan, *Venereal Disease*.
78 Rogers, *Grub Street*, 37f.
79 Welsh, *Bookseller of the Last Century*.
80 Porter, 'Language of quackery'.
81 Sells, *Oliver Goldsmith*, 186ff. The Walpole quotation is on p.187.
82 Nicolson, 'Ward's Pill and Drop'.
83 Young, *Gibbon*, 60.
84 Garlick and Macintyre (eds), *Diary of Joseph Farington*, II, 491. Farington

was well aware of the dangers of such nostrums: see ibid., II, 626.

85 Ibid., 491.
86 Fielding, *Journal of a Voyage to Lisbon*, 196. Fielding was also a great believer in the virtues of tar-water: ibid., 198.
87 Ibid., 196.
88 Ibid., 197
89 Ibid.
90 Ibid., 196.
91 Ibid., 197; Miller, 'Airs, waters and places'.
92 Nicolson and Rousseau, *This Long Disease My Life*, 297f.
93 Cross, quoted in ibid., 303.
94 Ibid.
95 Toynbee (ed.), *Walpole Letters*, II, 191–2.
96 Ibid.
97 Ibid.
98 Bynum and Porter (eds), *Medical Fringe and Medical Orthodoxy*.
99 All these issues are discussed at much fuller length in Porter, *Health for Sale*.

CHAPTER 7   THE ECONOMY OF MEDICINE

1 Brockbank and Kenworthy (eds), *Diary of Richard Kay*, 11.
2 Ibid.
3 Hill (ed.), *Lives of the English Poets by Samuel Johnson*, III, 415. Johnson wrote:

> A physician in a great city seems to be the mere plaything of fortune; his degree of reputation is, for the most part, merely casual: they that employ him know not his excellence; they that reject him know not his deficiency. By an acute observer, who had looked on the transactions of the medical world for half a century, a very curious work might be written on the Fortune of Physicians.

4 There is an excellent discussion in Harley, 'Honour and property'. John Haslam's *Illustrations of Madness* was, in effect, one long attack on his fellow practitioners, Drs Birkbeck and Clutterbuck. See Porter (ed.), *John Haslam, Illustrations of Madness*, 'Introduction'.
5 Waddington, 'Struggle to reform the Royal College of Physicians'; idem, 'General practitioners and consultants'.
6 Quoted in Porter, 'William Hunter'.
7 Bynum and Porter (eds), *William Hunter and the Eighteenth Century Medical World*, 32–3, 36–8.
8 Porter, 'William Hunter'; Brock, *William Hunter*; idem, 'Happiness of riches'.
9 See Jeaffreson, *Book About Doctors*, 85, for anecdotes of Radcliffe and Mead.
10 Brock, 'Happiness of riches', 40–1.

11 Abraham, *Lettsom*, 209.
12 Simpson (ed.), *Journal of Dr John Simpson*, 18.
13 Ibid.
14 Ibid., 3.
15 Loudon, *Medical Care and the General Practitioner*, 103–9.
16 Lewis, *In the Family Way*, 85ff.
17 Simpson, *Journal of Dr John Simpson*, 3.
18 Rodin, *Medical Casebook of Dr Arthur Conan Doyle*.
19 King-Hele (ed.), *Letters of Erasmus Darwin*, 206–7. Charles Darwin later remarked that his grandfather, Erasmus, could happily father two illegitimate daughters and not fear it would ruin his reputation. Charles used this as an example of changing mores.
20 Ibid.
21 Ibid.
22 Ibid., 139. He was even extremely anxious about publishing his medical writings: ibid., 76.
23 Butterfield (ed.), *Letters of Benjamin Rush*, I, 250–1.
24 Ibid.
25 Ibid., 284–5. This advice was given to a second student, William Claypoole, in 1782.
26 Ibid.
27 Ibid.
28 Loudon, *Medical Care and the General Practitioner*, 35f.; cf. Beier, *Sufferers and Healers*, 51f., who argues convincingly for the skill of seventeenth-century surgeons.
29 Burnby, *Study of the English Apothecary*.
30 Brockbank and Kenworthy (eds), *Diary of Richard Kay*, 70; S. Lawrence, 'Science and medicine at the London Hospitals'; C. Lawrence, 'Medicine as culture', Lane, 'Role of apprenticeship in eighteenth-century medical education'.
31 Ford (ed.), *Medical Student at St Thomas's*, 173f.
32 Ibid., 230.
33 Ibid.
34 For Bath see Rolls, *Hospital of the Nation*; Schnorrenberg, 'Medical Men of Bath'; Neve, 'Natural philosophy, medicine and the culture of science'.
35 N. C. Smith (ed.), *Letters of Sydney Smith*, 213.
36 Abraham, *Lettsom*; Corner and Booth (eds), *Chain of Friendship*.
37 Cave (ed.), *Diary of Joseph Farington*, IX, 3237.
38 Ibid.
39 Garlick and MacIntyre (eds), *Diary of Joseph Farington*, III, 712. For Sir Samuel Garth as a notorious drinker and coffee-house prescriber, see R. Cook, *Sir Samuel Garth*.
40 Brooks, *Sir Hans Sloane*.
41 Zuckerman, 'Dr Richard Mead'.
42 We owe this information to the kindness of Ernest Heberden.
43 Beattie, *John Arbuthnot*.

44 R. Cook, *Sir Samuel Garth*.
45 For science and scientific wrangling, see Posner, 'William Withering versus the Darwins', 51–7. Cf. MacNeil, *Under the Banner of Science*; for humane causes, see Abraham, *Lettsom*.
46 Cf. *Medicina Flagellata*; [Glyster], *Dose for the Doctor*; LaCasce, 'Swift on medical extremism'.
47 R. Cook, *Sir Samuel Garth*.
48 Abraham, *Lettsom*, 212–13. Other maxims Lettsom allegedly put into practice were: 'Engage in controversy with Eminent men, as a most excellent way of bringing a man into public notice'; 'Always pretend that you have a great deal of business on your hands, and the world will conclude that you are in a great practice'; and 'Force yourself into the Company of great men, and the world will think you are one of the number'.
49 Ibid.
50 Cave (ed.), *Diary of Joseph Farington*, X, 3535. For anecdotes of these fashionable physicians see Timbs, *Doctors and Patients*; Wadd, *Mems., Maxims, and Memoirs*; Jeaffreson, *Book about Doctors*. On fame, cf. Braudy, *Frenzy of Renown*.
51 Campbell, *London Tradesman*, 57.
52 Beresford (ed.), *Diary of a Country Parson*, II, 142.
53 Fitzgerald (ed.), *Correspondence of Emily, Duchess of Leinster*, III, 296.
54 A. Smith *Inquiry*, I, 137.
55 Ibid., 137–8.
56 Ibid., 138.
57 Percival, *Medical Ethics*, 115.
58 Burnby, *Study of the English Apothecary*.
59 Nelson, *Essay on the Government of Children*, 139.
60 Ibid., 140.
61 Ibid., 141.
62 Loudon, *Medical Care and the General Practitioner*, 65; idem, 'Nature of Provincial Medical Practice'.
63 Percival, *Medical Ethics*, 74.
64 Welsh, *Bookseller of the Last Century*, 25.
65 Archenholz, *Picture of England*, II, 156.
66 Butterfield (ed.), *Letters of Benjamin Rush*, I, 66.
67 Zwanenberg, 'The Suttons'.
68 Mitchell and Penrose (eds), *Letters from Bath*, 23; Beresford (ed.), *Diary of a Country Parson*, I, 191.
69 Home (ed.), *Letters and Journals of Mary Coke*, IV, 345–6. For Sutton's income – apparently over £6000 a year – see Baxby, *Jenner's Smallpox Vaccine*, 27.
70 Home (ed.), *Letters and Journals of Mary Coke*, IV, 345–6.
71 Ibid.
72 Ibid.
73 Welsh, *Bookseller of the Last Century*, 25.
74 Crellin, 'Dr James's fever powder'.

75 Bakewell, *Domestic Guide*.
76 Quoted in Sprott, *1784*, 286. For contemporary condemnation of Rowley as a medical exhibitionist, see Brock, *William Hunter*, 56f.
77 Johnson (ed.), *Letters from Lady Mary Wortley Montagu*, 361. The year was 1748.
78 Williams (ed.), *Swift, Journal to Stella*, 101.
79 Timbs, *Doctors and Patients*, 156. The story had a happy ending. Given over by the doctors, Pulteney drank some small beer and recovered.
80 Murray (ed.), *Newfoundland Journal of Aaron Thomas*, 158.
81 Cf. Hone, *Life of John Radcliffe*, 75, for some guesstimates.
82 Hunter and Macalpine, *Three Hundred Years of Psychiatry*, 26.
83 Hobhouse (ed.), *Diary of a West Country Physician*, 137.
84 Loudon, *Medical Care and the General Practitioner*.
85 Vaisey (ed.), *Diary of Thomas Turner*, 214. Compare William Holland's grumbles about surgeon Forbes: 'He is the very Deuce of a man for Visits, Physicks and Charges. I think I must put an end to this man's visits.' Ayres (ed.), *Paupers and Pig Killers*, 177.
86 Verney and Verney (eds), *Memoirs*, III, 191.
87 Climenson (ed.), *Passages from the Diaries of Mrs Philip Lybbe Powys*, 352: 'Mr Crook, the apothecary, only wish'd he could have a lease of this same influenza for eight years – he should not desire a better fortune.'
88 Woodward, *To Do the Sick No Harm*; Porter, 'Gift relation'.
89 Tröhler, 'Quantification in British medicine'.
90 Inkster, 'Marginal men'.
91 Lane, 'Provincial practitioner and his services'; Loudon, '"I'd rather have been a parish surgeon"'.
92 Holmes, *Augustan England*.
93 Ramsey, *Professional and Popular Medicine in France*.

CHAPTER 8   THE DOCTORS' POINT OF VIEW

1 Severn (ed.), *Diary of the Revd John Ward*, 244.
2 Quoted in Sheridan, *Doctors and Slaves*, 311.
3 Cheyne, *Essay of Health and Long Life*, 182.
4 Adair, *Essays on Fashionable Diseases*, 96.
5 Buchan, *Domestic Medicine*, 41.
6 Trotter, *View of the Nervous Temperament*, 110.
7 Beddoes, *Hygeia*, *passim*, but esp. Essay 5, Vol.II, 26ff.
8 Buchan, *Domestic Medicine*, 205.
9 Adair, *Essays on Fashionable Diseases*, 96.
10 Buchan, *Venereal Disease*, iii.
11 Mandeville, *Treatise of the Hypochondriack and Hysterick Diseases*; quoted in Turner, *Call the Doctor*, 61.
12 Mandeville, *Treatise of the Hypochondriack and Hysterick Diseases*.
13 Adair, *Essays on Fashionable Diseases*, 73ff. Adair singled out Buchan for attack: 105.

14 Saunders, *Edward Jenner*, 49.
15 J. M., *Letters to a Sick Friend*, 131.
16 Ibid.
17 Ibid., 118. Hellebore was the traditional remedy for insanity.
18 Morton, *Phthisiologia*, 8–9.
19 J.M., *Letters to a Sick Friend*, 131.
20 Ibid.
21 Ibid., 127.
22 Ibid.
23 Cheyne, *Essay of Health and Long Life*, 174. Cf. 173.
24 Willich, *Lectures on Diet*, 2.
25 Buchan, *Venereal Disease*, viii; G. Smith, 'Prescribing the rules of health'.
26 Shaw, *Doctor's Dilemma*, 'Preface', 67.
27 Eliot, *Middlemarch*, 204.
28 Percival, *Medical Ethics*, 72.
29 Ibid.
30 Hobhouse (ed.), *Diary of a West Country Physician*, 82.
31 Martineau, *Autobiography*, I, 255.
32 Buchan, *Venereal Disease*, xxix.
33 Ibid.
34 Ibid., viii.
35 Seward, *Memoirs of Dr Darwin*, 3.
36 Ibid.
37 Hankin (ed.), *Life of Mary Anne Schimmelpenninck*, I, 152.
38 Yorke (ed.), *Diary of John Baker*, 254; Chancellor (ed.), *Master and Artisan*, 87. Southam simply told Gutteridge to take lots of air and exercise.
39 Percival, *Medical Ethics*, 97.
40 Buchan, *Venereal Disease*, xv.
41 Percival, *Medical Ethics*, 84. The other side was that it was acknowledged that doctors could instigate procedures on poor and charity patients, especially in hospital, which private patients would never tolerate; above all, experimentation with new therapies. See Darwin, *Zoonomia*, IV, 436–7.
42 Trotter, *Essay on Drunkenness*.
43 Trotter, *View of the Nervous Temperament*, 289–90.
44 Quoted in Hunter and Macalpine, *Three Hundred Years of Psychiatry*, 463.
45 Ibid.
46 Quoted in Veith, *Hysteria*, 151.
47 Ibid.
48 Hone, *Life of Dr John Radcliffe*.
49 Quoted in Turner, *Call the Doctor*, 46.
50 Timbs, *Doctors and Patients*, 54.
51 Quoted in Thompson, *Unfit for Modest Ears*, 159.
52 Ford (ed.), *Medical Student at St Thomas's*, 171. 'Suaveter [*sic*] in modo', insisted Hampton Weekes to his brother, Dick: ibid., 248.
53 Timbs, *Doctors and Patients*, 53.

54 Buchan, *Venereal Disease*, 32.
55 Heberden, *Medical Commentaries*, 1.
56 Porter, 'Drinking man's disease'.
57 Porter, 'Introduction' to Trotter, *Essay on Drunkenness*.
58 Baur, *Hypochondria*; Fischer-Homberger, 'Hypochondriasis'; Porter and Porter, *In Sickness and in Health*, ch. 12.
59 MacDonald, *Mystical Bedlam*.
60 For detailed discussion see Porter, *Mind Forg'd Manacles*, especially chs 3 and 4; Scull, *Museums of Madness*; Parry-Jones, *Trade in Lunacy*.
61 Cf. Goubert (ed.), *Médicalisation*.
62 Cf. H. Cook, *Decline of the Old Medical Regime*.
63 'Tom Thumb, his Life and Death', in Butler (ed.) *Masterworks of Children's Literature*, I, 96.
64 Crawfurd, *Last Days of Charles II*.
65 Hone, *Life of Dr John Radcliffe*, 58; compare Sir Thomas Browne, 'To a friend, upon the occasion of the death of his intimate friend', 179. This work describes the slow quiet death of a man from consumption. See Finch, *Sir Thomas Browne*, 266.
66 R. Cook, *Sir Samuel Garth*, 37.
67 Beresford (ed.), *Diary of a Country Parson*, II, 224.
68 Hone, *Life of Dr John Radcliffe*, 58.
69 Verney and Verney (eds), *Memoirs*, II, 403.
70 Jeaffreson, *Book about Doctors*, 47.
71 King and Ryskamp (eds), *Letters and Prose Writings of William Cowper*, I, 216.
72 Dewhurst (ed.), *Willis's Oxford Casebook*, 99.
73 James, *Medicinal Dictionary*; cf. Ackerknecht, 'Death in the history of medicine'.
74 See Porter and Porter, *In Sickness and in Health*, ch. 14.
75 Illich, *Limits to Medicine*, 189f. For Bacon, see Rees, *Francis Bacon's Natural Philosophy*.
76 Hawkins, 'The history of resuscitation'; Payne, 'On the resuscitation of the apparently dead'; Bishop, *Short History of the Royal Humane Society*.
77 Ferriar, *Medical Histories*, III, 10. See also Noyes, 'The art of dying'.
78 Forbes, *Surgeons at the Bailey*.
79 Percival, *Medical Ethics*; Compare Gregory, *Observations on the Duties of a Physician*:

> Let me here exhort you against a barbarous custom of some physicians, the leaving your patients when their life is absolutely despaired of, and when it is no longer decent to take fees. It is as much the business of a physician to alleviate pain, and to smooth the avenues of death, as to cure diseases. Even in cases where his skill as a physician can be of no further avail, his presence and assistance as a man and as a friend may be highly grateful and useful, both to the patient and to his nearest relations. Neither is there any propriety in his going out at one door when the clergyman enters at the other; a quaint conceit of some of our faculty, more expressive of impiety than humour.

80 Ferriar, *Medical Histories*, III, 262.

81 Ibid., 273.
82 Gittings, *Death, Burial and the Individual*, 14f.
83 Brockbank and Kenworthy (eds), *Diary of Richard Kay*, 157. Kay often visited dying patients: ibid., 100, 158, 159.
84 Recorded by James Boswell: Brady and Pottle (eds), *Boswell in Search of a Wife*, 19 September 1769.
85 Munk, *Life of Sir Henry Halford*, 262. It is no accident that Munk also wrote *Euthanasia*.
86 Munk, *Life of Sir Henry Halford*, 264.
87 Ibid., 184.
88 Ibid., 264.
89 Ibid., 265.
90 Ibid., 97.
91 Buchan, *Domestic Medicine*, 143–4.
92 Fremantle (ed.), *Wynne Diaries*, III, 1.
93 Christie (ed.), *Diary of the Revd William Jones*, 128.
94 Butterfield (ed.), *Letters of Benjamin Rush*, 324.
95 Ferriar, *Medical Histories*, III, 265.
96 See Williams, *Age of Agony*.
97 See Berridge and Edwards, *Opium and the People*; Parssinen, *Secret Passions, Secret Remedies*; Hayter, *Opium and the Romantic Imagination*; Lefebure, *Samuel Taylor Coleridge*; Lindop, *Opium Eater*.
98 See Parssinen, *Secret Passions, Secret Remedies*.
99 Jones, *Mysteries of Opium Reveal'd*; Estes, 'John Jones's *Mysteries of Opium Reveal'd*'; Kramer, 'Opium rampant'.
100 Young, *Treatise on Opium*.
101 Crumpe, *Inquiry into the Nature and Properties of Opium*.
102 Cf. Risse, 'Brownian system of medicine', 45–51.
103 Butterfield (ed.), *Letters of Benjamin Rush*, 318–19.
104 King-Hele (ed.), *Letters of Erasmus Darwin*, 257, 245 and *passim*.
105 For the spread of these medicines see Bynum and Porter (eds), *Medical Fringe and Medical Orthodoxy*, and the literature cited there. On their dangers, see Adair, *Essays on Fashionable Diseases*, 235f.
106 Parssinen, *Secret Passions, Secret Remedies*, 16, quotes an early nineteenth-century source confirming its profitability: 'This is a very profitable business, the returns sometimes cent. percent, and seldom less than fifty; but it requires a capital of from £500 to £2000.'
107 Christie (ed.), *Diary of the Revd William Jones*, 27.
108 Parssinen, *Secret Passions, Secret Remedies*, 27.
109 Beresford (ed.), *Diary of a Country Parson*, I, 107.
110 Butterfield (ed.), *Letters of Benjamin Rush*, 327.
111 Paulshock, 'William Heberden and opium', 54.
112 Toynbee (ed.), *Letters of Horace Walpole*, III, 421.
113 Quoted in Wain, *Samuel Johnson*, 376.
114 Dittrick, 'Devices to prevent premature burial'.

CHAPTER 9   THERAPIES

1 Rosenberg, 'Therapeutic revolution'; Warner, 'Therapeutic perspective'.
2 Severn (ed.), *Diary of the Rev. John Ward*, 265.
3 Marrs (ed.), *Letters of Charles and Mary Lamb*, II, 3–4.
4 Norton (ed.), *Letters of Edward Gibbon*, III, 364.
5 See Beier, *Sufferers and Healers*, 149–50.
6 Porter, 'Quacks at court'.
7 Loudon, *Medical Care and the General Practitioner*, 73f.
8 Chapman (ed.), *Letters of Samuel Johnson*, III, 58.
9 Quoted in Macalpine and Hunter, *George III and the Mad Business*, 269.
10 King-Hele (ed.), *Letters of Erasmus Darwin*, 84; Corner and Booth (eds), *Chain of Friendship*, 134.
11 Cave (ed.), *Diary of Joseph Farington*, IX, 3235.
12 Jewitt (ed.), *Life of William Hutton*, 275.
13 Buchan, *Venereal Disease*, 7.
14 Heberden, *Medical Commentaries*, 21.
15 Porter, 'Drinking man's disease'.
16 Ayres (ed.), *Paupers and Pig Killers*, 173.
17 Porter, *Mind Forg'd Manacles*, 56.
18 Fitzgerald (ed.), *Correspondence of Emily Duchess of Leinster*, II, 347ff. Charlotte's illness highlights some of the ambiguities that could surround the 'sick role' in the eighteenth century. She was clearly shaken and bruised from the fall from her horse. She had given her head a severe knock and was laid low for a few weeks. The protracted nature of her 'decline', however, was treated with some suspicion by her relatives. Her aunt suspected that Charlotte was using her temporary 'sicknesses and pains' as an excuse for temperamental and selfish behaviour. Charlotte had a history of volatile spirits, and her emotional disequilibrium, especially around the time of her menstrual period, was anticipated and accommodated by her family. Louisa (Charlotte's aunt), writes to Emily (Charlotte's mother), specifically about these difficulties, which compounded the problem of dealing with her indeterminate sickness: 'Charlotte continues perfectly well; after the visit of the French lady [menstrual period] (which is expected this day or two) . . . Her temper to be sure is not good . . . I mean to [speak to her] as soon as ever the French lady's visit is over.' Her aunt further suspected that Charlotte's behaviour was influenced by the fact that she had an eye for Viscount Jocelyn, who ignored her: ibid., 335ff.
19 Ibid., 347ff.
20 Ibid.
21 Ibid.
22 See ch. 8 above.
23 Severn (ed.), *Diary of the Rev. John Ward*, 265.
24 Cf. Josten (ed.), *Elias Ashmole*, II, 606, 622, 626, 627, 631 ('whether my cousin Blagrave shall have any more children by his wife or not'), etc.
25 Nicolson (ed.), *Conway Letters*, 275.

26 Bessborough and Aspinall (eds), *Lady Bessborough*, 60.
27 Fitzgerald (ed.), *Correspondence of Emily, Duchess of Leinster*, I, 492.
28 Withering, *Account of the Foxglove*.
29 Cheyne, *Method of Cureing Diseases*, 24–5.
30 Matthews, *History of Pharmacy*; Poynter (ed.), *Evolution of Pharmacy*.
31 Griggs, *Green Pharmacy*; see discussion in Porter and Porter, 'Rise of the English drug industry'.
32 Clark, *History of the Royal College of Physicians*.
33 Loudon, *Medical Care and the General Practitioner*, 23f.; Burnby, *Study of the English Apothecary*.
34 McKendrick, Brewer and Plumb, *Birth of a Consumer Society*, 11f.
35 Porter, 'Enlightenment in England'.
36 King-Hele (ed.), *Letters of Erasmus Darwin*; Woodward, *To Do the Sick No Harm*.
37 Smith (ed.), *Selected Letters of Sydney Smith*, 6.
38 Adair, *Essays on Fashionable Diseases*.
39 Eaves and Kimpel, *Samuel Richardson*, 63. For Cheyne's advocacy of regular vomits, see *Essay of Health and Long Life*.
40 Porter, *Mind Forg'd Manacles*, ch. 4.
41 Buchan, *Domestic Medicine*, 151f.
42 See discussion in Wear, 'Puritan perceptions of illness'.
43 Griggs, *Green Pharmacy*, 109f.
44 Dover, *Ancient Physician's Legacy*; Dewhurst, *Quicksilver Doctor*.
45 Shorter, *Bedside Manners*. Cynics attacked this as a form of profiteering.
46 Beresford (ed.), *Diary of a Country Parson*, II, 122.
47 Hultin, 'Medicine and magic in the eighteenth century'.
48 King-Hele (ed.), *Letters of Erasmus Darwin*, 245–6. Janet was to die soon afterwards. 'Consumption' is not mentioned in the correspondence. Was it suspected by Watt and Darwin, but was there a gentlemen's agreement not to mention such an ominous disorder?
49 Ibid.
50 Ibid.
51 Ibid.
52 Ibid.
53 Cave (ed.), *Diary of Joseph Farington*, IX, 3221.
54 Ibid.
55 Cf. Warner, 'Therapeutic Perspective'.
56 Beier, *Sufferers and Healers*.
57 Porter and Porter, *In Sickness and in Health*, chs. 6 and 13.
58 De Moulin, 'Historical-Phenomenological study of bodily pain'; Wear, 'Historical and cultural aspects of pain'; Lewis, *Problem of Pain*; Keele, *Anatomies of Pain*.
59 Paulshock, 'William Heberden and opium'; Berridge and Edwards, *Opium and the People*; Parssinen, *Secret Passions, Secret Remedies*.
60 Cheyne, *Essay of Health and Long Life*, 213.
61 Upon which Coleridge dosed himself; cf. Porter and Porter, *In Sickness*

and in Health, ch. 12; Arthur (ed.), *Medicine in Wisbech and the Fens*.

62 Trotter, *Essay on Drunkenness*, 316.

63 Cheyne, *Essay of Health and Long Life*, 219.

64 Little and Kahrl (eds), *Letters of David Garrick*, I, 13.

65 Carswell, *Prospector*, 243.

66 King-Hele, *Erasmus Darwin*, 247.

67 Idem (ed.), *Letters of Erasmus Darwin*, 218.

68 Idem, *Doctor of Revolution*, 121.

69 Fremantle (ed.), *Wynne Diaries*, III, 11.

70 Shaw, quoted in Hunter and Macalpine, *Three Hundred Years of Psychiatry*, 314.

71 Cave (ed.), *Diary of Joseph Farington*, VIII, 3095–6.

72 Ibid.

73 Colp, *To Be An Invalid*; Crook and Guiton, *Shelley's Venomed Melody*.

74 Buchan, *Domestic Medicine*.

75 Brooks, *Sir Hans Sloane*, 85.

76 Cheyne, *Essay of Health and Long Life*, 71.

77 Brooks, *Sir Hans Sloane*, 78.

78 Cf. Aronson, *Account of the Foxglove*; King-Hele (ed.), *Letters of Erasmus Darwin*, 240f., for the use of digitalis.

79 Stansfield, *Thomas Beddoes*, 167.

80 Ibid.

81 Cave (ed.), *Diary of Joseph Farington*, XI, 3872–3.

82 Ibid.

83 Ibid.

84 C. Lawrence (ed.), *Essays in the History of Surgery*; Holmes, *Augustan England*.

85 Beresford (ed.) *Diary of a Country Parson*, II, 210.

86 Ford (ed.), *Medical Student at St Thomas's*.

87 Ibid., 12: this list was compiled by the editor.

88 Cave (ed.), *Diary of Joseph Farington*, X, 3672–3.

89 Ibid.

90 Ibid.

91 Vaisey (ed.), *Diary of Thomas Turner*, 65.

92 Ibid.

93 Chapman (ed.), *Letters of Samuel Johnson*, II, 394. Cf. ibid., 268, on taking valerian; Johnson refused to take it in a weak form, a decoction, as his doctor recommended: 'But I say, All or nothing'.

94 Porter, 'Hunger of imagination'.

95 Sorlein (ed.), *Diary of John Manningham*.

96 Lewis (ed.), *Extracts of the Journals and Correspondence of Miss Berry*, II, 15.

97 Fitzgerald (ed.), *Correspondence of Emily, Duchess of Leinster*, II, 323.

98 Paget (ed.), *Memoirs and Letters of Sir James Paget*, 21.

99 Weis and Pottle (eds), *Boswell in Extremes*, 154.

100 Bamford (ed.), *Dear Miss Heber*, 196.

101 Miller, *Adoption of Inoculation for Smallpox*; J. R. Smith, *Speckled Monster*, 9f.; Hopkins, *Princes and Peasants*.
102 Zwanenberg, 'The Suttons'.
103 King-Hele, *Doctor of Revolution*, 113.
104 Yorke (ed.), *Diary of John Baker*, 414–15.
105 Stansfield, *Thomas Beddoes*; Stansfield and Stansfield, 'Dr Thomas Beddoes and James Watt'; Neve, 'Natural philosophy'.
106 King-Hele (ed.), *Letters of Erasmus Darwin*, 262. Boulton responded that the manufacturer was Mr J. Schweppe, 141 Drury Lane. He assured Darwin, 'I am persuaded it has been of great use to me.'

CHAPTER 10   DOCTORS AND WOMEN

1 Prior, *Women in English Society*.
2 Shorter, *History of Women's Bodies*.
3 E. M. T., *Into the Silent Land*, 71.
4 Davidoff and Hall, *Family Fortunes*.
5 Craddock, *Young Edward Gibbon*, 20.
6 Shorter, *History of Women's Bodies*. Cf. Maclaren, *Reproductive Rituals*.
7 Shorter, *History of Women's Bodies*.
8 Shorter, 'Normal deliveries'. For male conceptions of the diseases of women see Astruc, *Treatise on Diseases Incident to Women*; Mauriceau, *Diseases of Women with Child*; Buchan, *Domestic Medicine*.
9 Ehrenreich and English, *Witches, Midwives and Nurses*; idem, *Complaints and Disorders*; idem, *For her own Good*; Versluysen, 'Midwives, Medical Men'; Donnison, *Midwives and Medical Men*.
10 Butterfield (ed.), *Letters of Benjamin Rush*, I, 617.
11 Davidoff and Hall, *Family Fortunes*. Cf. Fraser, *Weaker Vessel*; Jordanova, 'Natural facts'.
12 Anglesey (ed.), *Capel Letters*, 139.
13 Gallagher and Laqueur (eds), *Making of the Modern Body*; Showalter, *Female Malady*.
14 Marchand (ed.), *Byron's Letters and Journals*, III, 115–16.
15 Blackman, 'Popular theories of generation'; Porter, 'Touch of danger'; Ehrenreich and English, *For her own Good*.
16 See for example *Bath Journal*, 16 January 1786. For plenty of evidence of 'leech-women' in the early nineteenth century see Whitbread (ed.) *I know my own Heart*, 100f, 259f.
17 Fielding, *Journal of a Voyage to Lisbon*, 209.
18 Viseltear, 'Joanna Stephens'. Cf. Maggs, *Origins of General Nursing*; Wyman, 'The surgeoness'.
19 The view was William Hayley's, quoted in Craddock, *Young Edward Gibbon*, 33. Her purpose in doing this, it was alleged, was to conceal serious illnesses from the parents.
20 Bagley (ed.), *Great Diurnal of Nicholas Blundell*, II, 74.
21 Quoted in Rogers, *Feminism in Eighteenth-Century England*, 189.

22 Adair, *Essays on Fashionable Diseases*, 73f.
23 Mandeville, *Virgin Unmasked*, 123.
24 Maclaren, *Reproductive Rituals*; Griggs, *Green Pharmacy*; Chamberlain, *Old Wives' Tales*.
25 Pennington, *Mother's Advice to her Daughters*, 30.
26 See for instance Rowley, *Treatise of Female Diseases*; Laqueur, 'Orgasm, generation and the politics of reproductive biology'; Loudon, 'Chlorosis, anaemia and anorexia nervosa'; Figlio, 'Chlorosis and chronic disease'; Porter, 'Secrets of generation display'd'.
27 Veith, *Hysteria*; Trillat, *Histoire de l'Hystérie*.
28 Showalter, *Female Malady*.
29 Laqueur, 'Orgasm, generation and the politics of reproductive biology'.
30 Peterson, 'Dr Acton's Enemy'.
31 Trotter, *View of the Nervous Temperament*, 38.
32 Blair, 'Some observations', quoted in Hunter and Macalpine, *Three Hundred Years of Psychiatry*, 328.
33 Ibid.
34 Ibid.
35 Whitbread (ed.), *I know my own Heart*, 160; Porter, 'A touch of danger'.
36 Shorter, *History of Womens' Bodies*; Wilson, 'Participant or patient?'; idem, 'William Hunter'; Donnison, *Midwives and Medical Men*; Eccles, *Obstetrics and Gynaecology*; Versluysen, 'Midwives, medical men'; Lewis, *Politics of Motherhood*.
37 Shorter, 'Normal deliveries'; Eccles, *Obstetrics and Gynaecology*.
38 Ford (ed.), *Medical Student at St Thomas's*, 13.
39 Ehrenreich and English, *Witches, Midwives and Nurses*.
40 Quoted in Porter, 'A touch of danger', 229.
41 Shorter, 'Normal deliveries'.
42 King-Hele, *Doctor of Revolution*, 255.
43 Lewis, *In the Family Way*.
44 Sharp, *Compleat Midwife's Companion*, 'Preface'. Sharp goes on to insist, however, that in the whole development of civilization, women have generally made very satisfactory midwives, and that it would thus be preposterous and presumptuous for male practitioners to try to elbow out female ones: p. 3.
45 Wilson, 'Participant or patient?'.
46 Withers, *Observations on Chronic Weakness*, 98f.
47 Porter, 'A touch of danger'.
48 Cobbett, *Advice to Young Men*, 228.
49 Lewis, *In the Family Way*.
50 Loudon, *Medical Care and the General Practitioner*.
51 Verney and Verney (eds), *Memoirs*, IV, 256.
52 Plumb, 'New world of children'; Ariès, *Centuries of Childhood*; Bayne-Powell, *English Child in the Eighteenth Century*; Pollock, *Forgotten Children*; idem, *A Lasting Relationship*; Hardyment, *Dream Babies*.
53 Beekman, *Mechanical Baby*; Hardyment, *Dream Babies*.

54 Nelson, *Essay on the Government of Children*, 141.
55 Buchan, *Domestic Medicine*, 3.
56 Ibid.
57 Ibid., 6–7. Rosenberg has some excellent comments in his 'Medical text and medical context'.
58 Maloney, *George and John Armstrong*.

CHAPTER 11 MEDICAL KNOWLEDGE

1 Chapman (ed.), *Letters of Samuel Johnson*, III, 200–1; Crellin, 'Dr James's fever powder'.
2 Piozzi, *Anecdotes of Samuel Johnson*, 1, 2. He prescribed for himself, she remembered, 'with coolness and deliberation': 123.
3 Many of these issues are posed for medicine in Wright and Treacher (eds), *Problem of Medical Knowledge*, 'Introduction'; See also Woodward and Richards (eds), *Health Care and Popular Medicine*, 'Introduction'. For the wider issues see the discussion in Burke, 'Revolution in popular culture'.
4 See the illuminating remarks in Barry, 'Piety and the patient'. Fissell, 'Physic of charity', ch. 5 has been most helpful.
5 See discussion of Smollett in Rousseau, *Smollett*; Cheyne, *Essay of Health and Long Life*, xvi.
6 See Gay, *Enlightenment*; Porter, 'Was there a medical enlightenment?'; and discussion in Geyer-Kordesch, 'Cultural habits of illness'. For experience of the body, see Porter and Porter, *In Sickness and in Health*, chs 3–4, 12.
7 Temkin, *Galenism*.
8 See ch. 6 above; and Porter, *Health for Sale*.
9 De Beer (ed.), *Correspondence of John Locke*, III, 645.
10 Ibid.
11 Turner (ed.), *The Rev. Oliver Heywood*; Buchanan-Brown (ed.), *John Aubrey: Three Prose Works*, 44–90.
12 White, *Natural History of Selborne*, 53.
13 Ibid., 54.
14 Timbs, *Doctors and Patients*, 360; Tilley, *Dictionary of Proverbs*.
15 Robinson and Adams (eds), *Diary of Robert Hooke*, 311.
16 Chamberlain, *Old Wives' Tales*; Burke, *Popular Culture*. Bushaway, *By Rite*; Gladstone, 'English dialects, medicine and diet'; Fissell, 'Physic of charity'.
17 But see Leventhal, *In the Shadow of the Enlightenment*.
18 *Folklore Record*, III, 136; Hand, 'Folk-healer'; Black, *Folk Medicine*.
19 Helman, *Culture, Health and Illness*.
20 Thomas, *Religion and the Decline of Magic*; Buchanan-Brown (ed.), *John Aubrey: Three Prose Works*, 47; Porter, 'Medicine and the decline of magic'.
21 Ibid.; O'Keefe, *Stolen Lightning*.
22 Brand (ed.), *Observations on Popular Antiquities*, 731. The belief was widespread. In his *Natural History of Selborne*, 185, White called it a

'superstitious ceremony', which he believed had pagan origins. Cf. Linebaugh, 'Tyburn riot against the surgeons'.

23 Josten (ed.), *Elias Ashmole*, II, 580.
24 Contrast France, for which see Ramsay, *Professional and Popular Medicine in France*; Devlin, *Superstitious Mind*; Loux, *Sagesse du Corps*; idem, *Practiques et Savoirs populaires*.
25 Brookes, *General Practice of Physick*, I, 93. Buchan argued that so much of regular medicine and especially quack medicine was a charm in the eyes of its customers (*Domestic Medicine*, xix).
26 Griggs, *Green Pharmacy*; cf. Trimmer, 'Medical folklore and quackery'.
27 Palliser, 'Plants as wart cures'.
28 Bushaway, *By Rite*.
29 Quoted in Brand (ed.), *Observations on Popular Antiquities*, 727; MacDonald, 'Science, magic and folklore'.
30 Buchan, *Domestic Medicine*, xix.
31 Ibid.
32 Burton, *Anatomy of Melancholy*.
33 Bagley (ed.), *Great Diurnal of Nicolas Blundell*, II.
34 Zuckerman, 'Dr Richard Mead'; Porter, *Mind Forg'd Manacles*, ch. 2. Cf. Leventhal, *In the Shadow of the Enlightenment*.
35 Beresford (ed.), *Diary of Parson Woodforde*, III, 253.
36 Josten (ed.), *Elias Ashmole*, IV, 1680.
37 Quoted in Hunter (ed.), *John Aubrey*, 106.
38 Guthrie, 'Lady Sedley's receipt book'. See also the *Family Physician*.
39 For discussion, see Porter and Porter, *In Sickness and in Health*, ch. 8.
40 *British Apollo*, I, 137. Other readers' questions included 'What is the use of the spleen?' and 'What is the cause of the cholick?': ibid., 104, 335.
41 G. Smith, 'Prescribing the rules of health'; idem, 'Cleanliness'.
42 Capp, *Astrology and the Popular Press*.
43 Williams (ed.), *Sophie in London*, 296.
44 Porter, 'Lay medical knowledge'.
45 G. Smith, 'Cleanliness'. See for instance, *Family Companion of Health*; *Family Guide to Health*; Archer, *Every Man His Own Doctor*; and, above all, Reece, *Domestic Medical Guide*.
46 Wesley, *Primitive Physick*; Rousseau, 'Wesley's *Primitive Physick*'; Lawrence, 'William Buchan'; Rosenberg, 'Medical text and medical context'.
47 Buchan, *Domestic Medicine*; C. Lawrence, 'William Buchan'; Rosenberg, 'Medical text and medical context'.
48 Cheyne, *Essay of Health and Long Life*. Cf. Porter, 'Introduction' to George Cheyne, *English Malady*; Viets, 'George Cheyne'.
49 Wesley, *Primitive Physick*.
50 Archer, *Every Man his Own Doctor*, title-page; G. Smith, 'Prescribing the rules of health'.
51 Archer, *Every Man his Own Doctor*, 3; Niebyl, 'Non-naturals'.
52 Mandeville, *Treatise on the Hypochondriack and Hysterick Diseases*. For Profily, see Bynum, 'Treating the wages of sin'.

53 Cf. Bynum and Porter (eds), *Medical Fringe and Medical Orthodoxy*; Inglis, *Natural Medicine*; Porter, 'Before the fringe'; idem, *Health for Sale*; Wharton, *Crusaders for Health*.
54 Helfand, 'James Morison and his pills'.
55 Porter, 'Sexual politics of James Graham'; idem, 'Sex and the singular man'.
56 See above ch. 6.
57 Barry, 'Piety and the patient'.
58 Chancellor (ed.), *Master and Artisan*, 95.
59 Ibid., 131.
60 Ibid.
61 Ibid.
62 LeFanu, *British Periodicals of Medicine*.
63 Buchanan-Brown (ed.), *John Aubrey: Three Prose Works*, 339; Severn (ed.), *Diary of the Rev. John Ward*, 252. Hand-me-down female knowledge is well discussed in Chamberlain, *Old Wives' Tales*; and Fraser, *Weaker Vessel*, 46f.
64 J. R. Smith, *Speckled Monster*.
65 Razzell, *Conquest of Smallpox*.
66 Quoted from Withering's *Account of the Foxglove* in Chamberlain, *Old Wives' Tales*, 175. Cf. Aronson, *Account of the Foxglove*.
67 Burke, *Popular Culture*; idem, 'Revolution in popular culture'.
68 Helman, 'Feed a cold'.
69 Bynum and Porter (eds), *John Brown and Brunonianism*.
70 Cited in Baragar, 'John Wesley and medicine'.
71 Norton (ed.), *Letters of Edward Gibbon*, III, 141. Gibbon said he spent 'two hours *every day*' at these lectures.
72 Porter, 'Quacks at court'; idem, 'Sex and the singular man'.
73 Vaisey (ed.), *Diary of Thomas Turner*, 167.
74 Ibid., 210.
75 Sterne, *Tristram Shandy*, 104.
76 We are very grateful to Christine English for this information. Very slightly later, Sands' Circulating Library in Newcastle had these medical books:

> Adair on Human Body and Mind
> Ball's Treatise on Fevers
> Baylie on Use and Abuse of Bath Waters
> Bell's Principles of Animal Electricity and Magnetism
> Bell's System of Surgery
> John Clark Observations on Diseases of Long Voyages to Hot Countries
> Cornwell's Domestic Physician or Guardian of Health
> Duverney on the Ear
> Falconer on Influence of Passions on Disorders of Body
> Fordyce on Digestion of Food
> Gooch's Cases and Practical Remarks in Surgery
> Gravel and Gout
> John Gregory Elements of Practice of Physic
> Lectures on Duties of Physician
> Haller's Medical Cases
> Jenty Lectures on Human Structure

Jones on Distortion of the Spine
Kite's Essay on Recovery of the Apparently Dead
Leake on Efficiency of the Lisbon Diet Drink in Venereal Disease
Lynch's Guide to Health
Perfect's Cases in Insanity
Porterfield on Eye
Pott on Wounds
Rymer on Indigestion
Stevens Practical Treatise on Consumption
Stevens Practical Treatise on Fevers

77 Feather, *Provincial Book Trade*, 83; Looney, 'Advertising and society'.
78 Ferrier, *Marriage*, 108.
79 Ibid., 143.
80 Porter, '"Secrets of generation display'd"'; Blackman, 'Popular theories of generation'; Beall, '*Aristotle's Masterpiece* in America'.
81 John Cannon, 'Diary', Taunton Record Office. Note that James Lackington, the bookseller, stocked *Aristotle's Masterpiece* from early in his career: Feather, *Provincial Book Trade*, 39.
82 Martin, *Tennyson*, 3. One assumes she was not simply playing the innocent. Jaeger, *Before Victoria*; Purdon, *Dr. Bowdler's Legacy*.
83 Quoted in Dirckx, *Language of Medicine*, 119.
84 Rogers, 'Rise and fall of gout'.
85 King and Ryskamp (eds), *Letters and Prose Writings of William Cowper*, III, 91.
86 Cadogan, *Dissertation on Gout*; but contrast Heberden, *Medical Commentaries*, under Arthritis.
87 Wesley, *Journal*, IV, 110.
88 Macdonald (ed.) *Letters of Eliza Pierce*, 89.
89 Ibid.
90 Melville (ed.), *Lady Suffolk*, 34.
91 Climenson (ed.), *Elizabeth Montagu*, II, 73.

CHAPTER 12   SURVEY AND CONCLUSION

1 Wedgwood and Wedgwood (eds), *Wedgwood Circle*, 329.
2 Johnson (ed.), *Letters of Lady Mary Wortley Montagu*, 361. She added, 'nor is there any country in the world where doctors raise such immense fortunes'.
3 Quoted in Berridge and Edwards, *Opium and the People*, 11. Ball was arguing in favour of a massive increase in the home growing of opium.
4 Shorter, *Bedside Manners*.
5 Quoted in Percival, *Medical Ethics*, 204.
6 Ibid.
7 Jewson, 'Medical knowledge and the patronage system'; idem, 'Disappearance of the sick man'.
8 Jane Austen, *Sanditon*, 181.

9 Campbell, *London Tradesman*, 37.
10 Ibid.
11 Cobbett, *Advice to Young Men*, 160.
12 Garnett (ed.), *Novels of Thomas Love Peacock*, 114.
13 Willich, *Lectures on Diet*.
14 Trotter, *View of the Nervous Temperament*.
15 Beddoes, *Hygeia*, essay V, 40.
16 Buchan, *Venereal Diseases*, 26.
17 Illich, *Limits to Medicine*.

Bibliography

Abraham, J. J., *Lettsom: his Life, Times, Friends and Descendants* (London, Heinemann, 1933).

Ackerknecht, E. H., 'Death in the history of medicine', *Bulletin of the History of Medicine*, 42 (1968), 19–23.

Adair, J. M., *Essays on Fashionable Diseases . . .* (London, Bateman, 1790).

Aldington, B., *The Strange Life of Charles Waterton 1782–1865* (London, Evans, 1948).

Anglesey, The Marquess of (ed.), *Capel Letters* (London, Jonathan Cape, 1955).

Anning, S. T., 'A medical case book: Leeds, 1781–4', *Medical History*, 28 (1984), 420–31.

Appleby, A., *Famine in Tudor and Stuart England* (Stanford, Stanford University Press, 1978).

Arbuthnot J., *The History of John Bull*, ed. by A. W. Bower and R. A. Erickson (reprinted, Oxford, Clarendon Press, 1976).

Archenholz, J. W. von, *Picture of England* (London, [for the booksellers], 1797).

Archer, J., *Every Man his Own Doctor* (London, [for the author], 1671).

Ariès, P., *Centuries of Childhood: a Social History of Family Life* (London, Jonathan Cape, 1962).

——, *Western Attitudes towards Death: from the Middle Ages to the Present* (Baltimore, Johns Hopkins University Press, 1974; London, Marion Boyars, 1976).

——, *The Hour of our Death*, trans. by H. Weaver (London, Allen Lane, 1981).

——, *Images of Man and Death*, trans. by J. Lloyd (Cambridge, Cambridge University Press, 1985).

Armstrong, D., *The Political Anatomy of the Body* (Cambridge, Cambridge University Press, 1983).

Armstrong, G., *The Art of Preserving Health* (London, A. Millar, 1744).

——, *An Essay on the Diseases most Fatal to Infants. To which are added Rules to be Observed in the Nursing of Children* (London, T. Cadell, 1767).

——, *Medical Essays* (London, T. Davies, 1773).

——, *An Account of the Diseases Most Incident to Children* (London, T. Cadell, 1777).

Aronson, J. K., *An Account of the Foxglove and its Medicinal Uses, 1785–1985* (London, Oxford University Press, 1985).

Arthur, J. (ed.), *Medicine in Wisbech and the Fens 1700–1920* (London, Seagull Enterprises, 1985).

Aspinall, A. (ed.), *Letters of the Princess Charlotte, 1811–17* (London, Home & Van Thal, 1949).

Astruc, J., *A Treatise on all the Diseases Incident to Women* (London, Cooper, 1743).

Aubrey, J., *Aubrey's Brief Lives*, ed. by Oliver Lawson Dick (Harmondsworth, Penguin Books, 1972).

Austen, J., *Emma*, ed. by R. Blythe (Harmondsworth, Penguin, 1966).

——, *Sanditon*, ed. by M. Drabble (Harmondsworth, Penguin, 1974).

Ayres, J. (ed.), *Paupers and Pig Killers. The Diary of William Holland. A Somerset Parson 1799–1818* (Gloucester, Alan Sutton, 1984).

Bagley, J. J. (ed.), *The Great Diurnal of Nicholas Blundell*, transcr. and annot. by F. Tyrer, 3 vols (Record Society of Lancashire and Cheshire, 110 (1968); 112 (1970); 114 (1972)).

Bailey, M. (ed.), *Boswell's Column* (London, Martin Kimber, 1951).

Baird, J. D., and Ryskamp, C. (eds.), *The Poems of William Cowper*, vol. I, (Oxford, Clarendon Press, 1980).

Bakan, D., *Disease, Pain and Sacrifice: towards a Psychology of Suffering* (Chicago and Boston, Beacon Publications, 1971).

Bakewell, T., *The Domestic Guide in Cases of Insanity* (Hanley, T. Allbut, 1805).

Balderston, K. (ed.), *Thraliana, the Diary of Mrs Hester Lynch Thrale*, 2 vols (Oxford, Oxford University Press, 1941).

Balint, M., *The Doctor, the Patient and his Illness* (London, International Universities Press, 1957).

Ball, J., *The Female Physician, or Every Woman Her Own Doctor* (London, [n.p.] 1771).

Bambrough, J. B., *The Little World of Man* (London, Longman, Green, 1952).

Bamford, F. (ed.), *Dear Miss Heber* (London, Constable, 1936).

Baragar, C. A., 'John Wesley and medicine', *Annals of the History of Medicine*, 1st series, 10 (1928), 59–65.

Barbeau, A. (ed.), *Life and Letters at Bath in the Eighteenth Century*, ed. by A. Dobson (London, Heinemann, 1904).

Barkan, L., *Nature's Work of Art: the Human Body as Image of the World* (New Haven, Yale University Press, 1975).

Barker, F., *The Tremulous Private Body* (London, Methuen, 1984).

Barnes, B., and Shapin, S. (eds), *Natural Order: Historical Studies of Scientific Culture* (London, Sage, 1979).

Barrett, C. F. (ed.), *The Diary and Letters of Madame d'Arblay, Author of Evelina, Cecilia, etc. 1778–1840*, 7 vols (London, H. Colburn, 1842–46).

Barrett, C. R. B., *The History of the Society of Apothecaries of London* (London, Elliot Stock, 1905).

Barrett, M., and Roberts, H., 'Doctors and their patients: the social control of women in general practice', in C. Smart and B. Smart (eds), *Women, Sexuality and Social Control* (London, Routledge & Kegan Paul, 1978), 41–52.

Barry, J., 'Guide to sources and writings on the history of medicine in Bristol 1600–1900', *Bulletin of the Society for the Social History of Medicine*, 35 (1984), 48–52.

——, 'Piety and the patient: medicine and religion in eighteenth-century Bristol', in R. Porter (ed.), *Patients and Practitioners* (Cambridge, Cambridge University Press, 1985), 145–76.

——, 'Publicity and the public good: presenting medicine in eighteenth-century Bristol', in W. F. Bynum and R. Porter (eds.), *Medical Fringe and Medical Orthodoxy, 1750–1850* (London, Croom Helm, 1987), 29–39.

Baumgartner, L., 'John Howard (1726–90), hospital and prison reformer: a bibliography', *Bulletin of the History of Medicine*, 7 (1939), 486–534, 596–626.

Baur, S., *Hypochondria: Woeful Imaginings* (Princeton, Princeton University Press, 1988).

Baxby, D., *Jenner's Smallpox Vaccine. The Riddle of Vaccinia Virus and its Origin* (London, Heinemann, 1981).

Bayliss, W., *Practical Reflections on the Uses and Abuses of Bath Waters* (London, A. Millar, 1757).

Bayne-Powell, R., *The English Child in the Eighteenth Century* (London, John Murray, 1939).

Beall, O. T. jun., '*Aristotle's Masterpiece* in America: a landmark in the folklore of medicine', *William and Mary Quarterly*, 20 (1963), 207–22.

Beattie, L. M., *John Arbuthnot, Mathematician and Satirist* (Cambridge, Mass., Harvard University Press, 1935).

Beddoes, T., *Hygeia*, 3 vols (Bristol, Phillips, 1802–3).

Beekman, D., *The Mechanical Baby. A Popular History of the Theory and Practice of Child-Raising* (London, Dennis Dobson, 1977).

Beier, L. M., 'In sickness and in health: a seventeenth-century family experience', in R. Porter (ed.), *Patients and Practitioners* (Cambridge, Cambridge University Press, 1985), 101–28.

——, *Sufferers and Healers, The Experience of Illness in Seventeenth-Century England* (London, Routledge & Kegan Paul, 1987).

Bell, P., 'Early health care in Luton and Dunstable', *Bedfordshire Magazine*, 19 (1984), 229–35.

Benthall, J., *The Body Electric* (London, Thames & Hudson, 1976).

——, and Polhemus, T. (eds), *The Body as a Medium of Expression* (London, Allen Lane, 1975).

Beresford, J. (ed.), *The Diary of a Country Parson: the Rev. James Woodforde, 1758–1802*, 5 vols (reprinted Oxford, Oxford University Press, 1978–81).

Berliner, H., 'Medical modes of production', in P. Wright and A. Treacher (eds), *The Problem of Medical Knowledge. Examining the Social Construction of Medicine* (Edinburgh, Edinburgh University Press, 1982), 162–73.

Berridge, V., and Edwards, G., *Opium and the People* (London, Allen Lane, 1981).

Bessborough, Earl of, and Aspinall, A. (eds), *Lady Bessborough and her Family Circle* (London, Murray, 1940).

Bishop, P. J., *A Short History of the Royal Humane Society* (London, The Society, 1974).

Bishop, W. J., 'The evolution of the general practitioner in England', in E. Ashworth Underwood (ed.), *Science, Medicine and History: Essays on the Evolution of Scientific Thought and Medical Practice*, 2 vols (London, Oxford University Press, 1953), II, 351–7.

Black, C. (ed.), *The Cumberland Letters* (London, Martin Secker, 1912).

Black, W. G., *Folk Medicine: a Chapter in the History of Culture* (London, Folklore Society, 1883).

Blackman, J., 'Popular theories of generation: the evolution of Aristotle's Works. The study of an anachronism', in J. Woodward and D. Richards (eds), *Health Care and Popular Medicine in Nineteenth-Century England* (London, Croom Helm, 1977), 56–88.

Bliss, P. (ed.), *Reliquiae Hearnianae: the Remains of Thomas Hearne, M. A. of Edmund Hall . . .*, 3 vols (London, John Russell Smith, 1869).

Bloch, M., *The Royal Touch: Sacred Monarchy and Scrofula in England and France* (London, Routledge & Kegan Paul, 1973).

Blythe, R. (ed.), *William Hazlitt. Selected Writings* (Harmondsworth, Penguin, 1970).

Bond, D. (ed.), *The Spectator*, 5 vols (Oxford, Clarendon Press, 1965).

Bonnard, G. A. (ed.), *Edward Gibbon. Memoirs of My Life* (London, Nelson, 1966).

Boswell, J., *The Life of Samuel Johnson*, ed. by G. B. Hill, 6 vols (Oxford, Clarendon Press, 1934).

Bottomley, F., *Attitudes to the Body in Western Christendom* (London, Lepus Books, 1979).

Bottrall, M., *Every Man A Phoenix. Studies in Seventeenth-Century Autobiography* (London, John Murray, 1958).

Bourne, K. (ed.), *The Letters of the Third Viscount Palmerston to Laurence and Elizabeth Sulivan 1804–63* (London, Royal Historical Society, 1979).

Brady, F., and Pottle, F. A. (eds), *Boswell in Search of a Wife 1766–69* (London, Heinemann, 1957).

——, *James Boswell: the Later Years* (London, Heinemann, 1984).

Braithwaite, J. B. (ed.), *Memoirs of Anna Braithwaite, being a Sketch of her Early Life and Ministry and Extracts from her Private Memoranda, 1830–59* (London, Headley Brothers, 1905).

Brand, J. (ed.), *Observations on Popular Antiquities. Chiefly illustrating the Origin of our Vulgar Customs, Ceremonies and Superstitions* (London, Chatto & Windus, 1913).

Braudy, L., *The Frenzy of Renown* (Oxford, Oxford University Press, 1987).

Brian, T., *The Piss-Prophet, or Certain Piss-Pot Lectures* (London, R. Thrale, 1637).

Broadbent, J., 'The image of God or two yards of skin', in J. Benthall and T. Polhemus (eds), *The Body as a Medium of Expression* (London, Allen Lane, 1975), 305–26.

Brock, C. H., *William Hunter, 1718–83* (Glasgow, Glasgow University Press, 1983).

——, 'The happiness of riches', in W. F. Bynum and R. Porter (eds), *William Hunter and the Eighteenth-Century Medical World* (Cambridge, Cambridge University Press, 1985), 35–56.

Brockbank, W., and Kenworthy, F. (eds), *The Diary of Richard Kay (1716–51) of Baldingstone, near Bury* (Manchester, Chetham Society, 1968).

Brockliss, L. W. B., 'Taking the waters in early modern France: some thoughts on a commercial racket', *Bulletin of the Society for the Social History of Medicine*, 40 (1987), 74–7.

Brodum, W., *A Guide to Old Age or a Cure for the Indiscretions of Youth* (London, J. W. Myers, 1795).

Brody, H., *Stories of Sickness* (New Haven,.Yale University Press, 1987).

Brookes, R., *The General Practice of Physick*, 2 vols, 6th edn (London, T. Carnan & F. Newbery jun., 1771).

Brooks, E. St John, *Sir Hans Sloane* (London, Batchworth, 1954).

Brown, N. O., *Love's Body* (New York, Vintage Books, 1966).

——, *Life against Death. The Psychoanalytical Meaning of History* (London, Routledge & Kegan Paul, 1957).

Bryder, L., *Below the Magic Mountain. A Social History of Tuberculosis in Twentieth-Century Britain* (Oxford, Clarendon Press, 1988).

Buchan, W., *Domestic Medicine, or a Treatise on the Prevention and Cure of Diseases by Regimen and Simple Medicines* (Edinburgh, Balfour, Auld & Smellie, 1769).

——,*Observations Concerning the Prevention and Cure of the Venereal Disease* (London, Chapman, 1796).

Buchanan-Brown, J. (ed.), *John Aubrey, Three Prose Works* (Sussex, Centaur Press, 1972).

Burke, P., *Popular Culture in Early Modern Europe* (New York, Harper & Row, 1978).

——, 'Revolution in popular culture', in R. Porter and M. Teich (eds), *Revolution in History* (Cambridge, Cambridge University Press, 1986), 206–25.

Burkhardt, F., and Smith, S. (eds), *Correspondence of Charles Darwin*, vol. I (Cambridge, Cambridge University Press, 1985).

Burnby, J. G. L., *A Study of the English Apothecary from 1660 to 1760 (Medical History*, Supplement, no. 3 London, Wellcome Institute for the History of Medicine, 1983).

Burton, M. E. (ed.), *The Letters of Mary Wordsworth, 1800–15.* (Oxford, Clarendon Press, 1958).

Burton, R. *The Anatomy of Melancholy*, ed. by D. Floyd and P. Jordan-Smith

(New York, Tudor Publishing Company, 1948; 1st edn, London, H. Cripps, 1621).

Bushaway, B., *By Rite. Custom, Ceremony and Community in England 1700–1800* (London, Junction Books, 1982).

Butler, F. (ed.), *Masterworks of Children's Literature*, 6 vols (New York, Stonehill Publishing, 1983).

Butt, J. (ed.), *The Poems of Alexander Pope* (London, Methuen, 1963).

Butterfield, L. H. (ed.), *The Letters of Benjamin Rush*, 2 vols (Princeton, Princeton University Press, 1951).

Byles, C. E. (ed.), *Reminiscences of the Ministry of the Revd John Hawker, with a Brief Memoir of his Life by one of his Congregation* (London, Bodley Head, 1906).

Bynum, W. F., 'Health, disease and medical care', in G. S. Rousseau and R. Porter (eds), *The Ferment of Knowledge* (Cambridge, Cambridge University Press, 1980), 211–54.

——, 'Cullen and the study of fevers in Britain 1760–1820', in W. F. Bynum and V. Nutton (eds), *Theories of Fever from Antiquity to the Enlightenment* (*Medical History*, Supplement no. 1, London, Wellcome Institute for the History of Medicine, 1981), 135–48.

——, 'Treating the wages of sin: venereal disease and specialism in eighteenth-century Britain', in W. F. Bynum and R. Porter (eds), *Medical Fringe and Medical Orthodoxy, 1750–1850* (London, Croom Helm, 1987), 5–28.

——, and Nutton, V. (eds), *Theories of Fever from Antiquity to the Enlightenment* (*Medical History*, Supplement no. 1, London, Wellcome Institute for the History of Medicine, 1981).

——, and Porter, R. (eds), *William Hunter and the Eighteenth-Century Medical World* (Cambridge, Cambridge University Press, 1985).

——, and Porter, R. (eds), *Medical Fringe and Medical Orthodoxy 1750–1850* (London, Croom Helm, 1987).

——, and Porter, R. (eds), *Medicine and the Five Senses* (Cambridge, Cambridge University Press, forthcoming).

——, and Porter, R. (eds), *Brunonianism in Britain and Europe (Medical History* Supplement, no. 8, London, Wellcome Institute for the History of Medicine, 1988).

Cadogan, W., *A Dissertation on the Gout* (London, Dodsley, 1771).

Calder-Marshall, A., *Great Age of the Lady. Regency and Georgian Elegance in the Age of Romance and Revolution 1720–1820* (London, Gordon Cremonesi, 1979).

Campbell, C., *The Romantic Ethic and the Spirit of Modern Consumerism* (Oxford, Basil Blackwell, 1987).

Campbell, R., *The London Tradesman* (London, David & Charles, 1969; 1st edn, 1747).

Camporesi, P., *Bread of Dreams. Food and Fantasy in Early Modern Europe* (Cambridge, Polity Press, forthcoming).

——, *The Incorruptible Flesh. Bodily Mutation and Mortification in Religion and Folklore* (Cambridge, Cambridge University Press, 1988).

Capp, B., *Astrology and the Popular Press, English Almanacs, 1500–1800* (London and Boston, Faber & Faber, 1979).

Carpenter, K. J., *The History of Scurvy and Vitamin C* (Cambridge, Cambridge University Press, 1986).

Carroll, J. (ed.), *Selected Letters of Samuel Richardson* (Oxford, Clarendon Press, 1964).

Carswell, J., *The Prospector: being the Life and Times of R. E. Raspe* (London, Cresset Press, 1950).

Cartwright, A., *Patients and their Doctors: a Study of General Practice* (London, Routledge & Kegan Paul, 1967).

Cassell, E. J., *The Healer's Art. A New Approach to the Doctor-Patient Relationship* (Harmondsworth, Penguin, 1976).

——, *Talking with Patients*, 2 vols (Cambridge, Massachusetts, M.I.T. Press, 1985).

Castle, E. (ed.), *The Jerningham Letters (1780–1843)*, 2 vols (London, Bentley, 1896).

Cave, K. (ed.), *The Diary of Joseph Farington*, vols VII–XVI (New Haven, Yale University Press, 1982–84).

Chamberlain, M., *Old Wives' Tales: their History, Remedies and Spells* (London, Virago, 1981).

Chancellor, V. E. (ed.), *Master and Artisan in Victorian England* (London, Evelyn, Adams & MacKay, 1969).

Chaplin, A., *Medicine in England during the Reign of George III* (London, Henry Kimpton, 1919).

Chapman, A., 'Astrological medicine', in C. Webster (ed.), *Health, Medicine and Mortality in the Sixteenth Century* (Cambridge, Cambridge University Press, 1979), 275–300.

Chapman, R. W., (ed.), *The Letters of Samuel Johnson*, 3 vols (Oxford, Clarendon Press, 1984).

—— (ed.), *Jane Austen's Letters to her Sister Cassandra and Others* (London, Oxford University Press, 1952).

Checkland, S. G., *The Gladstones. A Family Biography 1764–1851* (Cambridge, Cambridge University Press, 1971).

Cherno, M., 'Feuerbach's "Man is what he eats": a rectification', *Journal of the History of Ideas*, 23 (1962), 397–406.

Cheyne, G., *An Essay on the True Nature and Due Method of Treating the Gout* (London, G. Strahan, 1722).

——, *An Essay of Health and Long Life* (8th edn, London, Strahan & Leake, 1734; 1st edn 1724).

——, *The English Malady; or, a Treatise of Nervous Diseases* (London, G. Strahan, 1733).

——, *An Essay on Regimen* (London, C. Rivington, 1740).

——, *The Natural Method of Cureing the Diseases of the Body and the Disorders of the Mind Depending on the Body* (London, G. Strahan, 1742).

——, *Account of Himself* (London, J. Wilford, 1743).

——, *Rules and Observations for the Enjoyment of Health and Long Life* (Leeds, G. Wright, 1770).

Christie, O. F. (ed.), *The Diary of the Rev'd William Jones, 1777–1821, Curate and Vicar of Broxbourne and the Hamlet of Hoddesdon 1781–1821* (London, Brentano's, 1929).

Clare, J., 'The autobiography, 1793–1824', in J. W. Tibble and A. Tibble (eds), *The Prose of John Clare* (London, Routledge & Kegan Paul, 1951).

Clark, G., *A History of the Royal College of Physicians of London*, 3 vols (Oxford, Clarendon Press, 1964–72).

Clark, R. W., *Benjamin Franklin* (London, Weidenfeld & Nicolson, 1983).

Clarkson, L., *Death, Disease and Famine in Pre-Industrial England* (Dublin, Gill & Macmillan, 1975).

Climenson, E. J. (ed.), *Passages from the Diary of Mrs Philip Lybbe Powys, 1756–1808* (London, Longmans, 1899).

——, *Elizabeth Montagu, the Queen of the Blue Stockings. Her Correspondence from 1720–61*, 2 vols (London, John Murray, 1906).

Cobbett, W., *Advice to Young Men, and (Incidentally) to Young Women in the Middle and Higher Ranks of Life*, ed. by G. Spater (Oxford, Oxford University Press, 1980; 1st edn, 1830).

Coburn, K. (ed.), *The Letters of Sara Hutchinson from 1800–35* (London, Routledge & Kegan Paul, 1954).

Cockshutt, A. O. J., *The Art of Autobiography in Nineteenth- and Twentieth-Century England* (New Haven, Yale University Press, 1984).

Collier, J. (ed.), *The Scandal and Credulities of John Aubrey* (London, Peter Davies, 1931).

Collins, K. E., 'Two Jewish quacks in eighteenth-century Glasgow and how they advertised their cures in the *Glasgow Advertiser*', *Jewish Echo*, 27 January 1984, 5.

Collison, R. L. W., *The Story of Street Literature: the Forerunner of the Popular Press* (London, Dent, 1973).

Colp, R., *To be an Invalid: the Illness of Charles Darwin* (Chicago, Chicago University Press, 1977).

Coltheart, P., *The Quacks Unmasked* (London, [the author], 1727).

Colvin, C. (ed.), *The Correspondence of Maria Edgeworth* (Oxford, Clarendon Press, 1974).

Comfort, A., *The Anxiety Makers* (London, Nelson, 1967).

The Compleat Herbal; or, Family Physician, giving an Account of all such Plants as are now used in the Practice of Physic (Manchester, 1787).

Cook, H., *The Decline of the Old Medical Regime in Stuart London* (Ithaca, Cornell University Press, 1986).

Cook, R., *Sir Samuel Garth* (Boston, Twayne, 1980).

Coope, R., *The Quiet Art: a Doctor's Anthology* (Edinburgh, Livingstone, 1952).

Cooter, R., 'Bones of contention? Orthodox medicine and the mystery of the bone-setter's craft', in W. F. Bynum and R. Porter (eds), *Medical Fringe and Medical Orthodoxy, 1750–1850* (London, Croom Helm, 1986).

Cope, Z., *William Cheselden 1686–1752* (Edinburgh, E. and S. Livingstone, 1953).

——, *The History of the Royal College of Surgeons of England* (London, Anthony Blond, 1959).

Corner, B. C., and Booth, C., (eds), *Chain of Friendship: Selected Letters of Dr John Fothergill* (Cambridge, Mass., Harvard University Press, 1971).

Cozens-Hardy, B. (ed.), *The Diary of Sylas Neville 1767–88* (London, Oxford University Press, 1950).

Craddock, P, *Young Edward Gibbon* (Baltimore, Johns Hopkins University Press, 1982).

Crawfurd, R. H. P., *The Last Days of Charles II* (Oxford, Clarendon Press, 1909).

——, *The King's Evil* (Oxford, Clarendon Press, 1911).

Crellin, J. K., 'Dr James's Fever Powder', *Transactions of the British Society for the History of Pharmacy*, 1 (1974), 136–43.

——, 'Pharmacies as general stores in the nineteenth century', *Pharmaceutical Historian*, 9, 1 (1979), [unpaginated].

——, and Scott, J. R., 'Lionel Lockyer and his pills', *Proceedings of the XXIII Congress of the History of Medicine* (1972) 2 vols (London, Wellcome Institute for the History of Medicine, 1974), II, 1182–6.

Cripps, E. C., *Plough Court: the Story of a Notable Pharmacy 1715–1927* (London, Allen & Hanbury's, 1927).

Crook, N., and Guiton, D., *Shelley's Venomed Melody* (Cambridge, Cambridge University Press, 1986).

Crumpe, S., *An Inquiry into the Nature and Properties of Opium . . .* (London, G. G. & J. Robinson, 1793).

Cumberland, R., *Memoirs of Richard Cumberland. Written by himself*, 2 vols (London, Lackington & Allan, 1806–7).

Curwen, E. C. (ed.), *The Journal of Gideon Mantell, Surgeon and Geologist* (London, Oxford University Press, 1940).

Darlington, A., 'The teaching of anatomy and the Royal Academy of Arts 1768–82', *Journal of Art and Design Education*, 5 (1986), 263.

Darwin, E., *Zoonomia*, 4 vols (London, J. Johnson, 1801).

——, *The Temple of Nature or the Origin of Society: A Poem with Philosophical Notes* (London, J. Johnson, 1803).

Darwin, F., and Seward, A. C. (eds), *More Letters of Charles Darwin* (London, J. Murray, 1903).

Davidoff, L., and Hall, C., *Family Fortunes. Men and Women of the English Middle Classes* (London, Hutchinson, 1987).

De Beer, E. S. (ed.), *The Diary of John Evelyn*, 6 vols (Oxford, Oxford University Press, 1955).

——, *The Correspondence of John Locke*, 8 vols (Oxford, Clarendon Press, 1976–81).

DeMause, L. (ed.), *History of Childhood* (London, Harper Torchbooks, 1975).

De Moulin, D., 'A historical-phenomenological study of bodily pain in western medicine', *Bulletin of the History of Medicine*, 48 (1974), 540–70.

Devlin, J., *The Superstitious Mind. French Peasants and the Supernatural in the Nineteenth Century* (New Haven, Yale University Press, 1987).

Dewhurst, K., *The Quicksilver Doctor. The Life and Times of Thomas Dover, Physician and Adventurer* (Bristol, John Wright, 1957).

——, *John Locke (1632–1704), Physician and Philosopher* (London, Wellcome Historical Medical Library, 1963).

——, *Thomas Willis as a Physician* (Los Angeles, University of California Press, 1964).

——, (ed.), *Willis's Oxford Casebook (1650–52)* (Oxford, Sandford Publications, 1981).

Dialogue Concerning Decency, A Philosophical (London, James Fletcher and J. J. Rivington, 1751).

Dick, O. L. (ed.), *Aubrey's Brief Lives* (Harmondsworth, Penguin, 1972).

Dirckx, J. H., *The Language of Medicine. Its Evolution, Structure, and Dynamics* (New York, Praeger, 1983).

Dittrick, H., 'Fees in medical history', *Annals of Medical History*, 10 (1928), 90–101.

——, 'Devices to prevent premature burial', *Journal of the History of Medicine*, 3 (1971), 161–71.

Doble, C. E. (ed.), *Remarks and Collections of Thomas Hearne*, 3 vols (Oxford, Clarendon Press, 1888–9).

Dobson, M. J., 'Population, disease and mortality in southeast England, 1600–1800' (University of Oxford, D.Phil. Thesis, 1982).

——, 'A chronology of epidemic disease and mortality in southeast England, 1601–1800' (*Historical Research Series*, 19, 1987).

——, *From Old England to New England: Changing Patterns of Mortality* (Oxford, School of Geography University of Oxford Research Paper 38, 1987).

[Dodsley, J.], *A Collection of Poems in Four Volumes by Several Hands* (London, J. Dodsley, 1783).

Doe, V. S. (ed.), *The Diary of James Clegg of Chapel-en-le-Frith, 1708–55*, 3 vols (Chesterfield, Derbyshire Record Society, 1978–81).

Donnison, J., *Midwives and Medical Men. A History of Interprofessional Rivalries and Women's Rights* (London, Heinemann Educational, 1977).

Doughty, O., 'The English malady of the eighteenth century', *Review of English Studies*, 2 (1929), 257–69.

Dover, T., *The Ancient Physician's Legacy to his Country* (London, A. Bettesworth & C. Hitch etc., 1732).

Durey, M., *The Return of the Plague: British Society and the Cholera 1831–2* (Dublin, Gill & Macmillan, 1979).

E. M. T., *Into the Silent Land* (London, Simpkin, Marshall Hamilton, Kent, [n.d.]).

Eaves, T. C. D., and Kimpel, B. D. (eds), *Samuel Richardson, a Biography* (Boston, Houghton Mifflin, 1971).

Eccles, A., *Obstetrics and Gynaecology in Tudor and Stuart England* (London, Croom Helm, 1982).

Ehrenreich, B., and English, D., *Witches, Midwives and Nurses* (New York, Old Westbury, 1973).

——, *Complaints and Disorders: the Sexual Politics of Sickness* (New York, Old Westbury, 1974).

——, *For her own Good: 150 Years of the Experts' Advice to Women* (London, Pluto Press, 1979).

Eland, G. (ed.), *Purefoy Letters*, 2 vols (London, Sidgwick & Jackson, 1931).

Elias, N., *The Civilizing Process* (Oxford, Basil Blackwell, 1983).

Eliot, G., *Middlemarch*, ed. by W. J. Harvey (Harmondsworth, Penguin, 1965).

Ellis, A. R. (ed.), *The Early Diary of Frances Burney, 1768–78*, 2 vols (London, George Bell, 1889).

Ellis, J. H. (ed.), *The Works of Anne Bradstreet in Prose and Verse* (Gloucester, Mass., Peter Smith, 1962).

Esher, Viscount (ed.), *The Girlhood of Queen Victoria. A Selection from Her Majesty's Diaries between the Years 1832–40*, 2 vols (London, John Murray, 1912).

Estes, J. W., 'John Jones's *Mysteries of Opium Reveal'd:* key to historical opiates', *Journal of the History of Medicine*, 34 (1979), 200–9.

Evans, M. (ed.), *The Letters of Richard Radcliffe and John James of Queen's College, Oxford, 1755–83* (Oxford, Oxford Historical Society, vol. 9, 1887).

Family Companion to Health (London, F. Fayram & Leake, 1729).

Family Guide to Health (London, J. Fletcher, 1767).

Family Receipt-Book (London, Oddy & C. La Grange, 1810–17).

Farr, A. D., 'Medical developments and religious belief, with special reference to the eighteenth and nineteenth centuries' (Open University PhD Thesis, 1977).

Faulkner, T. C. (ed.), *Selected Letters and Journals of George Crabbe* (Oxford, Clarendon Press, 1985).

Faust, B. C., *The Catechism of Health* (London, C. Dilly, 1794; Edinburgh, W. Creech, 1797).

Feather, J., *The Provincial Book Trade* (Cambridge, Cambridge University Press, 1986).

Ferriar, J., *Medical Histories and Reflections*, 3 vols (London, Cadell & Davies, 1792–8).

Ferrier, S., *Marriage, a Novel*, ed. by H. Foltinek (Oxford, Oxford University Press, 1977).

Fiedler, L., *Freaks* (Harmondsworth, Penguin, 1978).

Fielding, H., *Journal of a Voyage to Lisbon* (London, Dent, 1964).

Figlio, K., 'Chlorosis and chronic disease in nineteenth-century Britain: the social constitution of somatic illness in a capitalist society', *Social History*, 3 (1978), 167–97.

——, 'Sinister medicine? A critique of left approaches to medicine', *Radical Science Journal*, 9 (1979), 14–68.

Finch, J. S., *Sir Thomas Browne; a Doctor's Life of Science and Faith* (New York, Henry Schuman, 1950).

Fischer-Homberger, E., 'Hypochondriasis of the eighteenth century – neurosis of the present century', *Bulletin of the History of Medicine*, 46 (1972), 391–401.

Fissell, M. E., 'The physic of charity: health and welfare in the West Country, 1690–1834' (Philadelphia, University of Pennsylvania PhD Thesis, 1988).

Fitzgerald, B. (ed.), *Correspondence of Emily, Duchess of Leinster*, 3 vols (Dublin, Irish Manuscripts Commission, 1949–57).

Fletcher, G., and Harris, J. I., 'Pharmacy in Bath during the Regency period', *Pharmaceutical Historian*, 1, 5 (1970), 2–4.

Forbes, R., *Surgeons at the Bailey. English Forensic Medicine to 1878* (New Haven, Yale University Press, 1986).

Ford, J. M. T. (ed.), *A Medical Student at St Thomas's Hospital, 1801–2. The Weekes Family Letters* (*Medical History*, Supplement no. 7, London, Wellcome Institute for the History of Medicine, 1987).

Fothergill, B. (ed.), *Sir William Hamilton, Envoy Extraordinary* (London, Faber & Faber, 1973).

Foucault, M., *The Birth of the Clinic*, trans. A. M. Sheridan Smith (London, Tavistock, 1973).

——, *The History of Sexuality*, vol. 1, *Introduction* (London, Allen Lane, 1978).

Fox, R. H., *Dr John Fothergill and His Friends* (London, Macmillan, 1919).

Franklin, B., *The Life of Benjamin Franklin, written by Himself*, ed. J. Bigelow (Oxford, Oxford University Press, 1924).

——, *Poor Richard's Almanack* (New York, Paddington Press, 1976; 1st edn, 1733–58).

Fraser, A., *The Weaker Vessel* (London, Weidenfeld & Nicolson, 1988).

Fremantle, A. (ed.), *The Wynne Diaries*, 3 vols (London, Oxford University Press, 1935–40).

Gabbay, J., 'Asthma attacked? Tactics for the reconstruction of a disease concept', in P. Wright and A. Treacher (eds), *The Problem of Medical Knowledge* (Edinburgh, Edinburgh University Press, 1982).

Gallagher, C., and Laqueur, T. (eds), *The Making of the Modern Body. Sexuality and Society in the Nineteenth Century* (Berkeley, University of California Press, 1987).

Garlick, K., and Macintyre, A. (eds), *The Diary of Joseph Farington*, vols I–VI (New Haven, Yale University Press, 1978–9).

Garnett, D. (ed.), *The Novels of Thomas Love Peacock* (London, Rupert Hart-Davis, 1948).

Gay, P., 'The Enlightenment as medicine and as cure', in W. H. Barber (ed.), *The Age of the Enlightenment. Studies Presented to Theodore Besterman* (Edinburgh, St Andrews University Publications, 1967), 375–86.

——, *The Enlightenment: an Interpretation*, 2 vols (New York, Knopf, 1967–9).

Gazley, J. G., *The Life of Arthur Young* (Philadelphia, American Philosophical Society, 1973).

Gentleman's Magazine (London, Edward Cave, 1731–1907).

George, M. D., *England in Transition: Life and Work in the Eighteenth Century* (London, Penguin, 1953).

——, *English Political Caricature 1793–1832* (Oxford, Clarendon Press, 1959).

Geyer-Kordesch, J., 'The cultural habits of illness: the enlightened and the pious in eighteenth-century Germany', in R. Porter (ed.), *Patients and Practitioners* (Cambridge, Cambridge University Press, 1985), 177–204.

Gibbs, L. (ed.), *The Admirable Lady Mary. The Life and Times of Lady Mary Wortley Montagu (1689–1762)* (London, Dent, 1949).

Gibson, D. (ed.), *A Parson in the Vale of the White Horse* (Gloucester, Allan Sutton, 1982).

Gillow, J., and Hewitson, A. (eds), *The Tyldesley Diary* (Preston, A. Hewitson, 1873).

Ginzburg, C., *The Cheese and the Worms: the Cosmos of a Sixteenth Century Miller* (London, Routledge & Kegan Paul, 1980).

Gittings, C., *Death, Burial and the Individual in Early Modern England* (London, Croom Helm, 1984).

Gittings, R. (ed.), *Letters of John Keats: a Selection* (Oxford, Oxford University Press, 1979).

——, and Manton, J., *Dorothy Wordsworth* (London, Clarendon Press, 1985).

Gladstone, J., 'English dialects, medicine, and diet in the seventeenth and eighteenth centuries', in P. Burke and R. Porter (eds), *The Social History of Language*, II (Cambridge, Cambridge University Press, forthcoming).

Glyster, G., [pseud.] *A Dose for the Doctors; or the Aesculapian Labyrinth Explored* (London, Kearsley, 1789).

Goffman, E., *The Presentation of Self in Everyday Life* (Harmondsworth, Penguin, 1969).

Gomme, G. L., *The Gentleman's Magazine Library: Popular Superstitions* (London, Elliot Stock, 1884).

Goodwyn, E. A. (ed.), *Selections from Norwich Newspapers* (Ipswich, East Anglian Magazine, 1972).

Gosse, P., *Dr. Viper. The Querulous Life of Philip Thicknesse* (London, Cassell, 1952).

Goubert, J.-P. (ed.), *La Médicalisation de la Société Française 1770–1830* (Waterloo, Ontario, Historical Reflections Press, 1982).

Grange, J., 'Cambridgeshire Country Cures', *Cambridgeshire Life Magazine* (May 1985), 29.

Gregory, J., *Observations on the Duties of a Physician* (London, Strahan & Cadell, 1770).

Greig, J. Y. T. (ed.), *The Letters of David Hume*, 2 vols (Oxford, Clarendon Press, 1969).

Griggs, B., *Green Pharmacy. A History of Herbal Medicine* (London, Jill Norman & Hobhouse, 1981).

Griggs, E. L. (ed.), *Collected Letters of Samuel Taylor Coleridge*, 6 vols (Oxford, Clarendon Press, 1956–68).

Gunn, F., *The Artificial Face* (Newton Abbot, David & Charles, 1973).

Guthrie, L., 'The Lady Sedley's receipt book, 1686, and other seventeenth-century receipt books', *Proceedings of the Royal Society of Medicine*, 6 (1913), 150–70.

Halévy, E., *The Growth of Philosophical Radicalism* (London, Faber & Faber, 1924).

Hall, A. R., and Hall, M. B. (eds), *The Correspondence of Henry Oldenburg: 1641–73*, 9 vols (Madison, University of Wisconsin Press, 1973).

Hambridge, R. A., 'Empiricomany, or an infatuation in favour of empiricism, or quackery: the socio-economics of eighteenth-century quackery', in S. Soupel and R. A. Hambridge (eds), *Literature, Science, and Medicine* (W. A. Clark Memorial Library, University of California, Los Angeles, 1982), 47–102.

Hamilton, B., 'The medical professions in the eighteenth century', *Economic History Review*, 4 (1951), 141–69.

Hand, W. O., 'The folk-healer: calling and endowment', *Journal of the History of Medicine*, 26 (1971), 263–75.

Hankin, C. C. (ed.), *The Life of Mary Anne Schimmelpenninck*, 2 vols (London, Longmans, 1858).

Hardstaff, R. E., and Lyth, P., *Georgian Southwell* (Newark, Newark District Council, [n.d.]).

Hardyment, C., *Dream Babies. Child Care from Locke to Spock* (London, Jonathan Cape, 1983).

Harley, D., 'Religion and profesional interests in northern spa literature, 1625–1775', *Bulletin of the Society for the Social History of Medicine*, 35 (1984), 14–16.

——, 'Honour and property: the structure of professional disputes in eighteenth-century English medicine' (unpublished paper, 1987).

Harris, W., *Treatise on the Acute Diseases of Infants*, trans, by J. Martyn (London, T. Astley, 1742).

Hartshorne, A. (ed.), *Memoirs of a Royal Chaplain, 1729–63. The Correspondence of Edmund Pyle, D.D. Chaplain in Ordinary to George II, with Samuel Kerrich D.D., Vicar of Dersingham, Rector of West Newton* (London, John Lane: Bodley Head, 1905).

Hawkins, L. H., 'The history of resuscitation', *British Journal of Hospital Medicine*, 4 (1970), 495–500.

Haydon, B. R. *Autobiography and Memoirs*, ed. by A. Penrose (London, G. Bell, 1927).

Hayter, A., *Opium and the Romantic Imagination* (Berkeley, University of California Press, 1970).

Hayward, A. (ed.), *Life and Writings of Mrs. Piozzi* (London, Longmans, Green & Roberts, 1861).

[Heathcote, R.], *Sylva; or the Wood: being a Collection of Anecdotes, Dissertations, Characters, Apophthegms, Original Letters, Bons Mots, and Other Little Things* (London, T. Payne, 1786).

Heberden, W., *Medical Commentaries* (London, T. Payne, 1802).

Helfand, W. H., 'James Morison and his pills', *Transactions of the British Society of the History of Pharmacy*, 1 (1974), 101–35.

Helman, C., '"Feed a cold, starve a fever": folk models of infection in an English suburban community, and their relation to medical treatment', *Culture, Medicine and Psychiatry*, 2 (1978), 107–37.

——, *Culture, Health and Illness* (Bristol, Wright, 1984).

Hemlow, J. (ed.), *The Journals and Letters of Fanny Burney (Madame D'Arblay)*, 12 vols (Oxford, Clarendon Press, 1972–84).

Henry, M., *An Account of the Life and Death of Philip Henry by his Son* (London, John Lawrence, 1699).

Herbert, Lord (ed.), *Pembroke Papers (1790–94). Letters and Diaries of Henry, Tenth Earl of Pembroke and his Circle* (London, Jonathan Cape, 1950).

Herzlich, C., and Pierret, J., *Illness and Self in Society*, trans. E. Forster (Baltimore, Johns Hopkins University Press, 1987).

Heydon, J., *The English Physicians' Guide* (London, S. Ferris, 1662).

Heywood, T. (ed.), *The Diary of the Rev. Henry Newcome Sepr 30 1661 to Sepr 29 1663* (Manchester, Chetham Society, 1849).

Hill, A. W., *John Wesley among the Physicians* (London, Epworth Press, 1958).

Hill, G. B. (ed.), *Johnson's Lives of the Poets* (Oxford, Clarendon Press, 1905).

Hill, J., *The Useful Family Herbal* (London, W. Johnston & W. Owen, 1754).

——, *Hypochondriasis. A Practical Treatise on the Nature and Cure of that Disorder* (London, [for the author], 1756).

——, *The Old Man's Guide to Health and Longer Life*, 6th edn (London, E. & C. Dilly, 1771).

Hillam, F. C., 'The development of dental practice in the provinces from the late eighteenth century to 1855' (PhD Thesis, University of Liverpool, 1986).

Himmelfarb, G., *The Idea of Poverty* (London, Faber & Faber; New York, Knopf, 1984).

Hingston Fox, R., *Dr John Fothergill and His Friends* (London, Macmillan, 1919).

Hobhouse, E. (ed.), *The Diary of a West Country Physician, AD 1684–1726. Extracts from Dr. Claver Morris' Diary* (London, Simpkin Marshall, 1934).

Holmes, G., *Augustan England: Professions, State and Society, 1680–1730* (London, Allen & Unwin, 1982).

Home, J. A. (ed.), *Letters and Journals of Lady Mary Coke*, 4 vols (Bath, Kingsmead Reprints, 1970; 1st edn [privately printed], 1889–96).

Hone, C. R., *The Life of Dr. John Radcliffe 1652–1714. Benefactor of the University of Oxford* (London, Faber & Faber, 1950).

Hone, W., *The Table Book* (London, Hunt & Clarke, 1827).

Hopkins, D., *Princes and Peasants: Smallpox in History* (London and Chicago, University of Chicago Press, 1983).

Hughes, E., *North Country Life in the Eighteenth Century*, 2 vols (London, Oxford University Press, 1965–69).

Hultin, N. C., 'Medicine and magic in the eighteenth century: the diaries of James Woodforde', *Journal of the History of Medicine and Allied Sciences*, 30 (1975), 349–66.

Hunter, M., *John Aubrey and the Realm of Learning* (London, Duckworth, 1975).

——, and Gregory, A. (eds), *An Astrological Diary of the Seventeenth Century: Samuel Jeake of Rye 1652–99* (Oxford, Clarendon Press, 1988).

Hunter, R., and Macalpine, I., *Three Hundred Years of Psychiatry, 1535–1860* (London, Oxford University Press, 1963).

Ilchester, The Earl of (ed.), *Lady Holland's Journal*, 2 vols (London, Longmans & Green, 1908).

Illich, I., *Limits to Medicine. The Expropriation of Health* (Harmondsworth, Penguin, 1977).

Imhof, A. E., 'Methodological problems in modern urban history writing: twenty graphic presentations of urban mortality 1750–1850', in R. Porter and A. Wear (eds), *Problems and Methods in the History of Medicine. 1750–1850* (London, Croom Helm, 1987), 101–32.

Inglis, B., *Natural Medicine* (London, Collins, 1979).

Ingram, A. M., *Boswell's Creative Gloom* (London, Macmillan, 1982).

Ingram, R., *The Gout* (London, P. Vaillant, 1767).

Inkster, I., 'Marginal men: aspects of the social role of the medical community in Sheffield 1790–1850', in J. Woodward and D. Richards (eds), *Health Care and Popular Medicine in Nineteenth Century England* (London, Croom Helm, 1977), 128–63.

J.M., *Letters to a Sick Friend containing such Observations as may Render the Use of Remedies Effectual towards the Removal of Sickness and Preservation of Health* (London, T. Parkhurst, 1682).

Jackson, T. (ed.), *The Journal of the Rev. Charles Wesley* (London, John Mason, 1849).

Jaeger, M., *Before Victoria: Changing Standards and Behaviour, 1787–1837* (London, Chatto & Windus, 1956).

James, R., *A Medicinal Dictionary*, 3 vols (London, T. Osborne, 1743–5).

Jeaffreson, J. C., *A Book About Doctors* (London, Hurst & Blackett, [n.d.]).

Jenkins, J., *Observations on the Present State of the Profession and Trade of Medicine as practised by Physicians and Surgeons, Apothecaries, Chemists, Druggists and Quacks in the Metropolis, and throughout the Country of Great Britain* (London, [for the author], 1810).

Jewitt, L. (ed.), *The Life of William Hutton* (London, Frederick Warne, 1872).

Jewson, N., 'Medical knowledge and the patronage system in eighteenth-century England', *Sociology*, 8 (1974), 369–85.

——, 'The disappearance of the sick man from medical cosmology, 1770–1870', *Sociology*, 10 (1976), 225–44.

Johnson, R. B. (ed.), *Letters from the Right Honourable Lady Mary Wortley Montagu, 1709–62* (London, Dent, 1906).

Jones, J., *The Mysteries of Opium Reveal'd* (London, R. Smith, 1701).

Jordanova, L. J., 'Natural facts: a historical perspective on science and sexuality', in C. MacCormack and M. Strathern (eds), *Nature, Culture and Gender* (Cambridge, Cambridge University Press, 1980), 42–69.

——, 'The social sciences and history of science and medicine', in P. Corsi and P. Weindling (eds), *Information Sources in the History of Science and Medicine* (London, Butterworth Scientific, 1983), 81–98.

Josten, C. H. (ed.), *Elias Ashmole (1617–92). His Autobiographical and Historical Notes, his Correspondence*, 5 vols (Oxford, Clarendon Press, 1966).

Kanner, L., *Folklore of Teeth* (New York, Macmillan, 1928).

Keele, K., *Anatomies of Pain* (Oxford, Blackwell Scientific Publications, 1957).

Keynes, G. (ed.), *Complete Writings of William Blake* (Oxford, Clarendon Press, 1972).

King, J., and Ryskamp, C. A. (eds), *The Letters and Prose Writings of William Cowper*, 4 vols (Oxford, Clarendon Press, 1979–84).

King, L. S., *The Medical World of the Eighteenth Century* (Chicago, University of Chiacago Press, 1958).

——, *The Road to Medical Enlightenment, 1650–95* (London, Macdonald, 1970).

——, *The Philosophy of Medicine: the Early Eighteenth Century* (Cambridge, Mass., Harvard University Press, 1978).

King-Hele, D., *Erasmus Darwin* (London, Macmillan, 1963).

—— (ed.), *The Essential Writings of Erasmus Darwin* (London, McGibbon & Kee, 1968).

——, *Doctor of Revolution: The Life and Genius of Erasmus Darwin* (London, Faber, 1977).

—— (ed.), *The Letters of Erasmus Darwin* (Cambridge, Cambridge University Press, 1981).

Kleinman, A., *The Illness Narratives: Suffering, Healing, and the Human Condition* (New York, Basic Books, 1988).

Knox, R.A., *Enthusiasm* (London, Oxford University Press, 1950).

Kramer, J. C., 'Opium rampant: medical use, misuse and abuse in Britain and the West in the seventeenth and eighteenth centuries', *British Journal of Addiction*, 74 (1979), 377–89.

LaCasce, S., 'Swift on medical extremism', *Journal of the History of Ideas*, 31 (1970), 599–606.

Lain Entralgo, P., *Mind and Body. Psychosomatic Pathology: a Short History of the Evolution of Medical Thought* (London, Harvill, 1955).

Lane, J., 'The provincial practitioner and his services to the poor 1750–1800', *Society for the Social History of Medicine Bulletin*, 28 (1981), 10–14.

——, 'The medical practitioners of provincial England in 1783', *Medical History*, 28 (1984), 353–71.

——, '"The doctor scolds me": the diaries and correspondence of patients in eighteenth-century England', in R. Porter (ed.), *Patients and Practitioners* (Cambridge, Cambridge University Press, 1985), 207–47.

——, 'The role of apprenticeship in eighteenth-century medical education in England', in W. F. Bynum and R. Porter (eds), *William Hunter and the Eighteenth-Century Medical World* (Cambridge, Cambridge University Press, 1985), 57–104.

——, 'A provincial surgeon and his obstetric practice: Thomas W. Jones of Henley-in-Arden, 1764–1846', *Medical History*, 31 (1987), 333–48.

Laqueur, T., 'Orgasm, generation, and the politics of reproductive biology', *Representations*, 14 (1986), 1–14.

Laslett, P., *The World we have lost* (London, Methuen, 1965).

Latham, R., and Matthews, W. (eds), *The Diary of Samuel Pepys*, 11 vols (London, Bell & Hyman, 1970–83).

Lawrence, C., 'William Buchan: medicine laid open', *Medical History*, 19 (1975), 20–35.

——, 'The nervous system and society in the Scottish Enlightenment', in B. Barnes and S. Shapin (eds), *Natural Order* (Beverly Hills and London, Sage Publications, 1980), 19–40.

——, 'Medicine as culture: Edinburgh and the Scottish Enlightenment' (University of London, PhD Thesis, 1984).

——, 'Incommunicable knowledge: science, technology and the clinical art in Britain, 1850–1914', *Journal of Contemporary History*, 20 (1985), 503–20.

——, (ed.), *Essays in the History of Surgery* (London, Routledge, forthcoming).

Lawrence, S., 'Science and medicine at the London hospitals. The development of teaching and research 1750–1815' (PhD Thesis, University of Toronto, 1985).

——, 'Entrepreneurs and private enterprise: the development of medical lecturing in London, 1775–1820', *Bulletin of the History of Medicine* 62 (1988), 171–92.

——, 'Educating the senses. Students, teachers and medical rhetoric in eighteenth-century London', in W. F. Bynum and R. Porter (eds), *Medicine and the Five Senses* (Cambridge, Cambridge University Press, forthcoming).

LeFanu, W. (ed.), *Betsy Sheridan's Journal* (London, Eyre & Spottiswoode, 1960).

——, *British Periodicals of Medicine: A Chronological List* (Oxford, Wellcome Unit for the History of Medicine, 1984).

Lefebure, M., *Samuel Taylor Coleridge: a Bondage of Opium* (London, Victor Gollancz, 1974).

——, *A Bondage of Love* (London, Victor Gollancz, 1986).

Leventhal, H., *In the Shadow of the Enlightenment. Occultism and Renaissance Science in Eighteenth-Century America* (New York, New York University Press, 1976).

Lever, T. (ed.), *The Letters of Lady Palmerston* (London, Murray, 1957).

Levine, J., *Dr Woodward's Shield* (Berkeley, University of California Press, 1977).

Lewis, C. S., *The Problem of Pain* (London, Centenary Press, 1940).

Lewis, J., *The Politics of Motherhood: Child and Maternal Welfare in England 1930–9* (London, Croom Helm, 1980).

Lewis, J. S., *In the Family Way.Childbearing in the British Aristocracy 1760–1860* (New Brunswick, N. J., Rutgers University Press, 1986).

Lewis, Lady T. (ed.), *Extracts from the Journals and Correspondence of Miss Berry from the Year 1763–1852* (London, Longmans, 1865).

Lewis, T. T. (ed.), *Letters of The Lady Brilliana Harley, Wife of Sir Robert Harley* (London, Camden Society, 1854).

Lilly, W., *Christian Astrology Modestly Treated of in Three Books* (London, Partridge & Blunden, 1647).

Lindop, G., *The Opium Eater: a Life of Thomas de Quincey* (London, Dent, 1981).

Linebaugh, P., 'The Tyburn riot against the surgeons', in E. P. Thompson *et al.* (eds), *Albion's Fatal Tree* (London, Allen Lane, 1975), 65–118.

Little, D., and Kahrl, G. (eds), *The Letters of David Garrick*, 3 vols (London, Oxford University Press, 1963)

Lobban, J. H. (ed.), *Dr Johnson's Mrs Thrale* (Edinburgh and London, T. N. Foulis, 1910).

Looney, J. J., 'Advertising and society in England, 1720–1820: a statistical analysis of Yorkshire newspaper advertisements' (Princeton University PhD Thesis, 1983).

Loudon, I. S. L., 'Chlorosis, anaemia and anorexia nervosa', *Journal of the Royal College of General Practitioners*, 30 (1980), 1669–87.

——, 'Leg ulcers in the eighteenth and early nineteenth century', *Journal of the Royal College of General Practitioners*, 31 (1981), 263–73, and 32 (1982), 301–9.

——, 'A doctor's cash book: the economy of general practice in the 1830s', *Medical History*, 27 (1983), 249–68.

——, 'The origin of the general practitioner' (The James Mackenzie Lecture of the Royal College of General Practitioners for 1982), *Journal of the Royal College of General Practitioners*, 33 (1983), 13–18.

——, 'The concept of the family doctor', *Bulletin of the History of Medicine*, 58 (1984), 347–62.

——, 'The nature of provincial medical practice in eighteenth-century England', *Medical History*, 29 (1985), 1–32.

——, '"The vile race of quacks with which this country is infested"', in W. F. Bynum and Roy Porter (eds), *Medical Fringe and Medical Orthodoxy, 1750–1850* (London, Croom Helm, 1986), 106–28.

——, *Medical Care and the General Practitioner 1750–1850* (Oxford, Clarendon Press, 1986).

——, 'I'd rather have been a Parish surgeon than a Union one', *Bulletin of the Society for the Social History of Medicine*, 38 (1986), 68–73.

Loux, F., *Sagesse du Corps, Santé et Maladie dans les Proverbs réginaux Françaises* (Paris, Masionneuve et Larose, 1978).

——, *Practiques et Savoirs Populaires: le Corps dans la Societé Traditionnelle* (Paris, Berger-Levrault, 1979).

Lubbock, B. (ed), *Barlow's Journal of his Life at Sea in King's Ships, East and West Indiamen and other Merchantmen from 1654–1703* (London, Hurst & Blackett, 1934).

Lustig, J. S., and Pottle, F. A. (eds), *Boswell: the Applause of the Jury, 1782–85* (London, Heinemann, 1982).

—— (ed.), *Boswell: the English Experiment 1785–89* (London, Heinemann, 1986).

Lynch, B., *A Guide to Health through the Various Stages of Life* (London, [the author], 1744).

Macalpine, I., and Hunter, R., *George III and the Mad Business* (London, Allen Lane, 1969).

MacDonald, M., *Mystical Bedlam: Madness, Anxiety and Healing in Seventeenth-Century England* (Cambridge, Cambridge University Press, 1981).

——, 'Science, magic and folklore', in J. F. Andrews (ed.), *William Shakespeare: his World, his Work, his Influence* (New York, Charles Scribner's Sons, 1985), I, 175–94.

Macdonald, V. M. (ed.), *The Letters of Eliza Pierce (Eliza Taylor) 1751–75* (London, F. Etchells & H. Macdonald, 1927).

Macfarlane, A., *The Origins of English Individualism* (Oxford, Basil Blackwell, 1978).

——, *Marriage and Love in England* (Oxford, Basil Blackwell, 1986).

McKendrick, N., Brewer J. and Plumb J. H., *The Birth of a Consumer Society: The Commercialization of Eighteenth-Century England* (London, Europa, 1982).

MacLaren, A., *Reproductive Rituals: the Perception of Fertility in England from the Sixteenth Century to the Nineteenth Century* (London and New York, Methuen, 1984).

MacNeil, M., *Under the Banner of Science* (Manchester, Manchester University Press, 1987).

Maggs, C. J., *The Origins of General Nursing* (London, Croom Helm, 1983).

Maloney, W. J., *George and John Armstrong of Castleton. Two Eighteenth-Century Medical Pioneers* (Edinburgh and London, E. & S. Livingstone, 1954).

Mandeville, B., *A Treatise of the Hypochondriack and Hysterick Diseases* (2nd edn, London, Tonson, 1730; reprinted by George Olms Verlag, Hildesheim, 1981).

——, *The Virgin Unmask'd* (London, J. Morphew & J. Woodward, 1709).

——, *The Fable of the Bees*, ed. by P. Harth (Harmondsworth, Penguin, 1970).

Mandeville, G. F. (ed.), *Retrospections of Dorothea Herbert 1770–89*, 2 vols (London, Gerald Howe, 1929).

Marchand, L. A. (ed.), *Byron's Letters and Journals*, 12 vols (London, John Murray, 1973–81).

Marland, H., *Medicine and Society in Wakefield and Huddersfield* (Cambridge, Cambridge University Press, 1987).

Marrs, E. W. jun. (ed.), *Letters of Charles and Mary Lamb* (Ithaca, Cornell University Press, 1975–8).

Marshall, J. D. (ed.), *The Autobiography of William Stout of Lancaster 1665–1752* (Manchester, Chetham Society Publications, 3rd series, vol. 4; and New York, Barnes & Noble, 1967).

Martin, L. C. (ed.), *Thomas Browne. Religio Medici and Other Works* (Oxford, Oxford University Press, 1954).

Martin, R. B., *Tennyson: the Unquiet Heart* (Oxford, Clarendon Press, 1980).

[Martineau, H.], *Life in the Sick-Room. Essays by an Invalid* (2nd edn, London, Moxon, 1854).

Martineau, H., *Autobiography*, 2 vols (London, Virago 1983; 1st ed., 1877).

Matthews, H. (ed.), *Diary of an Invalid* (London, John Murray, 1835).

Matthews, L. G., *History of Pharmacy in Britain* (Edinburgh and London, E. & S. Livingstone, 1962).

Matthews, W. (ed.), *The Diary of Dudley Ryder* (London, Methuen, 1939).

Mauriceau, F., *The Diseases of Women with Child* (London, Andrew Bell, 1710).

Maynwaring, E., *The Method and Means of Enjoying Health, Vigour and Long Life* (London, Dorman Newman, 1683).

Mead, D. (ed.), *Diary of Lady Hoby* (London, Routledge, 1930).

Medicina Flagellata; or, the Doctor Scarify'd (London, J. Bateman & J. Nicks, 1721).

Melville, L. (ed.), *The Berry Papers: being the Correspondence hitherto unpublished of Mary Agnes Berry, 1763–1852* (London, John Lane, 1914).

—— (ed.), *Lady Suffolk and her Circle* (London, Hutchinson, 1924).

Miller, G., *The Adoption of Inoculation for Smallpox in England and France* (London, Oxford University Press, 1957).

——, 'Airs, waters and places in history', *Journal of the History of Medicine*, 17 (1962), 129–38.

Mills, H. (ed.), *George Crabbe, Tales, 1812, and Other Poems* (Cambridge, Cambridge University Press, 1967).

Mintz, S., *Sweetness and Power* (New York, Viking, 1985).

Mitchell, B., and Penrose, H. (eds), *Letters from Bath 1766–67 by the Rev. John Penrose* (London, Alan Sutton, 1983).

Modern Family Physician; or, The Art of Healing Made Easy (London, F. Newbery, 1775).

Moore, C. A., 'The English malady', in C. A. Moore (ed.), *Backgrounds of English Literature 1700–60* (Minneapolis, University of Minnesota Press, 1953), 179–235.

Moorman, M. (ed.), *Journals of Dorothy Wordsworth* (Oxford, Oxford University Press, 1971).

Morris, R. J., *Cholera, 1832. The Social Response to an Epidemic* (London, Croom Helm, 1976).

Morton, R., *Phthisiologia, or a Treatise of Consumptions* (London, Smith & Walford, 1694).

Mulhallen, J., and Wright, D. J. M., 'Samuel Johnson: amateur physician', *Journal of the Royal Society of Medicine*, 76 (1983), 217–22.

Munk, W., *The Life of Sir Henry Halford* (London, Longmans, 1895).

Murray, J. M. (ed.), *The Newfoundland Journal of Aaron Thomas, Able Seaman in H.M.S. Boston* (London, Longmans, 1968).

Nelson, J., *Essay on the Government of Children under Three General Heads: Health, Manners and Education* (London, R. & J. Dodsley, 1756).

Neve, M., 'Natural philosophy, medicine and the culture of science in provincial England: the cases of Bristol 1796–1850 and Bath 1750–1820' (University of London, PhD Thesis, 1984).

——, 'Orthodoxy and fringe: medicine in late Georgian Bristol', in W. F. Bynum and Roy Porter (eds), *Medical Fringe and Medical Orthodoxy,*

1750–1850 (London, Croom Helm, 1986), 40–55.

Nichols, J., *Literary Anecdotes of the Eighteenth Century*, ed. by C. Clair (Sussex, Centaur Press, 1967).

Nicolson, M., 'The metastatic theory of pathogenesis and the professional interests of the eighteenth-century physician', *Medical History*, 32 (1988), 47–70.

——, 'Stethoscopy in early nineteenth-century Edinburgh', in W. F. Bynum and R. Porter (eds), *Medicine and the Five Senses* (London, Routledge, forthcoming).

Nicolson, M. H. (ed.), *The Conway Letters* (New Haven, Yale University Press, 1930).

——, 'Ward's Pill and Drop and men of letters', *Journal of the History of Ideas*, 29 (1968), 173–96.

——, and Rousseau, G. S., *This Long Disease My Life. Alexander Pope and the Sciences* (Princeton, Princeton University Press, 1968).

——, and Rousseau, G. S., 'Berkeley and tar-water', in H. K. Miller, T. Rothstein and G. S. Rousseau (eds), *The Augustan Milieu* (Oxford, Clarendon Press, 1970), 102–37.

Niebyl, P., 'The non-naturals', *Bulletin of the History of Medicine*, 45 (1971), 486–92.

——, 'Old age, fever, and the lamp metaphor', *Journal of the History of Medicine*, 26 (1971), 351–68.

North, R., *General Preface and Life of Dr John North*, ed. by P. Millard (Toronto, University of Toronto Press, 1984).

Norton, J. E. (ed.), *The Letters of Edward Gibbon*, 3 vols (London, Cassell, 1956).

Noyes, R. jun., 'The art of dying', *Perspectives in Biology and Medicine*, 14 (1970), 432–47.

Oakley, A. F., 'Letters to a seventeenth-century Yorkshire physician', *History of Medicine*, 2 (1970), 24–8.

Ober, W. B., *'Boswell's Clap' and other Essays: Medical Analyses of Literary Men's Afflictions* (Carbondale, Southern Illinois University Press; London and Amsterdam, Feffer & Simons, 1979).

O'Keefe, D., *Stolen Lightning* (Oxford, Martin Robertson, 1982).

Oppenheimer, J., *New Aspects of John and of William Hunter* (London, Heinemann, 1946).

Owen, D., *English Philanthropy, 1660–1960* (Cambridge, Mass., Belknap Press, 1964).

Oxley, G. W., *Poor Relief in England and Wales 1601–1834* (Newton Abbot, David & Charles, 1974).

Paget, S. (ed.), *Memoirs and Letters of Sir James Paget* (London, Longmans & Green, 1902).

Palliser, S. M., 'Plants as wart cures in seventeenth- and eighteenth-century England', *Papers in Folk Life Studies*, 4 (Leeds Folklore Group, University of Leeds, 1983).

Parry-Jones, W., *The Trade in Lunacy. A Study of Private Madhouses in*

England in the Eighteenth and Nineteenth Centuries (London, Routledge & Kegan Paul, 1971).

Parsons, T., *The Social System* (London, Routledge & Kegan Paul, 1951).

Paston, G., *Little Memoirs of the Eighteenth Century* (London, Richards, 1901).

——, (ed.), *Mrs Delany (Mary Granville). A Memoir. 1700–1788* (London, Grant Richards, 1900).

Paulshock, B. Z., 'William Heberden and opium – some relief to all', *New England Journal of Medicine*, 308 (1983), 53–6.

Payne, J. P., 'On the resuscitation of the apparently dead: a historical account', *Annals of the Royal College of Surgeons*, 45 (1969), 98–107.

Pelling, M., *Cholera, Fever and English Medicine 1825–65* (Oxford, Oxford University Press, 1978).

——, and Webster, C., 'Medical practitioners', in C. Webster (ed.), *Health, Medicine and Mortality in the Sixteenth Century* (Cambridge, Cambridge University Press, 1979), 141–64.

——, 'Medicine since 1500', in P. Corsi and P. Weindling (eds), *Information Sources in the History of Science and Medicine* (London, Butterworth Scientific, 1983), 379–407.

——, 'Apothecaries and other medical practitioners in Norwich around 1600', *Pharmaceutical Historian*, 13 (1983), 5–8.

——, 'Old people and poverty in early modern towns', *Bulletin of the Society for the Social History of Medicine*, 34 (1984), 42–47.

——, 'Healing the sick poor: social policy and disability in Norwich, 1500–1640', *Medical History*, 29 (1985), 115–37.

——, 'Appearance and reality: barber-surgeons, the body and disease', in A. L. Beier and R. Finlay (eds), *London 1500–1700: the Making of the Metropolis* (New York, Longman, 1986), 82–112.

——, 'Medical practice in early modern England: trade or profession?', in W. Prest (ed.), *The Professions in Early Modern England* (London, Croom Helm, 1987), 90–128.

Penn, G. (ed.), *Memorials of the Professional Life and Times of Sir William Penn*, 2 vols (London, J. Duncan, 1833).

Penn, W., *Letter to his Wife and Children* (London, Tract Assocation of the Society of Friends, 1882).

Pennington, Lady S., *An Unfortunate Mother's Advice to her absent Daughters* (5th edn, London, J. & H. Hughes, 1770).

Percival, T., *Medical Ethics; or, a Code of Institutes and Precepts adapted to the Professional Conduct of Physicians and Surgeons* (Manchester, J. Johnson & R. Bickerstaff, 1803).

Perrin, N., *Dr Bowdler's Legacy* (New York, Atheneum, 1969).

Peterson, M. J., 'Dr Acton's enemy: medicine, sex, and society in Victorian England', *Victorian Studies*, 29 (1986), 570–90.

Pinkus, Philip, *Grub St. Stripped Bare* (Hamden, Conn., Archon Books, 1968).

Piozzi, H., *Anecdotes of Samuel Johnson* (reprinted, London, Alan Sutton, 1984).

Plumb, J. H., 'The new world of children in eighteenth-century England', *Past and Present*, 67 (1975), 64–95.

Polhemus, T. (ed.), *Social Aspects of the Human Body* (Harmondsworth, Penguin, 1978).

Pollock, L. A., *Forgotten Children. Parent-Child Relations from 1500 – 1900* (Cambridge, Cambridge University Press, 1983).

——, *A Lasting Relationship. Parents and Children over Three Centuries* (London, Fourth Estate, 1987).

Ponsonby, A. (ed.), *More English Diaries* (London, Methuen, 1927).

Ponsonby, D. A., *Call a Dog Hervey* (London, Hutchinson, 1949).

Porter, D. (see also Watkins, D.).

Porter, D., and Porter R., 'The politics of prevention: anti-vaccinationism and public health in nineteenth-century England', *Medical History*, 32 (1988), 231–52.

——, and Porter, R., 'What was social medicine? A historiographical essay', *Journal of Historical Sociology*, 1 (1988), 90–106.

Porter, R., 'The Enlightenment in England', in R. Porter and M. Teich (eds), *The Enlightenment in National Context* (Cambridge, Cambridge University Press, 1981), 1–18.

——, 'Was there a medical enlightenment in eighteenth-century England?', *British Journal for Eighteenth-Century Studies*, 5 (1982), 46–63.

——, *English Society in the Eighteenth Century* (Harmondsworth, Penguin, 1982).

——, 'The sexual politics of James Graham', *British Journal for Eighteenth-Century Studies*, 5 (1982), 201–6.

——, 'Sex and the singular man: the seminal ideas of James Graham', *Studies on Voltaire and the Eighteenth Century*, 228 (1984), 1–24.

——, 'Lay medical knowledge in the eighteenth century: the evidence of the *Gentleman's Magazine*', *Medical History*, 29 (1985), 138–68.

——, 'William Hunter: a surgeon and a gentleman', in W. F. Bynum and Roy Porter (eds), *William Hunter and the Eighteenth-Century Medical World* (Cambridge, Cambridge University Press, 1985), 7–34.

——, 'The patient's view: doing medical history from below', *Theory and Society*, 14 (1985), 175–98.

——, 'The hunger of imagination: approaching Samuel Johnson's melancholy', in W. F. Bynum, R. Porter and M. Shepherd (eds), *The Anatomy of Madness*, 2 vols (London, Tavistock, 1985), I, 63–88.

——, 'The drinking man's disease: the prehistory of alcoholism in Georgian Britain', *British Journal of Addiction*, 80 (1985), 384–96.

——, '"Under the influence": mesmerism in England', *History Today* (September 1985), 22–9.

——, 'Laymen, doctors and medical knowledge in the eighteenth century: the evidence of the *Gentleman's Magazine*', in R. Porter (ed.), *Patients and Practitioners* (Cambridge, Cambridge University Press, 1985), 283–314.

—— (ed.), *Patients and Practitioners. Lay Perceptions of Medicine in Pre-Industrial Society* (Cambridge, Cambridge University Press, 1985).

——, 'Making faces: physiognomy and fashion in eighteenth-century England', *Études Anglaises*, 38 (1985), 385–96.

——, 'Medicine and the decline of magic', *Strawberry Fayre* (autumn 1986), 88–94.

——, 'Before the fringe. Quack medicine in Georgian England', *History Today* (November 1986), 16–22.

——, '"I think ye both quacks": the controversy between Dr Theodor Myersbach and Dr John Coakley Lettsom', in W. F. Bynum and R. Porter (eds), *Medical Fringe and Medical Orthodoxy 1750–1850* (London, Croom Helm, 1986), 56–78.

——, 'Medical education in England before the teaching hospital: some recent revisions', in J. Wilkes (ed.), *The Professional Teacher* (London, History of Education Society, 1986), 29–44.

——, 'Medicine and religion in eighteenth-century England: a case of conflict?', *Ideas and Production*, 7 (1987), 4–17.

——, '"The secrets of generation display'd": *Aristotle's Masterpiece* in eighteenth-century England', in R. P. Maccubbin (ed.), *'Tis Nature's Fault. Unauthorised Sexuality during the Enlightenment* (Cambridge, Cambridge University Press, 1987), 7–21.

——, 'The language of quackery in England, 1660–1800', in P. Burke and R. Porter (eds), *The Social History of Language* (Cambridge, Cambridge University Press, 1987), 73–103.

——, *Disease, Medicine and Society in England 1550–1860* (London, Macmillan, 1987).

——, *Mind Forg'd Manacles. A History of Madness from the Restoration to the Regency* (London, Athlone, 1987).

——, *A Social History of Madness. Stories of the Insane* (London, Weidenfeld & Nicolson, 1987).

——, 'A touch of danger: the man-midwife as sexual predator', in G. S. Rousseau and R. Porter (eds), *Sexual Underworlds of the Enlightenment* (Manchester, Manchester University Press, 1988), 206–32.

——, 'Newspapers as resources for social historians', in E. Johansson (ed.), *Newspapers and the Press* (London, British Library, 1988).

——, *Edward Gibbon* (London, Weidenfeld & Nicolson, 1988).

——, and Porter, D., *In Sickness and in Health. The British Experience 1650–1850* (London, Fourth Estate, 1988).

——, 'Body politics: approaches to the cultural history of the body', in P. Burke (ed.), *Historiography Today* (Cambridge, Polity Press, forthcoming).

——, 'Barely touching', in G. S. Rousseau (ed.), *Mind and Body in the Enlightenment* (Los Angeles, University of California Press, forthcoming).

——, 'The gift relation: philanthropy and provincial hospitals in eighteenth-century England', in L. Granshaw and R. Porter (eds), *Hospitals in History* (London, Routledge, forthcoming).

——, 'The patient in eighteenth-century England', in A. Wear (ed), *History of Medicine in Society* (Cambridge, Cambridge University Press, forthcoming)

——, 'Quacks at court', in W. F. Bynum and V. Nutton (eds), *Medicine at* the *Royal Court* (London, Routledge, forthcoming).

——, *Health for Sale: Quack Medicine in Eighteenth-Century England* (Manchester, Manchester University Press, forthcoming).

——, 'The rise of the physical examination', in W. F. Bynum and R. Porter (eds), *Medicine and the Five Senses* (London, Routledge, forthcoming).

——, and Porter, D., 'The rise of the English drug industry: the role of Thomas Corbyn', *Medical History* (forthcoming).

——, and Porter, D., 'The enforcement of health: the English debate', in E. Fee and D. M. Fox (eds), *Aids: the Burdens of History* (Berkeley, University of California Press, 1988 forthcoming).

—— (ed.), 'Introduction' to Thomas Trotter, *An Essay on Drunkenness* (London, Routledge Reprint, forthcoming; 1st ed, 1804).

—— (ed.), 'Introduction' to George Cheyne, *The English Malady* (London, Routledge Reprint, forthcoming; 1st edn, 1734).

—— (ed.), 'Introduction' to John Haslam, *Illustrations of Madness* (London, Routledge Reprint, forthcoming; 1st edn, 1810).

Posner, E., 'Josiah Wedgwood's doctors', *Pharmaceutical Historian*, 3 (1973), 2–4.

——, 'William Withering versus the Darwins', *History of Medicine*, 6 (1975) 51–7.

Pottle, F. A. (ed.), *Boswell's London Journal* (London, Heinemann, 1951).

——, *James Boswell: the Earlier Years 1740–69* (London, Heinemann, 1966).

Poynter, F. N. L. (ed.), *The Evolution of Medical Practice in Great Britain* (London, Pitman, 1961).

—— (ed.), *The Evolution of Pharmacy in Britain* (London, Pitman, 1965).

—— (ed.), *The Evolution of Medical Education in Britain* (London, Pitman, 1966).

Praz, M., *The Romantic Agony* (London, Oxford University Press, 1951).

Prest, W. (ed.), *The Professions in Early Modern England* (London, Croom Helm, 1987).

Price, C. (ed.), *The Letters of Richard Brinsley Sheridan* 2 vols (Oxford, Clarendon Press, 1966).

Prior, M., *Matthaei Prioris Almae, Libritres Latino Versu Donati Opera . . . Thomae Martin* (Sarum, Typis E. Easton, 1763).

Prior, M., *Women in English Society* (London, Methuen, 1985).

Professional Anecdotes, or ANA of Medical Literature, 3 vols (London, John Knight & Henry Lacey, 1825).

Purdon, N., *Dr Bowdler's Legacy: a History of Expurgated Books in England and America* (London, Macmillan, 1964).

Quennell, P. (ed.), *The Private Letters of Princess Lieven to Prince Metternich, 1820–26* (London, John Murray, 1937).

Ramsey, M., 'Property rights and the right to health: the regulation of secret remedies in France, 1789–1815', in W. F. Bynum and R. Porter (eds), *Medical Fringe and Medical Orthodoxy* (London, Croom Helm, 1987), 79–105.

——, *Professional and Popular Medicine in France, 1770–1830. The Social World of Medical Practice* (Cambridge,Cambridge University Press, 1988).

Rathborne, Mrs Ambrose (ed.), *The Letters of Lady Jane Coke to her Friend Mrs Eyre at Derby 1747–58* (London, Swan Sonnenschein, 1899).

Rather, L., 'The "six things non-natural": a note on the origins and fate of a doctrine and a phrase', *Clio Medica*, 3 (1968), 337–47.

Razzell, P., *The Conquest of Smallpox* (Firle, Caliban Books, 1977).

Reece, R., *Domestic Medical Guide* (London, Longman & Reed, 1803).

Rees, G., *Francis Bacon's Natural Philosophy: a New Source* (Chalfont St Giles, British Society for the History of Science, 1984).

Reeve, H. (ed.), *The Greville Memoirs: a Journal of the Reigns of King George IV and King William IV by the Late Charles C. F. Greville*, 3 vols (London, Longmans, Green, 1875).

Reiser, S. J., *Medicine and the Reign of Technology* (Cambridge, Cambridge University Press, 1978).

Richardson, R., *Death, Dissection and the Destitute: a Political History of the Human Corpse* (London, Routledge & Kegan Paul, 1987).

Risse, G., 'Doctor William Cullen, physician, Edinburgh: a consultation practice in the eighteenth century', *Bulletin of the History of Medicine*, 48 (1974), 338–51.

——, *Hospital Life in Enlightenment Scotland: Care and Teaching at the Royal Infirmary of Edinburgh* (Cambridge, Cambridge University Press, 1986).

——, 'The Brownian system of medicine: its theoretical and practical implications', *Clio Medica*, 5 (1970), 45–51.

Ritson, J. (ed.), *Ancient Popular Poetry* (London, [privately printed], 1884).

Robinson, E. (ed.), *John Clare's Autobiographical Writings* (Oxford, Oxford University Press, 1983).

Robinson, H. W., and Adams, W. (eds), *The Diary of Robert Hooke (1672–80)* (London, Taylor & Francis, 1935).

Rodin, A. E., *Medical Casebook of Doctor Arthur Conan Doyle: from Practitioner to Sherlock Holmes and Beyond* (Florida, Krieger, 1984).

Rodgers, B., *Cloak of Charity* (London, Methuen, 1949).

Rogers, K. M., *Feminism in Eighteenth-Century England* (Brighton, Harvester Press, 1982).

Rogers, P., 'The rise and fall of gout', *Times Literary Supplement* (20 March, 1981), 315–16.

——, *Grub Street. Hacks and Dunces: Pope, Swift and Grub Street* (London, Methuen, 1980).

——, *Eighteenth-Century Encounters* (Brighton, Harvester Press, 1985).

Rolls, R., *The Hospital of the Nation. The Story of Spa Medicine and the Mineral Water Hospital at Bath* (Bath, Bird Publications, 1988).

Romilly, S., *Memoirs of the Life of Sir Samuel Romilly, written by himself; with a Selection from his Correspondence edited by his Sons*, 3 vols (London, John Murray, 1840).

Rosen, G., and Caspari-Rosen, B., *400 Years of a Doctor's Life* (New York, Schuman, 1947).

Rosenberg, C., 'The therapeutic revolution: medicine, meaning and social change in nineteenth-century America', in C. Rosenberg and M. J. Vogel (eds), *The Therapeutic Revolution: Essays in the Social History of American Medicine* (Philadelphia, University of Pennsylvania Press, 1979), 3–25.

——, 'Medical text and medical context; explaining William Buchan's *Domestic Medicine*', *Bulletin of the History of Medicine*, 57 (1983), 22–24.

Ross, E. D. (ed.), *The Diary of Henry Yeonge, Chaplain on Board H.M. Ships Assistance, Bristol and Royal Oak 1675–1679* (London, George Routledge, [n.d.]).

Rousseau, G. S., 'John Wesley's *Primitive Physick* (1747)', *Harvard Library Bulletin*, 16 (1968), 242–56.

Rowley, W., *A Treatise on Female, Nervous, Hysterical, Hypochondriacal, Bilious, Convulsive Diseases* (London, C. Nourse, 1788).

——, *Tobias Smollett. Essays of Two Decades* (Edinburgh, T. & T. Clark, 1982).

Ryskamp, C., and Pottle, F. A. (eds), *Boswell. The Ominous Years* (London, Heinemann, 1963).

Saunders, P. L. L. *Edward Jenner: the Cheltenham Years, 1795–1823* (London, University Press of New England, 1982).

Schnorrenberg, B. B., 'Is childbirth any place for a woman? The decline of midwifery in eighteenth-century England', *Studies in Eighteenth-Century Culture*, 10 (1981), 393–408.

——, 'Medical men of Bath', *Studies in Eighteenth-Century Culture*, 13 (1984), 189–203.

Schrank, B. G., and Supino D. (eds), *The Famous Miss Burney* (New York, John Day, 1976).

Schwartz, R. B., *Daily Life in Johnson's London* (Madison, University of Wisconsin Press, 1983).

Scull, A., *Museums of Madness* (London, Allan Lane, 1979).

Sedgwick, R. (ed.), *Lord Hervey's Memoirs* (London, Kimber, 1952).

Sells, A. L., *Oliver Goldsmith. His Life and Works* (London, Allen & Unwin, 1974).

Severn, C. (ed.), *Diary of the Rev. John Ward* (London, Colburn, 1839).

Seward, A., *Memoirs of the Life of Darwin* (London, J. Johnson, 1804).

Sharp, J., *The Compleat Midwife's Companion*, 4th edn (London, John Marshall, 1725).

Shaw, G. B., *Doctor's Dilemma* (London, Constable, 1926).

Sheridan, R. B., *Doctors and Slaves. A Medical and Demographic History of Slavery in the British West Indies, 1680–1834* (Cambridge, Cambridge University Press, 1985).

Shorter, E., *A History of Women's Bodies* (London, Allen Lane, 1983).

——, 'The management of normal deliveries and the generation of William Hunter', in W. F. Bynum and Roy Porter (eds), *William Hunter and the Eighteenth-Century Medical World* (Cambridge, Cambridge University Press, 1985), 371–83.

——, *Bedside Manners: the Troubled History of Doctors and Patients* (New York, Simon & Schuster, 1986).

——, 'Paralysis: the rise and fall of a "hysterical symptom"', *Journal of Social History*, 19 (1986), 549–82.

Showalter, E., *The Female Malady: Women, Madness, and English Culture, 1830–1980* (New York, Pantheon Press, 1986).

Silverman, K., *The Life and Times of Cotton Mather* (New York, Harper & Row, 1984).

Simpson, J., *The Journal of Dr John Simpson of Bradford, 1st January to the 25th July 1825* (Bradford, Metropolitan Bradford Libraries, 1981).

Singer, C., and Holloway, S. W. F., 'Early medical education in England', *Medical History*, 4 (1960), 1–17.

Slack, P., 'Mirrors of health and treasures of poor men: uses of the vernacular medical literature of Tudor England', in C. Webster (ed.), *Health, Medicine and Mortality in the Sixteenth Century* (Cambridge, Cambridge University Press, 1979), 237–74.

——, *The Impact of Plague in Tudor and Stuart England* (London, Routledge & Kegan Paul, 1985).

Slater, A. W. (ed.), 'Autobiographical memoir of Joseph Jewell 1763–1846', *Camden Miscellany*, 22 (1964).

Smith, A., *An Inquiry into the Nature and Causes of the Wealth of Nations*, 2 vols (London, W. Strahan & T. Cadell, 1776).

Smith, F. B., *The Retreat of Tuberculosis 1850–1950* (London, Croom Helm, 1988).

Smith, G., 'Thomas Tryon's regimen for women: sectarian health in the seventeenth century', in London Feminist History Group (eds), *The Sexual Dynamics of History* (London, Pluto Press, 1983), 47–65.

——, 'Prescribing the rules of health: self-help and advice in the late eighteenth-century England', in R. Porter (ed.), *Patients and Practitioners* (Cambridge, Cambridge University Press, 1985), 249–82.

——, 'The popularisation of medical knowledge: the case of cosmetics', *Bulletin of the Society for the Social History of Medicine*, 39 (1986), 12–16.

——, see also V. S. Smith.

Smith, J. R., *The Speckled Monster. Smallpox in England 1670–1970, with particular Reference to Essex* (Chelmsford, Essex Record Office, 1987).

Smith, N. C. (ed.), *Selected Letters of Sydney Smith* (Oxford, Oxford University Press, 1981).

Smith, V. S., 'Cleanliness: the development of an idea and practice in Britain 1770–1850' (University of London, PhD Thesis, 1985).

——, 'Physical puritanism and sanitary science: material and immaterial beliefs in popular physiology 1650–1840', in W. F. Bynum and R. Porter (eds), *Medical Fringe and Medical Orthodoxy* (London, Croom Helm, 1986), 174–97.

Smythson, H., *The Compleat Family Physician* (London, Harrison, 1781).

Solomon, S., *A Guide to Health, or, Advice to both Sexes in a Variety of Complaints*, 2nd edn (Stockport, [the author, c.1800]).

Sontag, S., *Illness as Metaphor* (New York, Farrar, Straus & Giroux, 1978; London, Allen Lane, 1979).

Sorlien, R. P. (ed.), *The Diary of John Manningham* (New Hampshire, University Press of New England, 1976).

Spence, J., *Observations, Anecdotes, and Characters of Books and Men*, ed. by James M. Osborn, 2 vols (Oxford, Clarendon Press, 1966).

Spilsbury, F.B., *Free Thoughts on Quacks and their Medicines* (London, J. Wilkie, 1776).

Spinckes, N., *The Sick Man Visited; or Meditations and Prayers for the Sick Room* (London, Freeman, 1712).

Spinke, J., *Quackery Unmask'd; or Reflections on the Sixth Edition of Mr Martin's Treatise on the Venereal Disease; . . . and the Pamphlet [by T. C. Surgeon] Call'd the Charitable Surgeon, containing a Detection and Refutation of Some Gross Errors etc of those Authors* (London, D. Brown, 1709).

——, *Venus's Botcher: or the Seventh Edition of Mr Martin's Comical Treatise or the Venereal Disease . . . Examin'd and Expos'd* (London, S.Popping, 1711).

Sprott, D. (ed.), *1784* (London, Allen & Unwin, 1984).

Stannard, D. E., *The Puritan Way of Death: a Study in Religion, Culture and Social Change* (New York and Oxford, Oxford University Press, 1977).

Stansfield, D. A., *Thomas Beddoes M.D. 1760–1808, Chemist, Physician, Democrat* (Dordrecht, Reidel, 1984).

——, and Stansfield, R. G., 'Dr Thomas Beddoes and James Watt: preparatory work 1794–6 for the Bristol Pneumatic Institute'. *Medical History*, 30 (1986), 276–302.

Staum, M. S., and Larsen, D. E. (eds), *Doctors, Patients and Society: Power and Authority in Medical Care* (Waterloo, Ontario, Calgary Institute of the Humanities, 1981).

Stein, D., *Ada: a Life and Legacy* (Cambridge, Mass., M.I.T. Press, 1985).

Stern, P., *Medical Advice to the Consumptive and Asthmatic People of England . . . And a New Easy Method of Cure* (London, J. Almon, 1767).

Sterne, L., *The Life and Opinions of Tristram Shandy*, ed. C. Ricks (Harmondsworth, Penguin, 1967).

Stevenson, L., '"New diseases" in the seventeenth century', *Bulletin of the History of Medicine*, 39 (1965), 1–21.

Strong, P. M., *The Ceremonial Order of the Clinic* (London, Routledge & Kegan Paul, 1979).

Szasz, T., *The Myth of Mental Illness* (New York, Paladin, 1961).

Temkin, O., *Galenism: Rise and Decline of a Medical Philosophy* (Ithaca, Cornell University Press, 1973).

——, 'Health and disease', *Dictionary of the History of Ideas*, 2 (1973), 395–407.

Thale, M. (ed.), *The Autobiography of Francis Place (1771–1854)* (Cambridge, Cambridge University Press, 1972).

Thomas, E. G., 'The Old Poor Law and medicine', *Medical History*, 24 (1980), 1–19.

Thomas, K., *Religion and the Decline of Magic: Studies in Popular Beliefs in Sixteenth- and Seventeenth-Century England* (London, Weidenfeld & Nicolson, 1971; reprinted, Harmondsworth, Penguin, 1978).

Thompson, R., *Unfit for Modest Ears* (London, Macmillan, 1979).

Thomson, E., 'The role of the physician in humane societies of the eighteenth century', *Bulletin of the History of Medicine*, 37 (1963), 43–51.

Thomson, G. S. (ed.), *Letters of a Grandmother 1732–35: being the Correspondence of Sarah, Duchess of Marlborough with her Granddaughter Diana, Duchess of Bedford* (London, Jonathan Cape, 1943).

Tilley, M. P. (ed.), *Dictionary of Proverbs in England* (Ann Arbor, University of Michigan Press, 1950).

Timbs, J., *Doctors and Patients; or Anecdotes of the Medical World and Curiosities of Medicine* (London, Bentley, 1876).

Todd, J., *Sensibility* (London, Methuen, 1986).

Tomaselli, S., 'The first person: Descartes, Locke and mind-body dualism', *History of Science*, 22 (1984), 185–205.

Townsend, J., *Guide to Health* (London, Cox etc., 1795).

Toynbee, P., and Whibley, L. (eds), *Correspondence of Thomas Gray*, 3 vols (Oxford, Clarendon Press, 1971).

Toynbee, Mrs Paget (ed.), *The Letters of Horace Walpole*, 16 vols (Oxford, Clarendon Press, 1903–25).

Toynbee, W. (ed.), *Diaries of William Charles Macready* (London, Chapman & Hall, 1912).

Trillat, E., *Histoire de l'Hystérie* (Paris, Seghers, 1986).

Trimmer, E. J., 'Medical folklore and quackery', *Folklore*, (1965), 161–75.

Tring, F. C., 'The influence of Victorian "patent medicines" on the development of early twentieth-century medical practice' (PhD thesis, University of Sheffield, 1982).

Tröhler, U., 'Quantification in British medicine and surgery 1750–1830; with special reference to its introduction into therapeutics' (University of London, PhD Thesis, 1978).

Trotter, T., *An Essay, Medical, Philosophical and Chemical on Drunkenness* (London, Longmans, 1804).

——, *A View of the Nervous Temperament* (London, Longman, Hurst, Rees & Owen, 1807).

Turner, B. S., *Medical Power and Social Knowledge* (London, Sage Publications, 1987).

Turner, E. S., *Call the Doctor. A Social History of Medical Men* (London, Michael Joseph, 1958).

——, *Taking the Cure* (London, Quality Book Club, 1967).

Turner, J. H. (ed.), *The Rev. Oliver Heywood B.A. 1630–1702. His Autobiographical Diaries, Anecdote and Event Books*, 4 vols (Brighouse, Bingley, T. Harrison, 1881–5).

Vaisey, D. (ed.), *The Diary of Thomas Turner* (Oxford, Oxford University Press, 1984).

Veith, I., *Hysteria* (Chicago, Chicago University Press, 1965).

Verney, Lady F. P., and Verney Lady M. M. (eds), *Memoirs of the Verney Family*, 4 vols (London, Tabard, 1970).

Verney, Lady M. M. (ed.), *Verney Letters of the Eighteenth Century from* the MSS at *Claydon House*, 2 vols (London, Ernest Benn, 1930).

Versluysen, M. C., 'Midwives, medical men and "poor women labouring of child": lying-in hospitals in eighteenth-century London', in H. Roberts (ed.), *Women, Health and Reproduction* (London, Routledge & Kegan Paul, 1981), 18–49.

Viets, H. R., 'George Cheyne, 1673–1743', *Bulletin of the Johns Hopkins Institute for the History of Medicine*, 23 (1949), 435–52.

Vigarello, G., *Le Corps Redressé: Histoire d'un Pouvoir Pédagogique* (Paris, J. P. Delarge, 1978).

Viseltear, A., 'Joanna Stephens and eighteenth-century lithontriptics; a misplaced chapter', *Bulletin of the History of Medicine*, 42 (1968), 199–220.

Wadd, W., *Mems., Maxims and Memoirs* (London, Callow & Wilson, 1827).

Waddington, I., 'The struggle to reform the Royal College of Physicians, 1767–71: a sociological analysis', *Medical History*, 17 (1973), 107–26.

——, 'General practitioners and consultants in early nineteenth-century England: the sociology of an intra-professional conflict', in J. Woodward and D. Richards (eds), *Health Care and Popular Medicine in Nineteenth-Century England: Essays in the Social History of Medicine* (London, Croom Helm, 1977), 164–88.

——, *The Medical Profession in the Industrial Revolution* (Dublin, Gill & Macmillan, 1984).

Wain, J., *Samuel Johnson* (London, Macmillan, 1980).

Ward, N., *The London Spy*, ed. by K. Fenwick (London, Folio Society, 1955).

Warner, J. H., 'The therapeutic perspective: medical knowledge, practice and professional identity in America, 1820–85' (Harvard University PhD Thesis, 1984).

Wear, A., 'Puritan perceptions of illness in seventeenth-century England', in R. Porter (ed.), *Patients and Practitioners* (Cambridge, Cambridge University Press, 1985), 55–99.

——, 'Historical and cultural aspects of pain', *Bulletin of the Society for the Social History of Medicine*, 36 (1985), 7–21.

Weatherill, L., *Consumer Behaviour and Material Culture in Britain, 1660–1760* (London, Routledge, 1988).

Webster, C. (ed.), *Health, Medicine and Mortality in the Sixteenth Century* (Cambridge, Cambridge University Press, 1979).

Wedgwood, B., and Wedgwood H., *The Wedgwood Circle* (London, Studio Vista, 1980).

Weindling, P. (ed.), *The Social History of Occupational Health* (London, Croom Helm, 1985).

Weis, C. McC., and Pottle, F A. (eds), *Boswell in Extremes* (London, Heinemann, 1970).

Welsh, C., *A Bookseller of the Last Century. Being some Account of the Life of John Newbery, and of the Books he published, with a Notice of the Later Newberys* (London, Griffith, Farran, Okeden & Welsh, 1885).

Wesley, J., *Primitive Physick: or, an Easy and Natural Method of Curing Most Diseases* (London, T. Trye, 1747).

——, *Journal of John Wesley* (London, Dent, [n.d.]).

West, J., *The Taylors of Lancashire: Bonesetters and Doctors* (Manchester, [the author], 1977).

Whitbread, H. (ed.), *I Know My Own Heart. The Diaries of Anne Lister (1740–1840)* (London, Virago, 1987).

White, G., *The Natural History of Selborne* (Harmondsworth, Penguin, 1981).

Whorton, J. C., *Crusaders for Fitness: the History of American Health Reformers* (Princeton, Princeton University Press,1982).

Williams, C.(ed.), *Sophie in London, 1786, being the Diary of Sophie v. La Roche*, (London, Jonathan Cape, 1936).

Williams, G., *The Age of Agony: the Art of Healing c.1700–1800* (London, Constable, 1975).

Williams, H. (ed.), *Jonathan Swift. Journal to Stella*, 2 vols (Oxford, Clarendon Press, 1948).

Williams, N., *Powder and Paint* (London, Longmans, 1957).

Willich, A. F. M., *Lectures on Diet and Regimen* (London, Longman & Rees, 1799).

Wilson, A., 'Participant or patient?', in R. Porter (ed.), *Patients and Practitioners* (Cambridge, Cambridge University Press, 1985), 129–44.

——, 'William Hunter and the varieties of man-midwifery', in W. F Bynum and R. Porter (eds), *William Hunter and the Eighteenth-Century Medical World* (Cambridge, Cambridge University Press, 1985), 343–69.

Withering, W., *An Account of the Foxglove and its Medical Uses* (Birmingham, Robinson, 1785).

Withers, T., *Observations on the Chronic Weakness* (York, Ward & Cadell, 1777).

Woodforde, J., *The Strange Story of False Teeth* (London, Routledge & Kegan Paul, 1968).

Woodward, J., *To do the Sick No Harm. A Study of the British Voluntary Hospital System to 1875* (London and Boston, Routledge & Kegan Paul, 1974).

——, and Richards, D. (eds), *Health Care and Popular Medicine in Nineteenth-Century England: Essays in the Social History of Medicine* (London, Croom Helm, 1977).

Woolf, V., 'On being ill', in *Collected Essays*, 4 vols, ed. by L. Woolf (London, Chatto & Windus, 1969), IV, 193–203.

Wright, P. W. G., 'The radical sociology of medicine', *Social Studies of Science*, 10 (1980), 103–20.

——, and Treacher, A. (eds), *The Problem of Medical Knowledge* (Edinburgh, Edinburgh University Press, 1982).

Wyman, A. L., 'The surgeoness. The female practitioner of surgery, 1400–1800', *Medical History*, 28 (1984), 22–41.

Wyndham, M., *Chronicles of the Eighteenth Century* (London, Hodder & Stoughton, 1924).

Yorke, C. (ed.), *The Diary of John Baker, 1751–8* (London, Hutchinson, 1931).

Young, G., *Treatise on Opium* (London, Miller, 1753).

Young, G. M., *Gibbon* (London, Rupert Hart-Davies, 1948).

Zuckerman, A., 'Dr Richard Mead (1673–1754): a biographical study' (University of Illinois, PhD Thesis, 1965).

Zwanenberg, D. van, 'The Suttons and the business of inoculation', *Medical History*, 22 (1978), 71–82.

Index